Taking Charge of Breast Cancer

Taking Charge of Breast Cancer

JULIA A. ERICKSEN

UNIVERSITY OF CALIFORNIA PRESS

Berkeley   Los Angeles   London

University of California Press, one of the most distinguished university presses in the United States, enriches lives around the world by advancing scholarship in the humanities, social sciences, and natural sciences. Its activities are supported by the UC Press Foundation and by philanthropic contributions from individuals and institutions. For more information, visit www.ucpress.edu.

University of California Press
Berkeley and Los Angeles, California

University of California Press, Ltd.
London, England

Library of Congress Cataloging-in-Publication Data

Ericksen, Julia A., 1941–.
    Taking charge of breast cancer / Julia A. Ericksen.
        p.   cm.
    Includes bibliographical references and index.
    ISBN 978-0-520-25291-2 (cloth, alk. paper)
    ISBN 978-0-520-25292-9 (pbk., alk. paper)
    1. Breast—Cancer—Patients—Interviews.   2. Breast—Cancer—
Psychological aspects.   I. Title.
RC280.B8E68   2008
362.196′99449—dc22   2007046303

Manufactured in the United States of America

17   16   15   14   13   12   11   10   09   08
10   9   8   7   6   5   4   3   2   1

This book is printed on New Leaf EcoBook 50, a 100% recycled fiber of which 50% is de-inked post-consumer waste, processed chlorine-free. EcoBook 50 is acid-free and meets the minimum requirements of ANSI/ASTM D5634-01 (*Permanence of Paper*).

For Gene

Contents

Tables

Acknowledgments

I have discussed my experiences with breast cancer and the reasons I came to write this book in the introduction, so I will not repeat them here. I will only add that writing about breast cancer is one of the most rewarding and difficult things I have done. As I told their stories, I could remember every woman I wrote about, and, indeed, as I write this I find myself wondering which women are no longer alive. The women I interviewed were in various stages of the disease, and I fear that not all of them will have survived to read what I said about them. Even so, for the most part, I believe this is an upbeat, not a sad, book. For this, I must share the credit with the ninety-six women who agreed to be interviewed about their experiences. In their responses to their breast cancer diagnosis, these women really underscore the concept of agency in that they all did take charge of their breast cancer and, in doing so, they did not always follow the same path. In the pages that follow some of their stories are described in more detail than others, but every woman I talked to enlightened my research.

I must also thank those individuals who helped my research by telling me about the many support services available to women once they are diagnosed. These generous people include Jean Sachs, executive director of Living Beyond Breast Cancer, who was kind enough to spend time with me explaining her organization. She also allowed me to put a flyer about my research in the package of materials handed out to attendees at an LBBC conference. This resulted in a number of interviews, particularly with women I call biomedical experts. Elaine Grobman, executive director of the Breast Health Institute, which was the local Philadelphia affiliate of the Susan G. Komen Foundation, not only agreed to an interview but invited me to a working meeting of the Race for the Cure, where I was able to recruit several activists to interview. I would also like to thank Patricia Wellenbach, former executive director of the Wellness Community, and Barbara De Luca, former executive director of the Linda Creed Breast Cancer Foundation, for helpful information about their programs.

Other women who freely gave me their valuable time to explain the variety of services available to breast cancer patients include Judy Wallace, education director of the National Breast Cancer Coalition; Bonnie Hay of the Women's Health and Environment Network; Nurit Shein, executive director of Philadelphia Community Health Alternatives (now renamed the Mazzoni Center); Helen Grotsky and Catherine Belt, a social worker and oncology nurse, respectively, at the Joan Karnell Cancer Center of Pennsylvania Hospital; Barbara Shapiro of Harriet's Inner Wear; Maria Scarduzio of Cuz'n Curl Company Salon and Spa; and Jane Antonowski, leader of a psychotherapeutic support group for breast cancer patients.

I also received help and advice from a number of colleagues. My friends in the Department of Sociology at Temple University listened to me expound on my topic and on the difficulties of running a department while writing a book. They even stayed away when I needed them to. Gretchen Condran and Gene Ericksen were helpful in finding and interpreting data on national trends in breast cancer and on demographic differences in breast cancer morbidity and mortality. Kevin Delaney and Sherri Grasmuck discussed issues of qualitative interviewing with me, and Kevin also advised me about where to publish. Outside the department, Sue Wells, Richard Immerman, and Bill Overton commiserated with me on the departmental chair problem and encouraged me to keep going. Rebecca Alpert had a number of conversations with me about my topic both before and after she was diagnosed. She also helped me locate lesbians who had had breast cancer. Denise O'Brien and Dolores Andy discussed their own experiences of breast cancer with me and helped me develop my questionnaire. Several anonymous reviewers provided helpful comments, and my book is better for following much of their advice.

I would like to thank the Department of Sociology for providing undergraduate and graduate student research assistants to transcribe and help code my data and to perform the many other tasks I assigned to them. These included Katy Seufert, Annalisa Synnestvedt, Amy Steinbugler, Rae Garrison, and Kelly McKormick. I would especially like to thank Rose Malinowski-Weingartner for her help in the months leading up to the final manuscript preparation. Rose did an amazing job of locating references, editing chapters, and taking care that the footnotes were all accurate and correctly formatted. My administrative assistant, Sharon Smith, helped me create the time to finish this book, and she kept people at bay when necessary.

Every few years, the media engage in collective angst about the problems of career and family for women. These stories always seem to start with the premise that professional women are leaving the workforce for the joys of raising a family, since it is so difficult to do both properly. It may be a measure of my dilettantish nature that I have found having a career and family to be the best of both worlds, with each providing a welcome balance to the demands of the other. My husband, Gene Ericksen, to whom this book is dedicated, has shared all aspects of this research with me, bringing both sociological and personal advice and support. My children, Polly, Andrew, and Monica, continue to shine in their own worlds and, in doing so, make me feel that I must be a successful parent. And I thank my three grandchildren, Miles, Drew, and Blake, for knowing little about my professional life. They take it for granted that I work, because they assume that all women do, but their interest in me is solely in my role as Grandma, and that too provides balance.

My list of thank-yous would not be complete without naming the doctors who provided excellent care as I dealt with my own breast cancer and who helped me in numerous ways with this research. Valerie Jorgensen, my gynecologist, got me in to see the surgeon immediately and was there every time I had a question or needed a second opinion. Allen Bar, my surgeon, took a great personal interest in me and my work, as did David Mintzer, my oncologist, and John Glassburn, my radiation oncologist. Lillian Cohn, my internist, who told me she never lets a pair of breasts leave the office without an exam, has remained interested and helpful in my research. Finally, John Lockart, my physical therapist, gave me the tools I needed to recover the full use of my arm after lymph node surgery and to avoid lymphedema. Although my book is about patients rather than doctors, I came to respect the difficulties of treating cancer—especially in helping patients juggle hope and realism—by my interactions with my own team of doctors.

Introduction

Writing a book about women's experiences with breast cancer allowed me to come to terms with my own diagnosis in December 1997. Like many of those I interviewed, I had not seen breast cancer on my horizon. My mother was still alive and physically robust in her nineties, as were my father and his sister. I had heard numerous stories of ancestors with similar longevity. So strong was this theme in my family that, although both my brother and I had experienced the same life-threatening illness as adolescents, I had long believed that old age was the only thing that would kill either of us.

Like many privileged women with access to good health care, I was health conscious. As part of my health regimen, I had annual mammograms and I performed monthly breast self-examinations. I did not do so out of a belief that I was at risk for breast cancer, and I never expected to find anything when I checked. I rarely thought about breast cancer and, if asked, would have said I knew almost no one who had had it. My only memory of thinking about it was during the 1970s. At this time, American surgeons were resisting evidence that lumpectomies gave women as good a chance of survival as the more drastic radical mastectomies. I viewed this resistance as an example of sexism in the medical profession but did not think the information concerned me personally. A politically aware feminist gynecologist performed my annual checkups, so I rarely interfaced with medical patriarchy. And anyway, I was not a candidate for breast cancer—or so I thought.

I retained this lack of engagement with the possibility of breast cancer for most of the period leading to my diagnosis, which started when I found a lump during a breast self-exam. I made an appointment for a mammogram, as I was due for one in any case. I expected that the lump would have to be biopsied but was confident it would prove benign, as is the case for most breast biopsies. In the interest of time management, I postponed the mammogram for three weeks in order to get an appointment for my annual gynecological checkup immediately afterward. Had I told the women scheduling my appointments that I had found a lump, they would have accommodated me sooner, but I had no fear and stayed silent.

To provide women with immediate feedback, and in most cases reassurance, the hospital I use for mammograms asks patients to wait until a radiologist reviews their pictures and gives them the results. In my case, the radiologist confirmed the presence of a lump and said that I needed a biopsy. As we arranged for her to contact my gynecologist, I told the radiologist, "Now, I'm not a worrying sort of person, so if you tell me this is probably nothing to worry about, I'm not going to worry." To her credit, she replied, "If I were you, I would worry." Had she not said that, I would have continued to assume the best until the shock of diagnosis. Because I told the radiologist that I had an appointment with the gynecologist immediately following her exam, she placed a call, and on my arrival at my gynecologist's office, I was ushered in promptly.

After examining my breast, my gynecologist called a surgeon whom she recommended highly, and he agreed to see me right away. Although

I had begun to realize that something might be wrong, a good part of me still resisted. As the surgeon performed a needle biopsy, he told me that sometimes these lead to false negatives. If mine was negative, he would not clear me unless a surgical biopsy also showed no malignancy. I replied that there was no history of breast cancer in my family, so I thought it unlikely I could have it, and he replied that the majority of women diagnosed have a similar story.

It takes time to absorb the idea of cancer. Going home alone after seeing these three doctors, one right after the other, I remember thinking, "I could possibly have breast cancer" and then thinking, "but there must be some kind of mistake." By the time the surgeon confirmed it the next day, I was no longer shocked or surprised. I do remember thinking that I did not want to die until my recently finished book was published, because I had worked so hard on it that I wanted to see it to fruition.

In the pages that follow, I describe the ways many different women experienced their diagnoses. Some, like me, gave little thought to their being diagnosed with breast cancer before it happened. Others had been more fearful. In listening to women describe their diagnoses, subsequent treatment decisions, and other experiences, I realized that there are several patterns of response to breast cancer. I describe these in chapter 1. When I describe these patterns to audiences, women often ask me to which category I belonged. The answer is that I became a biomedical expert. Biomedical experts are women who believe in the power of medicine to effect a cure and who want to gain as much knowledge about their disease as possible in order to partner with their doctors rather than to follow orders.

What did being a biomedical expert mean to me in practice? First, I had a strong desire to be a good patient. I wanted the doctors to like me and to think that I was handling my illness well. I wanted to continue working and to show everyone how strong I was. Showing great insight, my gynecologist sat me down shortly after diagnosis and told me that she had no worries about my falling apart. What worried her was that I would not take the time to grieve, or to acknowledge how tired I was, or to let others look after me. This astute observation fits a number of the women I interviewed. We are the women who want to get an A in handling breast cancer. We believe in medical science as the best route to a cure, even though in my case—and I suspect for others, too—we are less sure of scientific truths at an intellectual level.[1] We inform ourselves about the details of treatment alternatives. We treat doctors as partners, not as superiors. And most of all we exude an air of being able to handle the illness.

This way of responding to a diagnosis is not just the result of the patient's initiative. Usually, doctors treat educated, affluent career women with deference. When I was first diagnosed, I met with my surgeon— a kind and caring man who treats all his patients well—so he could explain my disease and the proposed treatment. He sat next to me with a pad and paper and confessed that he was nervous because, as he put it, "I have never had to teach a college professor before." A comment like that tells the patient that she is smart enough to understand everything and that the burden is on the doctor, not her. As is discussed in chapter 1, doctors have not always been so deferential, but clearly they have become less inclined to dismiss patients' rights to know.

In addition to their comfort in challenging doctors, patients functioning as biomedical experts take advantage of the variety of treatments available, and I was no exception. I had a number of treatments— lumpectomy, chemotherapy, radiation therapy, and hormone treatment, and I learned about each along the way. When I had treatment side effects, I solved them with more treatment. Sometimes it seemed like an endless array, one on top of another: chemotherapy for the cancer, antinausea medicine for chemotherapy side effects, stool softeners and fiber pills for the constipation resulting from the antinausea medicine, and so on.

Finally, like others in this category, I developed scientifically informed theories about why I got breast cancer: taking estrogen replacement therapy after a hysterectomy,[2] too many mammograms too early and before radiation levels were lowered, or too many chest X-rays when I had tuberculosis as a teenager.

Like many biomedical experts, I was fortunate in the support of my family and my friends. I have since learned that not all women have this level of support. My statistician husband became my scientific consultant. When I confronted chemotherapy, he obtained the latest research reports from the oncologist and helped me read and understand the statistical evidence about the benefits of chemotherapy for women in my age group and risk category. He was by my side every step of the way, asking questions of doctors and remembering the answers (I quickly discovered how hard it was to do both well). My three grown children called me all the time. When I had small emergencies, they were there to help. My younger daughter, the social worker, asked me professional questions about such things as my diet and my sleeping patterns to let me know she was monitoring me. In the end, however, I wanted to steer my own ship, to make my own decisions, and to feel I had done everything I could to increase my survival chances.

I did not question this way of responding, and it was not until I had interviewed other women that I found my approach to be only one of several possible types of response. I also found that other ways of responding were as helpful as mine in getting through the ordeal. Even women in the same general category differed from one another in the details. Some biomedical experts, for example, sought second, third, and even fourth medical opinions. I had one second opinion about whether to have chemotherapy, but in general, I was content to trust the doctors I first met, because I trusted the doctor who recommended them. I did not become as well informed about the details of my illness as many of the biomedical experts I interviewed.

Instead of focusing on my personal situation, I started to view my experience as if I were collecting research information and interpreting its larger meaning. For example, my radiation oncologist regularly told me what a great patient I was. Mindful of my gynecologist's warning to take things easy, I responded one day that it might be better were he to tell me to slow down and to take time off rather than rewarding me for stoicism. He looked at me and said, "I would never say that to a patient. I think it's good to be brave and to keep going." In repeating this to friends, instead of just telling the story, I explained his comments as indicative of the difficulties of being a cancer doctor and the need such doctors have—especially radiation oncologists who treat a lot of terminal cancers—to keep pain and despair at arm's length lest they drown in it.

It is probable that other women develop an intellectual interest in breast cancer in response to a diagnosis, but my training as an academic sociologist led me to do this in a particular way. Sociologists learn to step back from the world and take field notes about all kinds of encounters. It was understandable, therefore, that I would turn my sociological eye to the world of breast cancer by interviewing patients, listening to their stories, and writing about them. I attended numerous conferences and programs on the treatment of breast cancer, and I interviewed experts and other service providers from all walks of life. I told myself this was not because I personally wanted to know, but because I was doing research on breast cancer. This was true, but in doing so, it also helped me come to terms with and understand the meaning my breast cancer experience held for me. And I realized that others might also find it helpful to read about women like themselves as well as those who differed in their approaches to their breast cancer diagnoses.

I started this project about a year after my diagnosis and only a few months after treatment ended. I began by interviewing ninety-six women diagnosed with breast cancer. The interviewing began in the summer of 1999 and took about a year. In most cases, my respondents were diagnosed between 1994 and 1999.[3] To find respondents, I used a purposive technique, starting with women in one of the following categories: attendees at a conference on breast cancer, members of support groups, activists in breast cancer organizations, and women referred either by physicians or through personal contacts. These women then snowballed the sample by contacting others on my behalf. All lived in the Philadelphia area, including the outer suburbs, and they came from all walks of life.

Of the ninety-six women, the youngest was twenty-six at diagnosis and the oldest seventy-two. Two-thirds were between forty and fifty-nine years old, with a median age of fifty. Just over half the women had at least a college degree, and only three had completed less than high school. There were twenty African American women in the sample, which is more than might be expected randomly. This oversampling was deliberate, as is explained below. The African Americans had the lowest levels of education—although one-quarter had at least a college degree. Jewish respondents had the highest levels of education—four-fifths were college graduates. Median household income was seventy thousand dollars. Only six women had less than twenty thousand dollars in annual household income, while twenty-six lived in households with incomes over one hundred thousand dollars, in some cases considerably more. Thus the sample was largely but not exclusively middle to upper-middle class with a few very affluent women and a few very poor ones. Most respondents were married. About one-third were divorced or never married. Seven were lesbians, and each was in a relationship at diagnosis, although only three were in the same relationship at the time of the interview. Some lesbians had never been married; others were divorced. Most respondents had health insurance at diagnosis, including Medicare or Medicaid—only two reported none. However, I did not ask detailed questions about this and it is possible that I underestimated some women's difficulties. Some volunteered that they had not been able to have the doctor they wanted because of health insurance limits.

This sample is not a probability sample of women diagnosed with breast cancer and differs markedly from what such a sample would look like. This is true both because I used a snowball sample and because I deliberately oversampled certain groups. A comparison of these data with the National Health Interview Survey (NHIS) data from 2003 shows a number of differences. While African American women constitute 12 percent of all women in America, they are only 4 percent of women diagnosed with breast cancer. They were 20 percent of my sample. The women in my sample were, on average, younger than women who have had breast cancer nationally. This is in part because I mostly restricted my sample to women who had had breast cancer a few years before my interviewing them, whereas the NHIS asked about ever being diagnosed. It is also likely, however, that younger women were more interested in talking about it. My respondents were also better educated and had higher incomes than respondents to the NHIS. This is an important difference because the NHIS data show a negative relationship between breast cancer rates and both education and income. The one area of similarity between my data and that of the NHIS is that the NHIS data show that less than 1 percent of women with breast cancer had no health insurance.

This is undoubtedly because the majority of uninsured Americans are young, and the best predictor of breast cancer diagnosis is age.[4]

As is discussed in chapters 2–5, these four variables—race, age, education, and income—all vary by response group. It is important, therefore, for the reader to understand that the relative size of each response group cannot be generalized to the population. In addition, although I have analyzed my groups in terms of structural factors like race, education, and income, these findings must be treated with great caution given the small size and nonrandom nature of the sample.

In addition to my nonrandom method of sampling, I searched out specific groups, which had the effect of making my data even less representative. For example, I wanted to discuss the experiences of African American women, so I deliberately sought such interviews. African American women have lower rates of breast cancer diagnosis than white women, but higher mortality rates. Some have speculated that one reason for this is the discomfort African American women feel in dealing with the medical profession, causing them to avoid screening.[5] This made their presence essential in a study of women's responses to breast cancer diagnosis. And indeed, African Americans often responded quite differently than whites.

I also went to great lengths to interview lesbians. They often have difficulties with a medical system that expects significant others to be of a different gender. I wanted to understand how lesbians dealt with the medical profession when they faced a life-threatening illness, and I also wanted to compare their family support systems to those of the rest of the sample.

Finally, because so much has been written about the breast cancer movement, I wanted to interview a large number of activists. Many women do not want to make a career of breast cancer once treatment is over, so I recruited some of my respondents via breast cancer organizations. Doing so further distorted the sample, because such women are, on average, more affluent.[6] Activists are also more likely to be Jewish than are women who are not activists. As a result, I decided to treat Jews as a separate category from white non-Jewish women, which proved to be a useful strategy because the two groups differed in a number of respects.

Two groups not represented in the sample are Latinas and Asian Americans. This happened for reasons of both language and their communities still being reluctant to discuss breast cancer. The lack of these groups is a limit in the current study, as I suspect I would have found somewhat different responses. I did interview one Latina who came through one of the snowball chains, but she was from Argentina and had a high level of education, so she was not typical of Latinas in the United States.

A typical interview lasted about two hours and followed a respondent from before diagnosis to after treatment was over. We usually met in participants' homes though a few interviews were conducted in my university office or elsewhere. Respondents overwhelmingly reported that they found the interview to be worthwhile and even enjoyable. While I have no way of knowing who learned about my work and chose not to contact me, only four of the women I contacted refused an interview. Many who agreed to be interviewed told me that they did so because I had been through the same experience and so they felt a connection. Women frequently told me that they appreciated the opportunity to talk at length about having breast cancer. Family and friends, no matter how concerned, do not usually allow endless discussion. As a result, respondents were often pleased to recruit a friend to be interviewed. For some women, telling their story meant revisiting pain and trauma, but even so they appreciated the chance to talk. In spite of my own personal history, I believed I could maintain emotional distance during the interviews and, for the most part, I was able to. In three cases, young women had cancers that had metastasized, and, after the interview was over, I found myself emotionally devastated, but I felt privileged at their willingness to be interviewed and responsible for sharing their stories now in my care. These stories are told in the Conclusion.

Many women reported that they wanted their interviews to be used to help others who found themselves in similar circumstances. They hoped that telling their stories to me would allow others who read them to find solace. Laura Potts has noted that this is the motivation for many women who have written and published accounts of their experience with breast cancer.[7] In one of the most famous of these accounts, Audre Lorde's

Cancer Journals, the author wrote that she gave "voice" to her experiences so "that other women can take what they need from" her descriptions. She wanted to share her story "for use that the pain not be wasted."[8]

Since I wanted to know how women took charge of both diagnosis and the subsequent phases of the disease, I needed to understand the cultural milieus in which breast cancer patients find themselves. This necessitated immersing myself in the breast cancer support system. To learn about the messages women receive about breast cancer, I analyzed the contents of five years of the top-selling women's magazines in America as well as the two top-selling magazines geared toward African American women. I attended conferences on breast cancer treatment and on such related topics as alternative therapies, diet, exercise, and sexual response after diagnosis. Finally, I interviewed others: the leaders of many of the local and national breast cancer and general cancer organizations; providers of services to patients and survivors, including wig sellers and sellers of prostheses; women who ran support groups; and women who ran programs that target underserved groups.

My goal was to examine how women made sense of their breast cancer diagnosis and made decisions about their treatment. What I found was that they did this by developing narratives to explain their cancer to themselves and others. Many of their stories were of bravery and courage with the woman herself as the hero. Others recounted tragedies. With a beginning, a middle, and a resolution, each story helped its teller to cope with a terrifying diagnosis. Women constructed their stories using the images of breast cancer they saw around them—in media discourses, from the experiences of family and friends, and in their memories of others' experiences. And in doing so, they helped create visions of breast cancer for those who followed them. Each story told, in this book, is that of a real woman I interviewed, not a composite of different women. In the interest of confidentiality, I have changed all names and sometimes occupations. Where necessary, I occasionally changed other details, like geographic locale.

In chapter 1, I describe the world in which women find themselves upon diagnosis. This includes a discussion of the general cultural messages about breast cancer. I also describe the four categories into which I organized my respondents. Chapters 2 through 5 go into more detail about each category, telling the women's stories in their own words. In analyzing these narratives, I start with diagnosis and go through all phases of treatment. The second half of the book deals with the physical and emotional aspects of life after breast cancer, focusing on the breast in chapter 6, the body in chapter 7, and breast cancer activism in chapter 8. The main reason for giving separate chapters to bodies and breasts was that all women regardless of group found the changes difficult to deal with and the options limited. And, since sociologists have written so extensively on activism, I wanted to have a chapter devoted to this topic rather than fragmenting my findings. Finally, the concluding chapter summarizes the book's findings and their implications, including a discussion of the ways in which advanced breast cancer transforms women's experiences.

Along the way, we visit the many issues women face when coping with breast cancer—making decisions about breast reconstruction, attending support groups, handling family responses, and becoming breast cancer activists, to name but a few. The one thing almost all the women had in common was not becoming a victim of breast cancer. It is a testament to the human spirit that ordinary women can be so extraordinary when faced with a life crisis. In this sense the experiences of the women I talked to are inspirational.

ONE Telling Stories

Jo-Ellen's breast cancer story takes the form of a woman's worst nightmare. Her adoptive mother was a forty-year survivor, so Jo-Ellen knew the disease was something that women might get but could also recover from.[1] Upon finding a lump at age twenty-eight, Jo-Ellen went to a gynecologist who told her that it was only a cyst, so she did not go for a mammogram and ultrasound until a year later when the lump was still there. After that, things moved pretty quickly through a double mastectomy, breast reconstruction, chemotherapy, and tamoxifen.[2] Jo-Ellen was newly married with her life ahead of her, and, to ensure her future, she chose the most aggressive treatment, including prophylactic removal of her second breast. Tamoxifen put her into menopause by age thirty-three, a serious consequence for a woman who desperately wanted children. Even more serious was the discovery, a year after the original diagnosis, that the cancer had metastasized to her bones.

Jo-Ellen had lots of social support. Her new husband remained devoted through the loss of her breasts, her baldness, her weight gain, her loss of interest in sex, and the realization that she would never give birth. Her mother went with her for appointments, taking long lists of questions to supplement Jo-Ellen's own. Family and friends encouraged her to talk about her illness openly and to share her fears. She remained optimistic. When I interviewed her two years after the first diagnosis, she still believed she would survive in the face of several new masses, and she was hoping that her situation would not prevent her from gaining approval as an adoptive parent.

In openly facing her illness and talking about it to all who would listen, Jo-Ellen's response is a modern tale. In the second half of the twentieth century, breast cancer was transformed from an illness mentioned in hushed tones, if at all, to a huge public presence supporting a massive industry.[3] Jo-Ellen's story is unusual because she was younger than most women at diagnosis and her disease progressed more rapidly. Breast cancer is commonly more virulent among the young. Most breast cancer does not metastasize, and, according to the American Cancer Society, 88 percent of victims live at least five years and 63 percent live at least twenty.[4] Why then is the image of breast cancer so associated with death and so vivid in most women's minds? In her book *Illness as Metaphor*, Susan Sontag noted that the idea that "cancer = death" has been around for a long time and still continues to exert a strong influence.[5]

The only other illness with an equally visible profile is HIV/AIDS. Like breast cancer, HIV/AIDS has spawned a mass of organizations devoted to its management and cure.[6] However, the two diseases differ greatly. Most people who contract HIV feel the stigma of a disease that is associated with a "wrong" lifestyle.[7] In contrast, few breast cancer sufferers nowadays feel ashamed of having cancer, and most talk openly or even write about their illness.[8] In addition, AIDS severely shortens life expectancies, and, to beat the odds, patients must henceforth, and forever, organize their behavior around complex drug treatments and behavioral restrictions. With breast cancer, although medical treatment is debilitating, doctors rarely make recommendations about lifestyle changes, and most women, once treatment is finished, may return to their former lives with impunity.[9] While cancer always brings the threat of a horrible death, the high survival rate for breast cancer means a large group of women have lived to tell their tales. Most American women know others, including family members, in this category. However, those who have survived diagnosis and treatment still live with the threat of a reoccurrence or worse, and they form a potential army of activists to keep the disease in the public eye.

Threats of reoccurrence and of metastasis to other areas of the body remain permanent possibilities for women diagnosed with breast cancer, even if these threats diminish over time. In the 1920s, physicians decided to use five-year survival rates as a benchmark for determining a cure. This benchmark has remained in place, as medical historian Barron Lerner has noted, even though there is no particular significance to the five-year time frame when it comes to breast cancer. However, both the American Cancer Society and the major cancer hospitals have long believed that emphasizing high levels of curability would promote the benefits of early detection.[10]

Women have not always been as willing to discuss their experience with breast cancer as they are now. For many years, the stigma of breast cancer usually meant that the disease's existence was kept in the closet.[11] Ellen Leopold examined the correspondence from 1960 to 1964 between Rachel Carson, the author of the best-selling book *The Silent Spring*, and her surgeon, George Crile. Even Carson, a woman who battled the scientific establishment, was private about her breast cancer. She did not see it as something to share with other women. Rather, she handled it alone with the aid of her surgeon and a close friend.[12] She strove not to be angry but to bear up with courage. Crile, whose own wife had died of breast cancer, was ahead of his time in his willingness to reveal a cancer diagnosis to Carson, something her first surgeon would not do.[13]

In the 1970s, several prominent women broke the silence, including Shirley Temple Black in 1972.[14] The first woman to write about her own breast cancer experience, Rose Kushner, was diagnosed in June 1974. Kushner was a pioneer in insisting that she not be subjected to the then ubiquitous one-step operation. In this procedure, surgeons would perform a surgical biopsy, and, after examining the results, husbands and surgeons would make the final decision as to what further surgery to perform, while the patient was still under anesthesia. Women would go to sleep not knowing if they would still have a breast when they awoke. In fighting this, Kushner became one of the earliest breast cancer activists. When Betty Rollin was diagnosed in 1976, she was an NBC news correspondent. Rollin's book about her bout with breast cancer, *First You Cry*, became a best seller.[15] But none of these events produced the publicity occasioned when First Lady Betty Ford announced her breast cancer in 1978 and received an outpouring of public sympathy for her plight plus admiration for her bravery. Nancy Brinker, in her account of the death of her sister, Susan Komen, in whose memory she founded the Komen Foundation, cited Betty Ford as having inspired her sister to finally speak about her own illness.[16] And the Komen Foundation, with its annual Race for the Cure in cities across America, has continually encouraged women to publicly acknowledge their diagnoses.

Increased openness also resulted from the women's health movement. In the 1970s, feminist health activists began questioning the way American surgeons continued to perform debilitating radical mastectomies when European doctors were switching to less invasive lumpectomies.[17] Faced with growing evidence that the more limited surgery did not lower survival rates, a few American physicians had begun to perform lumpectomies or to modify radical mastectomies.[18] Yet most women, including those—like Betty Ford—with access to the most prominent surgeons, still had the more invasive surgery. This typically occurred because most women consented to a one-step procedure, as did Betty Ford.[19] In their best-selling book *Our Bodies, Ourselves,* members of the Boston Women's Health Collective made the case that radical mastectomies were abusive, and this idea was picked up by women's magazines.[20] In 1979, as a result of pressure from both inside and outside the medical profession, the Consensus Development Conference at the National Institutes of Health (NIH) agreed that the radical mastectomy was no longer the accepted procedure, and most surgeons switched to the newer surgery.[21]

The National Breast Cancer Coalition (NBCC), founded in 1991, has taken a more explicitly feminist position than the Komen Foundation.[22] It lobbies Congress to increase funding for breast cancer research and educates survivors to participate in allocating this funding. By copying the model of AIDS activism, the organization has successfully increased funding for breast cancer research and trained thousands of activists.[23] These two strands of breast cancer activism, represented by the NBCC and the Komen Foundation, continue to exist side by side along with other more militant organizations such as Breast Cancer Action as well as numerous support and educational groups.

The attention and public discussion mobilized by these groups have led to an increase in symbolic representations of the disease, particularly in the media. These images include, among others, the danger to the sexualized breast; death and dying; sacrifice, especially to family; and the miracles of modern scientific medicine. When diagnosed, a woman has to deal with the disparate imagery of her plight as she works her way through the frightening and tedious steps of decision-making and treatment. Of all cancers, that of the breast is currently the best publicized with the greatest resource allocation.[24] In much of the Western world, breasts are the single most important symbol of women's femininity, and, even though many women feel ambivalent about their actual breasts, surgical removal or partial removal of the breast is traumatic, an attack on womanhood itself.[25] Not only do breasts signify women's facility for nurturing, they are prime sexual ornaments.[26] In the current era, the ideal female body is seen as a slender figure with large breasts. Since most women cannot expect to achieve this shape without assistance, it is not surprising that liposuction and breast augmentation have become two of the three most common plastic surgeries for women.[27]

The media, particularly women's magazines, frequently run stories about breasts.[28] Most of these stories are about breast cancer. A search of top-selling women's magazines published during a five-year period produced an average of almost one article per issue on some aspect of the disease.[29] In studying the representation of breast cancer in the media, Cherise Saywell and colleagues described it as having the most visible press coverage of all cancers.[30] When Jennifer Fosket and colleagues examined breast cancer stories in popular women's magazines, they found that the overriding message was women's personal responsibility for detection, prevention, and survival.[31] Describing the various faces of breast cancer portrayed in the media and elsewhere, and the fears created in women, helps us understand how women respond to a diagnosis and how they cope during their months of treatment.

For the media, breast cancer is a sexy subject. Although the majority of sufferers are over fifty years old, magazines frequently portray it as a young woman's illness.[32] And even where writers note the actual age distribution, they emphasize youth indirectly. *Self* magazine's annual section on breast cancer for 1999 noted that this "has never been primarily a young women's disease" but undermined this point by illustrating the section with portraits of young survivors.[33] The magazine's selection of photographs, which emphasized youth and ongoing reproductive lives, showed a woman diagnosed at age twenty-eight who gave birth four years later, a thirty-three-year-old writer who "wants young women to pay attention to their bodies because their symptoms can be easily overlooked," a "fitness enthusiast" diagnosed at thirty-one, and a woman diagnosed at twenty-nine who subsequently married and gave birth. The visual message, that breast cancer is a disease of young women, was underscored by the inclusion in the issue of an advertisement for Ford Motor Company, which showed a little girl being hugged by her mother; the caption read:

> My breast cancer hero is my mommy. In April 1993, at the age of 27 and six weeks before her wedding day, she discovered a lump in her right breast. She survived lumpectomy and lymph node dissection. In June of that year, she married my daddy. . . . [When] I was conceived . . . she decided she had to live. She would not allow me to grow up without her. . . . She promised me that she would make it to my fourth birthday so that I would remember her if nothing else. I turned five this year. . . . Through her love for me and my Daddy, she survived.

Such images have great emotional appeal and stress the idea that surviving breast cancer is a matter of courage and perseverance. By implication, therefore, women who do not survive lack these attributes.

A titillating image of breast cancer appeared in the annual fall fashion promotion, "Fashion Targets Breast Cancer." For the four days of this event, 2 percent of Saks Fifth Avenue's sales went to breast cancer charities.[34] An eight-page spread in the *New York Times* told the story.[35] On the first page, three very young fashion models wore their tresses long and full, much of their skin bare, tight jeans, and the campaign T-shirt, the logo of which is a bright blue and navy bull's eye surrounded by "Fashion Targets Breast Cancer" and "Council of Fashion Designers of America." This T-shirt was designed by Ralph Lauren, one of many prominent supporters of breast cancer research.[36] Other similarly dressed young women adorned subsequent pages, in every case wearing full sets of perfect breasts, not breasts already altered by disease. These were threatened breasts, threatened because even beautiful, vibrant young women might succumb. The use of the bull's eye positioned on their chests and the word "Targets" underscored the danger.

These newer images of breast cancer, portrayed in the media and by cancer organizations, compete with older ones of death and disability. There remains an overwhelming fear of dying. Many women grew up in families where breast cancer was rarely mentioned. Memories of older relatives with the disease frequently involve debilitating surgery or painful death. This image of silence and death still appears in the media. Indeed, Brinker's account of Komen's death is in this tradition. Brinker described her sister as a hometown girl who trusted her family doctor and questioned neither his advice nor that of the surgeon to whom the doctor sent her. It was too late by the time Komen switched to competent treatment.

Other accounts make a different point. A number of descriptions of courageous and independent women who still died have appeared, among them Sandra Butler and Barbara Rosenblum's account of their shared experience of Rosenblum's diagnosis and eventual death from breast cancer.[37] Sometimes stories of death in top-selling women's magazines describe courage in death's face. For example, a woman with metastatic breast cancer told how she taught her daughter important lessons about life and death. More frequently, articles with titles such as "Will I Inherit My Mother's Disease?" contain frightening implications of dying too young. In one account, a woman's mother, grandmother, and great-grandmother had all died of breast cancer; after much hesitation about undergoing genetic testing, the story's subject tested positive for one of the known breast cancer genes and chose prophylactic breast removal to increase her chances of beating the survival odds.[38]

Another immediate concern for many women upon receiving a diagnosis of breast cancer is how family members will cope with their diagnosis. Here, too, images of death and disfigurement abound. Many women are the main caregivers in their families, the person around whom family life revolves. Family members do not always know how to respond when this caregiver becomes seriously ill, and their fears for her survival mix with concerns about their own potential loss of support. Women often anticipate such problems, both because of previous personal experiences and because of the cultural expectations about wives, mothers, and daughters. Newly diagnosed women may find themselves having to provide emotional support to family members, rather than focusing on their own treatment.

Women's magazines present stories lauding the choices women make. In these tales, motherhood is woman's central imperative, and accounts abound of survivors who risked their lives for their families. The most common story, in this genre, has been of the woman diagnosed with breast cancer either while pregnant or even before she had a chance to become pregnant. Chemotherapy's danger to fetuses may postpone urgently needed treatment, and pregnancy can cause estrogen-receptor positive tumors—the great majority of tumors—to grow more rapidly. In these accounts, doctors often advised pregnant women to have abortions and childless young women to avoid pregnancy. But, in most of the stories, the natural desire to be a mother overcomes the fear. Most such stories ended with a beautiful baby and a triumphant mother. Only one account described a woman choosing to have an abortion rather than risk worsening her cancer. This woman lost a badly wanted baby and was angry with doctors who missed her early symptoms. Furthermore, her abortion was not to protect herself but to ensure that her existing child would not grow up motherless. Many stories make the point that "A pregnant woman with breast cancer confronts agonizing choices."[39] The message here tells women that self-sacrifice is their role even when their lives are at stake.

Once women enter the formal medical system, scientific images of breast cancer overshadow private ones. Arthur Frank has described the modern experience of illness as beginning when "popular experience" is "overtaken by technical expertise." Where sick people used to go to bed at home to be cared for by family, they now go to paid professionals who "reinterpret their pain as symptoms, using a specialized language that is unfamiliar and overwhelming."[40] Both science and medicine are accorded high status in our culture.[41] Women with breast cancer quickly learn that theirs is a complex disease with each treatment phase bringing its own specialist. Bruno Latour has argued that scientific truth is established when scientific "facts" become accepted. When this happens, further developments in a field of discovery are constrained. So knowledge production involves more than a disinterested accumulation of evidence. Instead, some knowledge is reified, while some falls by the wayside. Furthermore, science becomes the place where the truth is determined.[42] The presentation of scientific truth and the circulation of these truths become important in framing breast cancer and its treatment, even if, as Charles Bosk has stated, illness definitions depend more on everyday values than on scientific expertise.[43]

Continued prospects of medical miracles in cancer treatment receive widespread media attention. Such stories are told in technical language, which may serve to mystify science and medicine.[44] These stories are not about death but about cures and the lifesaving benefits of early detection. Newspapers, women's magazines, television, and the Web sites of organizations like the American Cancer Society all report on treatment options, especially new potential breakthroughs. They portray the quest for a breast cancer cure as involving courageous, humanitarian genius searching for truths that will inevitably be revealed with time. Well-publicized mass events such as the Race for the Cure position breast cancer as a deadly plague whose spread will only be arrested by increasing the pace of medical discovery.

The image of the imminent cure has been around since the 1930s and continues to the present day.[45] The following statement, appearing at the end of the National Cancer Institute's (NCI) Breast Cancer Progress Review Group report in 1998, could have been written at any time between 1930 and the present:

The past two decades of painstaking research and substantial national investment have yielded major advances in our ability to care for women with breast cancer and for those at risk . . . by charting the course and implementing the recommendations described in this report, the nation will take the next crucial steps toward the ultimate goal of removing the threat of breast cancer from the lives of women and their families.[46]

This statement contains the standard optimism and priorities—basic biology, diagnosis, and treatment. In other words, scientists have made progress and, with increased funding in the right areas, will soon find a solution. As Susan Sontag noted, if cancer is a "killer," the only appropriate response is a "fight" or a "crusade" against it. For almost a hundred years, this fight has continued and the repeated announcements of imminent victory are reminiscent of government pronouncements in times of actual war.[47]

The media also emphasize the position long taken by organizations such as the American Cancer Society that breast cancer mortality rates are declining due to both early diagnosis and improved treatment options. This information is presented as unvarnished truth, when the story is more complicated.[48] If the cure for cancer involves early diagnosis and constantly improving medical intervention, this creates a dilemma for women. On the one hand, the newly diagnosed woman is expected to acquiesce in the face of medical expertise. The long-standing tradition of male surgeons possessing unquestioning authority over subservient and unknowing female patients still holds sway, even in an era where many women have entered medicine, including surgery. On the other hand, women feel considerable pressure to take charge of their interactions with doctors and to stay informed about treatment innovations.

Rachel Carson knew more about her disease and its progress than most women at the time. Yet she knew little compared to today's patients. In the modern era, the widespread availability of books, articles, and other materials and the ready accessibility of the Internet mean that doctors no longer have a monopoly on information about breast cancer. For example, typing the word "tamoxifen"—until recently the most widely used hormone treatment for breast cancer—into the search engine

Google produced 2,420,000 hits.[49] Many patients educate themselves about every aspect of their illness including diagnosis, types of malignancies, stages of the disease, treatment options, and support services. They engage their doctors with long lists of questions and use medical language with ease.

This readily available information, coupled with trends in the medical profession, in particular the proliferation of malpractice suits, has had a profound impact on doctor-patient relationships. In theory, at least, doctors must now educate patients about tumor type and stage of development and explain the resulting treatment options. As a result, the doctor no longer possesses all the wisdom about the patient's needs; rather, doctor and patient are partners.

Doctors' increased concern for patients' rights can be partially explained by the growth of the health promotion movement. This movement has its roots in the nineteenth century, when health activists like William Kellogg promulgated the idea that the right diet could improve health. However, it grew rapidly in the last few decades in reaction to the long-accepted, conventional medical/scientific model of "Doctor knows best." Now the focus is on prevention and on personal responsibility for health. The health promotion movement's image of breast cancer is well represented in women's magazines. Titles such as "The Nine Top Ways to Prevent Breast Cancer," "Your Best Self-Defense against Breast Cancer," or "The Anti–Breast Cancer Diet" have clearly communicated the message that by eating right, exercising, staying thin, and taking special action when risk is high, women can keep breast cancer at bay.[50] This is also underscored in popular health books.[51]

Twenty years ago, Marshall Becker complained that the rising health promotion movement was leading to a situation where patients were being blamed for getting sick, that is, for having a disease-inducing lifestyle.[52] Susan Yadlon has even argued that the dominant discourse around breast cancer assigns women personal responsibility for getting the disease, especially by eating the wrong diet.[53] While this is not the only message in the media, it is a common one, and it has been influential, even though Susan Sherwin has noted that there is a lack of concrete evidence that diet, especially the level of dietary fat, makes a difference.[54]

The implication of this message is that those who get breast cancer have not taken personal responsibility and therefore have failed at protecting their own health. Among the most commonly emphasized failures are poor diets, lack of exercise, excess weight, smoking, alcohol consumption, and high stress.

Almost any woman can find reasons to blame herself for her illness and to think that lifestyle changes could prevent a reoccurrence.[55] Best-selling books testify to this. Bernie Siegel's *Love, Medicine, and Miracles* has described the "typical" personality profile of those who get cancer as "compulsively proper and generous people . . . because they put other people's needs ahead of their own" but who "are giving love only in order to receive love." Adding that "there are no incurable diseases, only incurable people," Siegel described "exceptional" patients who cured themselves by their determination to fight and to embrace healing techniques.[56] Magazine articles have made the same point with titles such as "Boost Your Immunity: The Seven Traits That Keep People Healthy," "A Woman of Valor," or "Think Yourself Well." Only one article, of those that I analyzed, acknowledges a lack of empirical evidence that the causes of breast cancer lie in the mind.[57]

In addition to emphasizing personal failure, the health promotion model reinforces women's personal responsibility for recovery. The patients' rights movement and the women's health movement have further promoted this idea by demanding that patients be given access to complete information about their illnesses and that patients should participate in treatment decisions. And the replacement of the radical mastectomy with less drastic surgery, in conjunction with the use of radiation, chemotherapy, and hormones, means that women no longer face one all-powerful surgeon but a team of doctors, each of whom may offer choices. This has increased women's sense of involvement in decision-making about treatment.

The idea of patients as partners has created its own problems for women. The easy availability of masses of information, often coupled with separate decisions at each doctor's office, makes decisions more confusing. Much of this information is highly technical, and women must struggle to understand, let alone decide on, the options open to them. Furthermore, in spite of the rhetoric of patients' rights, many doctors do not treat breast cancer patients as partners. Instead, they may resist what they see as intrusions on their expertise. This is especially true for male physicians, who are particularly likely to be patronizing to women patients.[58] The percentage of women physicians has increased; in 1970, women constituted less than 8 percent of physicians in the United States but were almost 25 percent by 2001.[59] However, they are concentrated in general medicine and in specialties such as obstetrics, gynecology, and dermatology. Even as late as 1999, only 21 percent of surgical residents were women compared with 67 percent of obstetrical and gynecological residents.[60] A woman diagnosed with breast cancer will have exclusively female physicians only if she puts considerable effort into doing so. Among the ninety-six women I interviewed, over two-fifths had an all-male team of doctors and only four women had an all-female team. The rest had teams of mixed gender; in most cases, one woman was on a team with two or three men.

Much has been written about the ways in which problems faced by Westerners have been increasingly medicalized. This has happened in part because of the tendency of the medical profession to increase its sphere of influence. In addition, the respect accorded medicine leads groups to want their problems to be designated as medical problems and thus treatable. This idea of medicalization is closely associated with Peter Conrad, who has described numerous concerns—overeating, alcoholism, hyperactivity—that once were seen as behavior problems but now are treated as medical conditions.[61]

Clearly breast cancer did not have to struggle for inclusion in the illness lexicon. However, some writers have expanded Conrad's arguments to focus on the medicalization of women's bodies. Emily Martin, who first propounded this viewpoint, and other writers have taken the position that women's bodies are increasingly seen as pathological and that female functions formerly viewed as normal—menstruation, reproduction, menarche—are now viewed as medical conditions requiring expert intervention and management.[62] The resulting sense of bodily estrangement has led women to view their bodies as in need of constant surveillance and to anticipate that things might go wrong, particularly with those body parts that are exclusively female.[63] Thus women feel under great pressure to check their breasts, to subject themselves to regular examinations, and to fear for their futures. Furthermore, as Nora Jacobson has shown, with the introduction of breast implant techniques, a whole industry has emerged involving plastic surgeons, manufacturers of implants, and complicit women. This industry has helped change a woman's breast into an idealized version of itself.[64]

Like other aspects of medicine, medicalization has resulted not only from doctors' expansionist tendencies but from patients' desires for the best that medicine can offer. However, this has not always been a smooth relationship. Medicalization can be both empowering and repressive to women, depending on the relationship they have with their doctors.[65] Frequently, patients' desires for involvement in decision-making have collided with autocratic doctors. This has sometimes led to resentment about doctors, which is reflected in women's magazines to a surprising degree. In clear, nontechnical terms, readers have been told that they must select carefully, since some doctors mask incompetence with authority. Doctors' reported failures have included saying "not to worry about a small hard spot in your breast because it hasn't shown up on your mammogram," prescribing mastectomies where lumpectomies are appropriate, claiming "You're too young to have breast cancer," performing breast exams improperly, not warning that fertility treatments increase breast cancer risks, and not informing women that mammograms may produce false positives.[66] With these stories of doctors as ordinary mortals, the media demystify the practice of medicine. Yet simultaneously, they exalt biomedical science with miraculous tales of medical breakthroughs.[67]

If women feel ambivalent about organized medicine, they sometimes pursue alternative treatments. Magazines abound with stories of women who have aided their recovery with techniques such as hypnotherapy, visualization, or Chinese medicine.[68] So popular have these "fringe" methods become that mainstream hospitals now offer information sessions and classes on alternative practices. One hospital in suburban Philadelphia even opened a wellness center with furniture and facilities arranged according to feng shui principles.[69]

Most of the cultural images of breast cancer in women's magazines evoke individual pathologies and treatments as opposed to risk factors that are beyond individual control.[70] In recent years, however, some activists have taken the position that breast cancer is a disease outside an individual's control or personal history. Breast cancer, these advocates have argued, is produced by modern industrial life, particularly by pollutants and pesticides, and the cure for cancer involves government action and even a restructuring of social life. Proponents of this view, first articulated in the 1960s by Rachel Carson, have interpreted its relative lack of attention from the media as resulting from the corporate pressures of industry, the medical profession, and university researchers.[71] In this model, the disease's "cause" is not to be found in the individual woman or her history, but in the environmental toxins she cannot avoid because they are all around her.[72] Genetic traits or other risk factors may increase a woman's potential for breast cancer, but the trigger is a sick society bent on profit without regard for its citizens' health. This image is at odds with the medical community's view, where the emphasis is on finding a cure rather than on promoting prevention. In the late 1980s, the director of the National Institutes of Health, Harold Varmus, stated that "You can't do experiments to see what causes cancer. It's not an accessible problem. It's not something that scientists can afford to do."[73] When prevention has been discussed, it has been usually at the level of the individual woman rather than of society as a whole.

Women's magazines pay little attention to the idea of breast cancer as anything other than an individual pathology. A lone story on estrogen in *Self*, in 1994, noted the high rate of cancer on Long Island and included information on environmental estrogens, but such stories are rare.[74] However, in recent years, both the National Cancer Institute and the Environmental Protection Agency have started to collect epidemiological data on incidence in an attempt to measure which pollutants might be to blame for breast cancer's apparent increase. This is a difficult task relying on possibly spurious ecological correlations, but pressure from environmental activists and from some breast cancer activists to undertake this type of research has pushed government agencies forward. A number of recent books on breast cancer have argued that environmental toxins account for an increase in the rates.[75] Several of these books are by breast cancer survivors with a history of political activism.

Some activist organizations have taken a militant position on breast cancer and the environment. Most notable among these is the San Francisco–based organization Breast Cancer Action, whose Web site states that, in spite of massive research funding for cancer ("$23 billion"), "Environmental factors have been largely ignored by science as possible explanations for the escalation of the incidence of breast cancer."[76] Taking the existence of a breast cancer epidemic for granted, Breast Cancer Action has argued that if breast cancer is to be contained, exposure to toxins must be reduced. And at the international level, the Women's Environment and Development Organization has made breast cancer and its environmental connections into a central issue. This organization has held two world conferences on breast cancer, and each included numerous sessions on the environment.

Breast cancer is not the only disease where activist and expert interpretations of data have led to a struggle over the meaning of scientific evidence. In his study of leukemia in Woburn, Massachusetts, Phil Brown demonstrated how activists forced the debate over the relationship between a toxic water supply and higher than average levels of leukemia. And Steven Epstein has documented the ways in which AIDS activists questioned the scientific basis of clinical trials in testing the efficacy of AIDS drugs.[77]

So women with breast cancer face competing images as they struggle to understand what is happening to them. Each image is gendered in important ways. Women know that breast cancer can lead to death, but they may also believe that women should put aside their own fears and focus on what will happen to their families should they get seriously ill or even die. Individual women may reject this theme of sacrifice, but it resonates loudly in our culture and in the media. Patients must put their faith in the ability of doctors to cure them, yet they also receive loud messages that they themselves are responsible for getting well. And they may question themselves about how they allowed cancer to happen. Women are responsible for the health of themselves and their families, and to get too sick to be the family caregiver is to fail miserably at this task. Even those who deny the truth of this cultural mandate are not indifferent to it. Neither are women who distrust the medical profession indifferent to its power and authority. Finally, for some women, their diagnosis confirms the sorry state of society and the lack of power women face in trying to create change.

Women diagnosed with breast cancer not only struggle to understand and respond to the crisis but typically must make difficult choices among an array of options. In the majority of cases the tumor is small, and women may choose between two surgical procedures: a mastectomy or a lumpectomy plus radiation. In some cases there is no choice; the size and type of tumor necessitate a mastectomy. When treatment involves a mastectomy, decisions must be made about breast reconstruction.

Depending on a woman's age and the type and stage of her tumor, a further series of decisions involve chemotherapy. Sometimes women are given a choice about whether or not to undergo chemotherapy; in other cases, doctors strongly recommend or even insist on it. When women have chemotherapy, doctors often present options about type. In addition, while women who have lumpectomies are prescribed radiation, it may also be recommended for mastectomy patients, especially where there is extensive lymph node involvement.

To further complicate matters, new treatments appear frequently. There have been recent changes in, for example, the preferred method of diagnosis, the order of surgery and chemotherapy, and the chemotherapy protocols. One of the most difficult decisions has been whether or not to take hormones, and here too recommendations have changed. In the past, the hormone of choice was tamoxifen. Tamoxifen is generally taken for five years, and its unpleasant and potentially dangerous side effects make it controversial, especially for premenopausal women, as it typically puts them into menopause.[78] More recently, the dominance of tamoxifen has been challenged by a new set of hormones—aromatase inhibitors—taken either in conjunction with tamoxifen or instead of it.

As a result of the constant treatment changes, it is not uncommon for a woman who seeks a second or third opinion to receive more than one set of treatment recommendations. So how do women who have just received the devastating diagnosis of breast cancer work through their choices? As Sherwin has noted, while women's health activists fought hard for the right of patient autonomy in decision-making, this right assumes that patients are independent agents and in control of other aspects of their lives and that they feel entitled to have opinions.[79] Furthermore, the information necessary to understand and to make a decision is highly technical, and most women start out ill-equipped to make decisions that may have life or death consequences. In addition to learning about tumor size and type, women must learn about their lymph nodes and the meaning of lymph node involvement. They learn that some of their treatments are intended to minimize chances of a reoccurrence in the breast while others lessen the chance of metastases. Many treatments have dangerous side effects, and it is not easy to weigh the health benefits of treatment against these. Women who have mastectomies must not only decide whether or not to undergo breast reconstruction but also, if they choose to undergo it, what type to have.

In most cases there is no particular urgency to decide on the course of treatment, yet women feel tremendous pressure to decide quickly. They perceive untreated breast cancer to be a killer, so they want treatment to start as soon as possible. This pressure is in part a result of medical and media messages that cancer diagnosis and survival cannot tolerate delay.[80]

While they are processing this new information and making these terrifying decisions, women must sort through the various faces of breast cancer and make sense of their diagnosis. At the same time, they must decide whom to tell and how to tell them. And there are other struggles: whether or not to continue working, whether or not to go for second opinions, whether or not to use alternative treatments and if so which ones, and the biggest struggle of all: how best to cope with chemotherapy and radiation.

These decisions and struggles form the basis of what many women experience as a journey through cancer treatment and recovery. This journey has a number of stages, not always the same, and each brings its own set of issues. Patricia Kaufert has described each stage as "another rite in the passage from being the 'well' woman to being this other woman, the cancer patient."[81] And all women must decide how well informed they will become, and how involved they will be in their treatment.

The first stage in the breast cancer narratives of the women I interviewed involved their beliefs and practices before diagnosis. This often included accounts of their ideas about cancer and their history of self-examinations and mammograms. The second stage was diagnosis, starting with an account of how they found out something was wrong. To make sense of their diagnosis, most women created a theory about why they had developed cancer. At diagnosis, patients not only want to know the name of their disease, they want to understand its cause. In her sample of working-class women in Scotland taken over twenty years ago, Mildred Blaxter discovered that they viewed cancer as a random fate.[82] It is most likely a testament to the increased optimism about cancer treatment that almost all the women in the current study had a theory to explain why they got cancer.

Once diagnosed, women had to decide what to do next—whether to seek second opinions and whether to obtain treatment at a local hospital, a comprehensive cancer center, or a teaching hospital. And they had to decide about the myriad of possible treatments. These decisions did not occur in a vacuum. While some women gave priority to helping those around them, others who had expected their loved ones to provide support had not received it and felt outraged that it was not forthcoming. Next, women had to undergo difficult and debilitating treatment. With breast cancer, it is usually the treatment and not the disease that makes the patient ill. Going through treatment involved dealing with side effects and coping with the consequences of treatment such as hair loss and weight gain.

Finally, after cancer treatment was over, women had to get on with their lives. They also had to live with increased feelings of vulnerability caused not only by the events they had lived through but also by fears of reoccurrence or metastasis. Furthermore, some were permanently disfigured after surgery. Some experienced significant weight gain. These, in turn, had profound implications for intimate relations. After treatment, in facing the future, women had to decide whether to stay focused on breast cancer in some way or to try and put their illness behind them. Some remained involved with breast cancer as activists and volunteers, while others tried to go back to the lives they had lived before diagnosis.

Either way, many saw themselves as permanently changed psychologically. Such women needed to feel that their illness was not completely in vain but had had a profound and generally positive effect on them as individuals.

At each stage of the journey, the various images of breast cancer portrayed in the media were important in helping women I interviewed frame the issues. And just as these images varied, these women's views about their treatment did also. There were two major dimensions to this: their attitudes toward biomedicine and the extent to which they wanted to take charge of the decision-making.

A majority of women believed in the message that, in the modern world, biomedicine works miracles. They thought that they had the best doctors, and they saw medical science as their salvation. These were women who supported the extension of medical authority into more and more areas of life.[83] Adele Clarke and colleagues have described an extension of medicalization that they call "biomedicalization." This involves the commodification of health and the use of ever-expanding technologies and treatments.[84] Women who believed in biomedicine wholeheartedly embraced this notion of ever-expanding medical miracles.

However, some of the women I interviewed had more critical views of biomedicine; they did not completely trust doctors or the medical establishment, and in some cases not at all. Such women sought alternatives or supplements to the established health care system when they were diagnosed with breast cancer. And many felt critical of their treatment by the medical system, describing insensitivity, insults, and even incompetence. This finding that some women were ambivalent or hostile is similar to that of Martha Balshem in her study of cancer and community. Many of Balshem's working-class respondents did not accept the biomedical explanations for cancer that they were given.[85] This division between those who embraced biomedicine and those who looked outside can be understood by viewing medicine as both a resource to people facing serious illness and as a constraint on coming to terms with the deeper meaning of the illness.[86]

In addition to their attitudes toward biomedicine, the women I interviewed varied in the level of personal responsibility they took for their own recovery. Some believed that, to get better, they must put themselves in others' hands. Such women frequently had family responsibilities or personal fears that led them to minimize their own involvement and levels of learning. They were often intimidated by the medical establishment. Others felt they must make decisions themselves, usually with the aid of experts but never by deferring to another's judgment without thorough consideration of the issue. This division is similar to that made by other researchers. In an Australian study, Deborah Lupton divided patients into consumers and passive patients, based upon their relationships to doctors. The former saw themselves as autonomous actors in making medical decisions, while the latter were more dependent on the doctors' recommendations.[87] In a study of doctor and breast cancer patient encounters, Tovia Freedman found that while some patients wanted doctors to tell them what to do, others wanted to believe they had made all the decisions themselves.[88]

Christy Simpson has described three types of ideologies in talking about health and disease. While one ideology operates at the level of the social—that is how societies promote or inhibit the achievement of health—the other two take place at the level of the individual patient. They concern "the belief in technological and pharmacological solutions to problems of health and disease" and "the promotion of personal or individual responsibility for health."[89]

These two distinctions in types of response—attitudes toward biomedicine and level of personal involvement in decision-making—led me to identify four groups of respondents in my interviews. These groups help us understand the variations in women's interpretations of the meaning of breast cancer and in their coping strategies. These four groups are described briefly below and in more detail in chapters 2 through 5.

Two groups put their faith in doctors, hospitals, and medicine. The first of these—the traditional responders—believed in biomedicine and also believed that the doctor knows best and should be deferred to. These women rarely questioned a doctor's decision or recommendation. They often remained uncritical of their doctors, even as they told stories of less than stellar care. They learned little about their illness because they found knowledge frightening and instead tried to get on with their lives with as few interruptions as possible. This was one of the two largest groups, comprising one-third of the women I interviewed.

The other largest group of responders—the biomedical experts—also believed in biomedicine. However, these women saw themselves as responsible for their own health and sought partnerships with their doctors rather than deferring to superior medical expertise. They obtained numerous second opinions in their quest to find the best experts, they read about all aspects of their disease, and they became conversant with the technical language of breast cancer. Biomedical experts were also one-third of the total sample.

In contrast to those who believed in biomedicine—whether in a traditional way or by becoming an expert—were two groups with less faith in its powers. The first of these, the religious responders, generally did what their doctors asked but believed that, if they were to get better, they must put their ultimate faith in God and not in doctors. So while they deferred to a higher power, this was a power outside the medical profession and, in these women's opinions, superior to it. They used prayers, their own and those of others of similar faith, to help them safely through their illness. They found support in organized religion both while they were receiving medical treatment and afterward. This was the smallest group—just over 10 percent of the total sample.

A final group consisted of women who wanted to take charge of their own recovery but did not place great faith in doctors. While no one turned their backs completely on biomedicine, women in this group used alternative practices to supplement or replace some aspects of the standard medical treatment; thus they are called the alternative experts. They viewed doctors as dictatorial and often as in league with corporate capitalism in profiting from patients' desperate needs. In looking outside their own individual behaviors to explain breast cancer, this was the only group that also embodied Simpson's other health ideology—that of the social. They believed they were beating the medical system by taking their search for a cure elsewhere. They often chose to wholly or partly reject doctors' recommendations. One-sixth of respondents fell into this category.

Table 1   Response Groups by Race and Ethnicity*

Race/Ethnicity	Traditional responders	Biomedical experts	Religious responders	Alternative experts
White (not Jewish)**	19	21	2	10
Jewish	5	9	0	5
African American	8	2	8	2
Total	32	32	10	17

* Five interviewees had mixed responses, including the three with metastatic cancer, and so are not included in this tally.

** Includes one Latina.

As can be seen from table 1, traditional responders were the most racially and ethnically mixed of the groups. Biomedical experts had an overrepresentation of Jewish women but only two African American women. The group most different in race and ethnicity from biomedical experts was the religious responders. While less than half of all black respondents were religious responders, almost all the religious responders were African American. Had I not made a decision to interview enough African American respondents to generalize about their experience, I would not have found this group. None of the religious responders were Jewish. This does not mean that Jewish respondents found no comfort in faith but rather that relying on faith first and foremost was not their main response. Finally, alternative experts were similar in race and ethnicity to biomedical experts.

In the following chapters, I expand on the differences among these four groups as we join the women I interviewed in their journeys through the land of breast cancer. We also see how many aspects of treatment differed for the women in these four groups. The stories of how these different groups of women made sense of their experiences are told to a great extent in the women's own words. The stories follow Martin's injunction that we need to provide a forum to show the variety of ways in which women understand their bodies and the meanings they give to the physical events in their lives.[90] I should note that five of the women were not easy to categorize into groups. Two had simultaneously tried many different responses and the other three had moved between categories at some point. These issues are discussed in the Conclusion.

Illness narratives take a particular form because the speaker is telling a story about a major disruption in her everyday life. While everyday accounts are easily understood by both speaker and listener, telling the illness narrative takes more work. It must be constructed in a way that makes sense to the woman and to her audience, and it must include previously unthinkable possibilities like imminent death.[91] The sufferer has to categorize and explain the progress of the disease and its treatment as well as the ways in which it causes pain.[92] In a study of rheumatoid arthritis patients, Gareth Williams found that the experience of chronic illness forced its victims to reconstruct events in order to explain how the illness happened at the particular moment in history and to reaffirm the belief in life as purposeful.[93] The breast cancer survivors I interviewed needed to do this also.

The ways in which individuals talk about their illnesses tell us both about personal experience and about the cultural context in which the experience occurred. Culture shapes the experience of illness and gives it meaning.[94] In analyzing the narratives of sufferers of TMJ,[95] Linda Garro described patients as struggling because their illnesses deviated from an existing cultural model of how illness was supposed to progress and be understood.[96] Women who have had breast cancer have a different experience. Unlike TMJ, their illness has enormous visibility and an established language that all understand.

The narratives about illness and sickness that appear in subsequent chapters tell the reader what the tellers wanted the world to hear. Many times, women commented that they agreed to an interview so I would share their stories with others. In her book on cancer and culture, Jackie Stacey has described such narratives as carrying a "health warning." By this she meant that the reader should beware of "the certainties they promise" and "the truths they guarantee."[97] As Lucy Yardley argued in her essay on discourses of health and illness, we can only explain our experiences to ourselves and others by using the language and the human concepts that are accessible to us.[98] A woman who tells the interviewer about her breast cancer is engaging in impression management and directing her responses to support the way she wants to present herself.[99] Catherine Kohler Riessman illustrated this point by describing how a man interviewed about divorce was able to structure the conversation in a way that protected his masculine identity in the face of multiple sclerosis.[100]

In the end, the reader has to make of these narratives what she or he will. When the women I interviewed told me their stories, they most likely had a larger audience in mind, at least some of the time. I as the writer must necessarily change their stories by setting them in a context and by selecting which voices and segments to recount. Many of these women wanted their voices to be part of the public face of breast cancer. Yet, while we need to accept that their narratives are a kind of story, we should also realize that, to the narrators, they represent breast cancer's truth. I have tried to honor that truth in the pages that follow.

TWO Following the Doctors' Orders

Like most of the women I interviewed, Carla, a single mother of three young children, told a well-rehearsed story, beginning with the time before she was diagnosed, moving through treatment, and ending with life after breast cancer. Such accounts often reflected the stories about cancer that women had seen in the media or heard described by others. But where some women featured themselves as heroines, Carla's story described a victim to whom bad things happened, either as a result of her own irresponsible behavior or because of circumstances that she could not prevent. Women such as Carla, who gave accounts of victimhood and passivity in the face of crisis and hardship, I call "traditional responders." In this chapter I describe the traditional responders, explain why they responded as they did, and examine the consequences of the paths they took.

I interviewed Carla in her small and tidy row house in a working/lower-middle-class neighborhood just outside the Philadelphia city limits. Self-conscious about her weight and her breasts, she wore a loose sweat suit to hide her figure. She told her story with a great deal of emotion. She was still experiencing the trauma of breast cancer and lived in fear of a reoccurrence. When the taped interview was over, she asked me lots of questions about both my cancer experience and hers, and she told me confidences that she did not want on tape about why she felt cancer was her just reward.

Carla learned she had breast cancer at age forty. She decided to check her breasts when she heard that a neighbor was having a breast biopsy after discovering a lump. Carla had already had a biopsy, and she firmly believed she should be checking her breasts diligently. When asked to pray that her neighbor's biopsy would prove benign, Carla's immediate thought was, "My goodness, I haven't done [a breast exam] in a while." When she did so, she found a mass and called her gynecologist, who thought it was probably nothing but arranged for a precautionary mammogram. Carla was overdue for a mammogram because she had switched her medical insurance and the new procedures were complex. When Carla's mammogram led to a diagnosis of breast cancer, the surgeon found three malignant lymph nodes in addition to the cancerous breast.[1] Carla blamed herself for this because she had delayed getting checkups. Yet, for a single parent of three young children, it is understandable that Carla might delay attending to tasks such as getting a mammogram.

The behavior described here is typical of traditional responders. Carla's story reflects two of the cultural messages about breast cancer discussed in chapter 1. Carla believed that women must take on the task of detecting cancer, and she blamed herself for not doing this. She also had faith that regular checkups, both medical and by self-examination, were her best protection, that is, that biomedicine could keep her well. These themes appeared repeatedly with traditional responders. Although some of the women in this group had been more conscientious about checkups, because of their fears about developing cancer, many had not.

Gina, age forty-six and a divorced secretary who lived a few blocks away from her father in one of the city's Italian American neighborhoods, was typical. When asked how she envisioned breast cancer before diagnosis, she replied:

> I was always frightened of it. I had been asking my gynecologist for many years about my chances, and he said one in eight, because I had no reasons. . . . Once I heard on the television that women who have miscarriages were more apt to develop breast cancer, because of something to do with the milk ducts not being able to fulfill what they were supposed to do, and, at that one moment in my life, I knew that I was doomed because I had a miscarriage when I was 38, and sure enough it happened.

As can be seen from these two stories, traditional responders believe that they have little control over the onset of breast cancer. They also believe they cannot themselves improve their chances of a recovery, so a breast cancer diagnosis is terrifying. In a study of published accounts of breast cancer, Rosenbaum and Roos noted how frequently women equated breast cancer with death.[2] This was Carla's response when she was diagnosed; her first thought was, "Who's going to take care of my children. . . . I'm a single mom. Their father is not involved in their lives." Carla was burdened by her day-to-day responsibilities of work and family and believed that these had prevented her from looking after herself more carefully. Yet, although she realized that life was difficult for a single parent, she blamed herself for not taking better care. It would be her fault if she did not survive, and her thoughts of death related to another cultural message that resonated with traditional responders. For a woman with three young children and no husband, the future was frightening.

Gabrielle, a forty-seven-year-old teacher and mother of two sons living in the outer suburbs of the city, also described herself as terrified when she was diagnosed. She thought women usually died when they had breast cancer. Calling herself "kind of a fatalist," she reported that she "just knew this was gonna happen." In a similar vein, Gina reported that, after diagnosis, she thought that "it would spread and I would die. That was all I kept thinking about."

At the same time, traditional responders often believed that their failure to live up to a proper standard of performance was the reason they got cancer in the first place.[3] In a study of cervical cancer screening,

Kavanagh and Broom described three types of risk factors women used to explain illness: environmental risk factors, lifestyle factors, and a category Kavanagh and Broom call embodied factors, by which they mean a risk contained in the body over which the woman may have no control.[4] Traditional responders blamed lifestyle factors for their illness, that is, they saw cancer as the result of something they had or had not done.

Carla's litany of self-blaming reasons for her breast cancer can be seen in the following quotes. In the first place, she explained:

> I've always had a weight problem. It was always a crash diet. So before I was diagnosed, all I basically had during the day was eat some hard pretzels, smoke cigarettes, and drink soda. I really believe that contributed to my cancer—and the stress with work and children.

Later in the interview, she saw herself as creating her cancer through fear:

> It was always a concern in the back of my head . . . when I was in my late thirties—that forty was going to be the year I got cancer. And it happened. And now I have fifty in my head, because I'm a little superstitious that way, and I really think that you can think yourself into things.

Finally, she blamed herself for finding life so stressful and for her inadequacy as a mother:

> I was so stressed out in a depression. . . . I took care of [my children] and I loved them, but that's all I wanted to do was love them. To take care of them was such a chore. . . . To me, it was a wake-up call from God saying, "Look, you're working, you're going out dancing."

At the same time as she blamed herself, Carla recognized she was overburdened by guilt, which, she explained, was the result of an upbringing that told her, "Don't do this or you'll go to Hell." She had absorbed the cultural messages that she received with her Catholic upbringing, which told her that good women do not lose their husbands and that, if they do, they must not have any dancing pleasure.

Traditional responders were the group most likely to blame themselves for cancer, and some of the reasons given by Carla—in particular, stress and depression—were the most common sins described by this group.

Gabrielle, for example, reported that she got breast cancer because she "just stressed herself," and Gina blamed her diagnosis on depression. Self-blame appears to be a common response of traditional responders to times when their bodies fail them. Linda Layne has described how women who experience miscarriages, stillbirths, or infant deaths frequently blame themselves for their inability to ensure a positive outcome.[5]

When we look at the responsibilities of the women in this group, we can understand that many of them led stressful lives. Almost all had extensive family responsibilities, and a number were single parents trying to manage with limited financial resources. Present-day American society is not particularly forgiving of women who find themselves in such a predicament, and traditional responders appear to have internalized the judgments of others. To the reader there might be a different analysis focused around the lack of government support for families, but traditional responders instead accept the common American norm of personal responsibility. Yet they felt unable to live up to this imperative. They assumed that they could not control their destinies, but they blamed themselves for this fatalism. Guilt as a cause of breast cancer was a common theme.

Susan Sontag, in *Illness as Metaphor,* described a "growing literature and body of research" supporting the idea that cancer has an emotional cause. Much of this literature uses interview data with cancer patients to show that many had been depressed or unsatisfied with their lives. However, Sontag noted that this would also be true, no doubt, for individuals without cancer. Since most studies of stress do not use control groups, it is hard to assess a relationship between emotions and cancer even though there is some evidence for the hypothesis.[6] These ideas have found their way into general consciousness, supported by popular medical writers like Bernie Siegel, who has argued strongly for the existence of such a relationship.[7]

Traditional responders not only believed that they were to blame for developing cancer but also thought there was little they could do personally to effect a recovery.[8] After the first panic about death, they decided that their only hope was to put themselves in their doctors' hands and to follow orders. They strongly believed in the cultural messages that doctors could perform miracles. Their view of doctors as persons who could cure cancer led traditional responders to trust those assigned to them and to accord them great respect and deference. Gina was devastated by the cancer diagnosis but enthused, "The doctors involved in my life made a difference. You just fall apart when you hear this, but if you have a good doctor it means everything." Gina added that her surgeon had been very kind to her in making sure she understood everything. She described him as a "beautiful man [who] explained everything—that he could fix this for me and he would take me step by step through what I had to go through."

Carla's desire to believe in her doctors' competence made her excuse her oncologist when she found his explanations confusing. She commented, "Even when you ask him to come down to your level, you don't understand what he is saying," but she explained this away by adding that he "is an extremely intelligent person." In her view, his intelligence made it impossible for him to simplify things to a level that she could understand. Her twelfth-grade education led her to believe that she could not challenge doctors and that she would not be able to understand the treatment.

Gabrielle also did as her doctors told her. As she put it, "I didn't question a lot. I kind of felt like a pinball . . . and whoever told me what to do, I did it. . . . I was very overwhelmed." This pattern of women deferring to doctors has a long tradition. When Deborah Lupton interviewed sixty laypersons in Sydney, Australia, about their experiences with medical practitioners, she found that some of the respondents believed strongly that doctors had high social status and deserved respect. As a result, the interview subjects felt they should not challenge them. She called these people "passive patients," and they are similar to the traditional responders described here.[9]

This pattern of deference occurs not only because women are socialized into dependence, but because doctors assert authority over them. Ann Dally, in her study of the history of gynecological surgery, argued that doctors in the nineteenth century "worked hard to keep women in their place" and, in doing so, set themselves up as the medical authority over women's lives.[10] In a study of doctor-patient encounters, Sue Fisher reported that the doctors made assumptions that women patients needed guidance, which made it difficult for women to be partners in decision-making.[11] It is this combination of their belief in biomedicine and, at the same time, following doctors' orders with little question (as women have for generations), that makes this group into traditional responders. And since many of them had to keep caring for families throughout their treatment, we can see that turning their medical care over to doctors, and having faith that the doctors they went to would heal them, is a rational decision.

Another reaction that traditional responders had in common was their eagerness to start treatment immediately and to get it over with quickly. Like Carla, these women believed the standard biomedical argument that, to maximize the chances of survival, diagnosis should be early and treatment should occur promptly. While this was believed by many women regardless of the response group they fell into, the traditional responders were more anxious about even small delays. They thought that, without treatment, death was imminent; that only biomedicine could prevent this; and that the cure should start immediately. Gabrielle said she "wanted it out the very next day" after hearing the bad news. During the week and a half between diagnosis and surgery, she kept thinking, "How can you be walking around knowing you have cancer? This is not healthy. . . . They should have you in the very next day. This should not be allowed to be in your body this long." This unhappiness over delays was one of the few areas where traditional responders were somewhat critical of the medical profession, although they blamed the system rather than their own doctors.

The idea that medical attention for breast cancer must occur immediately after diagnosis dates back to the beginning of the twentieth century, and, while it was challenged from the 1960s on, it remains the most common cultural message.[12] Traditional responders were particularly prone to this belief, both because of their reliance on doctors to effect a cure and because of their unwillingness to challenge conventional medical protocols.

These twin patterns of self-blame for cancer and of dependence on doctors to perform a medical miracle are the distinguishing features of traditional responders. I chose this label because this group most closely mirrored the traditional doctor-patient relationship of responding to the doctor rather than initiating treatment. Yet, while this appears to be a result of female passivity, there is more to the story. Traditional responders were typically lower to middle class with family incomes concentrated between twenty thousand dollars and seventy thousand dollars. They also had fairly low levels of education; 40 percent had completed high school or less compared to less than twenty-five percent of the total sample. As women have become more assertive in general, it is not surprising that the ones least likely to challenge doctors are those with lower levels of education. No doubt doctors are more likely to talk down to them than they would to more educated women. In terms of income and education, they were similar to the religious responders and lower than the other two groups. This suggests that taking charge of one's own illness is a more common practice among affluent, highly educated women than their less affluent and less well-educated sisters.

In addition, the traditional responder group contained the largest number of young women—over half the women under age forty were traditional responders. Almost all of these were mothers of young children and so had considerable mothering responsibilities that continued when they became ill. This provided another reason to rely on doctors rather than taking the time to make independent judgments. Only half the group was married at the time of the interview, which is lower than for the sample as a whole, and one-third were divorced compared to less than a quarter of the total sample. This group of women had fewer than average resources and greater than average responsibilities, so it is not surprising that they chose to put their faith in doctors and did not feel they had the power to challenge biomedicine. Since there is so little institutional help in American society for women who become seriously ill, women with few resources and extensive family responsibilities have to scrounge around for support in coping with their illness.

Traditional responders followed traditional women's roles in other ways also. Few of them had professional careers, and those who did had careers like teaching, which have long been assumed to be suited to women and their nurturing abilities. The group contained most of the homemakers in the sample, and a number of the others worked part-time

Table 2   Traditional Responders by Selected Variables

	White (not Jewish)	Black	Jewish	Total
Age				
Less than 40	5	2	0	7
40–49	5	0	3	8
50–59	3	5	2	10
60 and over	6	1	0	7
Family income				
Less than $20,000	0	0	0	0
$20,000–$39,999	7	2	1	10
$40,000–$69,999	7	4	0	11
$70,000–$99,999	3	1	2	6
$100,000 and over	1	1	2	4
Missing	1	0	0	1
Education				
12 years and less	10	2	1	13
13–15	1	4	2	7
16–17	3	1	0	4
18 and over	5	1	2	8
Marital status*				
Currently married	11	3	3	17
Divorced	6	2	2	10
Never married	2	1	0	3
Widowed	0	2	0	2
Total	19	8	5	32

* The marital status of lesbians was cataloged as either "never married" (4) or "divorced" (3). Three lesbians were cohabiting at the time of the interview. Cohabiting heterosexuals were treated similarly.

or from the home. They tended to take on nurturing roles for those around them, roles often exacerbated by particularly stressful family situations or family demands such as small children.

As a result of the successes of the women's health movement, all women have read messages about the importance of participating in treatment decisions when they are sick. Given their reliance on doctors, their fear and guilt, and their lack of education, how did traditional responders cope with making decisions after breast cancer diagnoses? Like most women in this group, Carla did not really make choices. The surgeon first suggested a mastectomy because of "an enlarged lump" under her armpit, and she agreed. However, when she went to see him again, he changed his mind and performed a lumpectomy. She did not question him about this change. After the lumpectomy, the surgeon called her and said she would need a mastectomy after all, because "we found three cancer cells in the surrounding tissue." So Carla returned for a second surgery. Carla described these events without any indication that she was given a choice at any stage of the process or that she expected to make such a choice. Nor did she complain that the surgeon's vacillation had caused her to undergo extra surgery. While the description of the doctor's behavior comes in the form of an indirect account from the point of view of the patient, it is likely that Carla was not a patient the doctor felt he had to defer to.

Although Gina's surgeon gave her a choice between a lumpectomy and a mastectomy, he pushed her into a lumpectomy, telling her that she "did not by any means need a mastectomy." Gabrielle's doctor gave her no choice at all. He told her he would not "know til they went in" because "it would depend on what he found" but that "if a full mastectomy needed to be done, it was going to be done." Apparently, he was using a version of the discredited one-step procedure that pioneering activists such as Rose Kushner had fought against in the 1970s.[13]

After surgery, Carla was taught the standard series of exercises to do at home in order to regain the full use of her arm. This was to prevent postoperative lymphedema, a painful swelling in the arm and hand caused by the removal of lymph nodes and the consequent inability of lymph fluids to drain from the arm. Carla was required to maintain a regimen of uncomfortable and boring exercises, and she did not do them conscientiously. When she developed lymphedema, her surgeon prescribed three additional physical therapy sessions. The physical therapist put her through a more complex exercise program and taught her how to do the exercises at home. Carla reported that she "was amazed at the movement I had in my arm afterwards." However, she did not even then maintain the exercise program on her own because "I'm just like, I don't even think of doing it. I'm supposed to use a wrap on my hand. I don't do that." Her only solution to the swelling and discomfort she was having in her arm at the time of the interview was to say she needed to go back to physical therapy and learn again. Had Carla had better health insurance, she would have been able to go for more than three sessions and would have, perhaps, maintained more discipline.

Gabrielle also developed lymphedema, a condition about which her doctor was apparently indifferent. When she asked him about it, he told her, "When I'm watching TV at night, I should be propping it up with a pillow." He also suggested, if it bothered her, "to wrap it . . . with an ace bandage, but I haven't done that yet." Gabrielle noted that her arm swelled whenever she used it a lot, and she added, "I'm kind of out there, not knowing what to do with this arm." This was not the only way in which Gabrielle suffered from her surgery:

> The drains[14] were taken out too early, and I filled with fluid, and the pain had been terrible, but no one had ever mentioned to me that the fluid could build up in there. . . . I thought when the drains came out, that would be it. Oh, the pain was terrible, and I didn't know why. And I finally called the office . . . and then that's when they took me in and drained it. . . . It built up again, but by this time I knew and I went back in.

This is a woman who described her doctors as "very sensitive to your needs." Her story, along with others, illustrates not only the unwillingness of traditional responders to challenge their doctors but also the authority the doctors assume over women they most likely see as not their social or intellectual equals.

Reliance on medical authority rather than personal action typifies traditional responders. For example, Gina still lived close to her father and siblings and relied on them for almost everything, even though she was in her forties. When she was diagnosed, she talked about it only to her family and her boss, and she never questioned her doctors. She saw no reason for questions because, she said, "I loved every one of my doctors."

For many women in this group, the dependence on the doctors' authority frequently occurred because other aspects of their lives were burdensome. Women in this situation needed the doctor to take care of their cancer, while they took care of other things. Myra, an affluent stay-at-home mother who was divorced and engaged to a physician, blamed her breast cancer on the stress caused by raising a daughter with serious developmental problems. In addition, she had a mother who "flipped out" when Myra was diagnosed. Her daughter was traumatized by Myra's illness, and her mother was so difficult that Myra and her brother used to joke about whether "Mom's going to make it through my next treatment." These family problems caused Myra to depend more on her doctors than she might have done otherwise. She even recognized the fallacy in her dependence, saying about her surgeon, "Even before the surgery . . . he was full of it, but I didn't care; he said, 'We're going to make you better.'" In addition to her problems with her family, Myra explained that she did whatever the doctors told her because "I felt I had no choice."[15] Myra was unusual among traditional responders because she had an MBA and one of the highest incomes of anyone I interviewed. Had it not been for her family situation, she might have acted like a biomedical expert, a group that was more involved in medical decision-making. Myra's life was too difficult for her to give her full attention to breast cancer, but she retained her belief in biomedicine while turning her illness over to her doctors.

Carla's reliance on the advice of her doctors caused several problems. After the failed lumpectomy, she went to arrange for her mastectomy. The surgeon scheduled this and sent her to a plastic surgeon who would reconstruct her breast—a procedure she did not question—while she was still under anesthesia from the mastectomy. This is a common procedure when women have breast reconstruction. However, the plastic surgeon refused to operate on a smoker. Carla stopped smoking—an act that is difficult at the best of times and no doubt more difficult at times of great stress—but she had to wait an additional three weeks to get the nicotine out of her system.[16] By that time, she could not coordinate the plastic surgeon's schedule with the breast surgeon's. She went ahead with the breast surgery, because of her anxiety to have the cancer removed as soon as possible, and she had the plastic surgery after she completed radiation, which entailed a third surgery. Her reconstruction was a tramflap, which is the most painful type and consists of pulling stomach muscle and fat up through the chest muscle to replace the breast. Although the plastic surgeon would not operate on smokers, he had no such concerns about surgery after radiation, even though problems are common.[17] In Carla's case, radiation caused her skin to stick to her chest wall, making the surgery even more painful and the result visually disappointing. Even so, Carla described this as just another medical problem that had happened to her because of her own bad habits, rather than holding her doctors even partially responsible for the poor results. Like other traditional responders, she held doctors in high esteem, so high that she found it difficult to say anything critical. Given the class differences between themselves and their doctors, it may not be surprising that traditional responders would be hesitant to issue challenges even if they wished to. However, the extent to which they described themselves as not wanting to challenge doctors is striking and suggests they had internalized social-class values and did not feel entitled to issue such challenges. Their lack of entitlement contrasts markedly with other groups.

These ways of relating to doctors on the part of traditional responders are quite rational given the difficulty these women would have had getting doctors to listen. Traditional responders did not struggle to get the respect of doctors and instead focused on the other burdens in their lives, burdens that often increased when they became ill.

Because breast cancer treatment has numerous side effects, patients must rely on family and friends for support. Carla's need was particularly strong, because she was raising three young daughters by herself. These problems were made worse because she had a somewhat strained relationship with her strict Catholic mother, who had not forgiven Carla for her divorce. Her mother believed that, no matter how badly husbands behaved, "You made your bed, so lay in it." Before she had cancer, Carla "had to fight for some of my family members to help out with my children." And now, "Because I have cancer, suddenly everybody cares." Carla's resulting anger, particularly toward her mother for the earlier neglect, meant that she wanted help to be confined to the minimum. "I didn't want her hugging me. I didn't want her with me for my doctors' appointments. . . . I just wanted to do it by myself, because I did before."

In this story we see that when Carla acted in her own interests—leaving an abusive and neglectful husband—she was punished for her actions. This lesson resonated strongly with many traditional responders and helped give rise to their frequent belief that, when they did things for themselves, they messed up in some way. They did not recognize the institutionalized reasons for this—poor single mothers are one of the most powerless groups in society. Instead they blamed themselves.

Carla experienced problems during treatment and had to turn to her mother and her twin sister for help with child care for two weeks each time she had chemotherapy, because she became too ill to cope with three little girls on her own. In addition, her oncologist's office told her that someone must come with her when she had treatment, and thus she had to take her mother. Her mother, who lived nearby, took in the oldest child for the worst week of each round of chemotherapy, because this daughter was in second grade and Carla did not want her to miss school. Carla's twin sister, who lived fifty miles away, took the middle child out of kindergarten each time. Carla's next-door neighbors looked after the youngest child, age three, so that Carla could be near her. The complications of these child-care arrangements were a sufficient burden to Carla and left no time for questioning treatment.

Greater financial resources to pay for assistance or a state that helps during emergencies would have helped the family stay together, and Carla told me that her children still suffered from the aftereffects of repeatedly leaving their sick mother and imagining she was going to die. They were shuffled back and forth from their home to the various other houses and even to additional houses when the primary arrangements fell through. At the time of the interview, the middle child, who had to celebrate her birthday while away from her mother, was still fearful of going to sleep at night because of her anxiety that Carla might die of cancer before the morning.

An additional problem that Carla had with her family was the tendency of her mother and sister to interject themselves between Carla and her doctors, by calling to ask the doctors' assistants how she was doing. Carla needed help, not interference, and she became so incensed about this that she instructed the doctors' offices not to tell her family anything. This pattern of relying on family, but finding their involvement prob-

lematic and tension producing, was common among traditional responders. They simply felt unable to let families take on the burden of their illness, because the type of help they received was not always what they
wanted, so they relied on doctors instead. It is no accident that many of
the women without husbands became traditional responders. As is discussed in the next chapter, when women became seriously ill, the presence of husbands generally enabled them to focus on their disease.

About half of the traditional responders were married, but these married women often had other difficult family situations. When this happened, they had to take on the burden of helping their families cope with
the diagnosis and treatment. Gabrielle, who had a supportive husband,
described problems with both her younger son and her mother:

> My younger son was in the eighth grade at the time, and he had the
> most horrendous year. He failed classes. This is an extremely bright
> kid. . . . We told him I would be fine, that the prognosis was good,
> but he watched me going through the chemo and getting weaker and
> weaker and weaker. And he thought we were lying to him, that I was
> gonna die. And so he was probably the biggest emotional burden of
> everything.

Gabrielle was so worried about her son that she asked the school counselor to talk to the boy. The counselor asked Gabrielle's son if he would
like to talk and, upon receiving a negative reply, did not pursue it further.
Gabrielle then turned to a friend who reassured the boy that his mother
was going to get better, but the son continued to agonize.

In addition to problems with her son, Gabrielle struggled with her
mother:

> My mom had a real hard time with this, because her next-door neighbor's
> daughter died of breast cancer. So my mom would call and say, "Edna
> said . . ." throughout the whole thing. . . . And when I was on Compazine
> and Ativan, and my mother said, "Those drugs are addictive and you—
> Edna said . . ." And at some point I hung up on my mother. . . . I thought,
> "I can't deal. I just can't deal with my mother's problems."

Because Gabrielle felt guilty for hanging up on her mother, she continued
to listen to her mother's concerns about the prognosis, even though she

found it stressful to do so. While her family problems were different than Carla's, Gabrielle also found them burdensome enough that relying on her doctors provided great comfort.

Gina described herself as someone whose depression had caused her illness. She had a great desire to trust her doctors, but at the same time, she found herself taking care of family members' reactions to her illness. Her mother had died of cancer three years prior to Gina's diagnosis, so she found telling her father hard, because "he watched my mother suffer so badly." Although she reported that "I wish I could just be sick and not have to worry about anything else," she did not feel able to do this. In addition to her father, her younger sister "went totally bonkers. She suffered so much because of me." Gina kept control of her own feelings throughout her illness, holding a different standard for herself than for the other members of her family:

> I never let them see any bad parts of me, except one night when I lost control and I was vomiting something fierce. . . . I never let them see me irritable, or tired, or unhappy, nothing. And you know what? It not only worked for them. It worked for me. I couldn't afford the luxury of being down.

Gina was divorced and had no children, so her family of origin was very important to her. Since her mother's illness and death, she had taken on the role of family caregiver, a task many grown women must still shoulder. She cooked for her father every day and did not return home until he had eaten and she had cleaned up. But as can be seen from the preceding quote, Gina's reliance on her doctors and their decisions was not only caused by her need to focus on her family. It was also facilitated by a desire to repress her own worries about the possibility of death. Thus she described not being able to afford "the luxury of being down" as therapeutic.

In spite of problems with family members, traditional responders relied on family support even if it was not always provided in the form they wanted. Myra had her brother's help in dealing with her difficult mother, and he also helped her in a practical way. The husband of Myra's housekeeper worked for the family business. Myra's brother, who ran the business, made this man available to Myra on a full-time basis while she was having treatment. Myra's fiancé gathered information about doctors for her, and he accompanied her to doctors' visits. She found this helpful, because "being a doctor, he was able to ask questions about the treatment." Gabrielle also had some expert help. Her older son was a premed college student, "taking all kinds of courses right then that were relevant. . . . At school, he would do research, and he would bring me things home. [He] was probably my main source of information."

In addition to family and friends, as we saw in chapter 1, the modern world has many other sources of support for women, including masses of information in the media and on the Internet.[18] Anthony Giddens has argued that, in our information-rich society, individuals must negotiate decisions and plans through a confusing mass of contradictory facts and opinions.[19] In a study of patients diagnosed with familial hyperlipidemia—having too many lipids in the blood—Helen Lambert and Hilary Rose found that while all those diagnosed had a "good enough" level of knowledge to manage the complicated dietary needs of their illness, what constituted good enough varied from patient to patient.[20]

For traditional responders, "good enough" information meant not very much. Because they were so fearful about their diagnoses and because they wanted doctors to make decisions, traditional responders dealt with the mass of information on breast cancer by avoiding certain kinds of material. They particularly avoided medical facts about their disease, since this led them to imagine the worst possible outcome. This is only partly explained by their level of education. Carla reported that, while she read little of the medical material available about cancer, other women's stories of survival encouraged her to go forward with treatment, by reassuring her that she was right in her faith that doctors could indeed cure this life-threatening disease. Myra decided she was getting enough information from her doctors, so she read nothing about cancer and watched nothing about it on television. She was still deliberately avoiding learning anything about breast cancer when I interviewed her a year after her treatment ended. This pattern of avoidance was typical of traditional responders. Gina reported that "I should have read Marisa Weiss's book very many times, and yet I can't pick up the book. . . . I just don't like to read anything to do with breast cancer."[21] Traditional responders found many types of media presentation just too painful to watch. Carla watched some television shows on breast cancer, but they always made her cry. Gabrielle reported that she had tried to watch a breast cancer show on the women's television channel, but as soon as it started, she began crying and had to walk away. Again and again, traditional responders told me of having to turn off such shows because they found them to be too upsetting. Traditional responders were women whose class and gender rendered them powerless to deal with biomedicine. Since they did not see a way to organize their own recovery, they chose not to learn about things that would increase their fear.

Traditional responders had an additional reason for avoiding learning too much. Women who read a lot for themselves often began to question what their doctors were telling them. Traditional responders had many reasons to want to maintain a harmonious and trusting relationship with their doctors, and they found it better not to learn too much independent information.

In recent years, one common source of help for women diagnosed with breast cancer has been support groups. These have grown in response to research suggesting that women attending such groups live longer than those who do not.[22] This research is often cited as a rationale for support groups but is based on therapeutic support groups run by clinical psychologists. In practice, most support groups are organized more loosely and with less professionally trained leaders. Some women I interviewed found support groups to be useful in getting them through their treatment and in helping them come to terms with their fears of a reoccurrence after treatment ended. Although some did join these groups, most traditional responders tended to find support groups unhelpful because they found being around other women with breast cancer frightening and depressing, especially since someone in the group was inevitably in metastasis. Traditional responders had enough to cope with in their own lives and wisely chose not to dwell on the frightening possibilities of their illness.

Carla was one of the few traditional responders who attended a support group for a while, but she found that it often left her feeling scared. Myra spoke for many of the women in this group when she said that "I did go a couple of times. The first time I was a little overwhelmed because it was all show and tell. I saw a tramflap. I saw a prosthesis. I saw someone's bald head. . . . I did go a couple more times, but I found it depressing."

Like many of the traditional responders I interviewed, Gina did not even try support groups. She told me that she did not like talking about breast cancer, and she added, "I told my dad tonight, when I left him, that I was doing this interview, and I said to him, 'I really don't want to talk about it, but . . . if it will help someone else, then I need to do it.'" That Gina overcame her hesitation testifies to the power of illness narratives in our culture. Gina's motivation to help others also testifies to the meaning illness narratives have for their owners.

In addition to discomfort with medical knowledge, traditional responders found the insensitivity of those around them upsetting. Carla told of a woman who babysat her children one time and who, when Carla went to pick them up, said, "Oh, my sister had breast cancer, and she died." Although Carla tried to laugh this off, because "that's just how this woman is," she added that she "did not need to be told that." Another source of annoyance was gratuitous advice; for example, Gabrielle became annoyed at "people telling me what I already knew, that I should be eating right and getting plenty of rest, where I didn't have any control over that."

So what was helpful to this group of women who felt overwhelmed by their illness and who focused on survival, while avoiding discouraging evidence? In addition to believing that their doctors were among the best and that they could be cured, they liked hearing this hopeful message from others. Carla spoke for many when she said the most helpful things were when people told her that she would be all right:

> Basically, the doctors reassuring me that everything looked fine. My survival rate and stuff like that. People telling me, when I was going through my chemo treatments, you wouldn't know I was sick.

These comments show great insight on the part of traditional responders. They knew they were frightened by their illness. They were facing the possibility of death, so they had reason to be nervous. This was exacerbated by a lack of resources and by tremendous responsibilities for others, particularly young children. Even Myra, who had lots of places to turn for help, knew that if anything happened to her it would be difficult for her disabled child to get the level of attention that she got from Myra. So by turning their attention to the other things in their lives and by avoiding learning or hearing anything frightening, they managed to make it through treatment.

After the bulk of the treatment was over and the only remaining therapy was their daily dose of tamoxifen, which many women took, how did traditional responders rebuild their lives and what changes did they make? In general, all women wanted to make some changes in their lives in order to feel they were actively warding off a cancer reoccurrence. The most typical change made by the women I interviewed was dietary. In a study of white middle-class men and women, Robin Saltonstall found that food was usually the first item listed by women in response to her question, "What kind of things do you do to be healthy?"[23] However, diet is something that cancer doctors almost never speak about, and unlike the other groups, most traditional responders did not change their diet in any significant way. When asked what she now ate in a typical day, Carla responded:

> Yesterday was a bad day, because all I had was a turkey and cheese sandwich at noon. And then I didn't eat again until eight o'clock, and then it was like leftover stuffing, leftover mashed potatoes. And then later on I was eating Frosted Flakes out of the box to snack.

The lack of resources that had made women like Carla struggle throughout their adult lives did not change because cancer was over.

Nor did traditional responders exercise very much. Like diet, this is something women frequently start doing after having breast cancer, as a way of regaining control over their lives. It is also something that is recommended in the popular breast cancer literature.[24] In Saltonstall's study, exercise was women's second most common way of staying healthy. Robert Crawford has argued that self-control, self-discipline, self-denial, and willpower are all seen as keys to the pursuit of health in modern society, and that exercise embodies these values. At the same time, individuals face pressure to consume and to let go of restraint.[25] Many traditional responders resolved the tension inherent in these two opposing mandates in favor of letting go, but this was in part because they were holding on so fiercely elsewhere.

As a group, traditional responders tended to make minimal lifestyle changes, if any at all. For example, Myra described her food sins and, in doing so, showed great awareness of the cultural rules about a good diet:

> I don't drink enough water. For lunch, I try to eat salads, but some-times I don't, and, a lot of times, I could eat fast food, and I don't forget the French fries, and a Quarter Pounder with cheese is not out of the ordinary. . . . I feel bad when I have to eat fast food, I really do. I never felt bad about doing it before, now I do.

Myra also confessed that she was not doing any exercise but said she was planning to.

When traditional responders tried to change their diet in ways that might prevent breast cancer, they sometimes received contradictory mes-sages. Gabrielle, who had long tried with mixed success to keep her weight down by going to Weight Watchers and eating healthy food, stated:

> The doctor said I had to cut back on the caffeine. I used to be a big iced tea drinker, now I'm seeing on TV that I should be drinking my teas again—my green teas. So I don't know what I'm supposed to do here now, 'cause I stopped doing that and came home from school and was drinking herbal teas every day. Now, I'm thinking I need to go back, but, then, I'm getting caffeine, and I don't know.

Gabrielle had also been hoping to start walking for exercise, but subse-quent medical problems made it difficult to do so. This bothered her. She said, "That is my problem, my major problem."

As noted, women find breast cancer treatment more debilitating than the cancer itself. Treatment can make women feel they have lost control over their lives. Looking back on their experience, traditional responders were particularly likely to report this feeling. Gabrielle was one such woman. Even when people would tell her, "Oh, you're doing wonder-fully," she would think to herself:

"I have no idea what I'm doing . . . . I am reacting only. . . ." In between, I was so tired and so overwhelmed, I didn't even have time to think. . . . I'd teach, come home, and go to bed. And [my husband] would wake me at like seven, and we would have dinner. And I might sit down here for an hour, and after that I was back in bed again.

This feeling of living in a haze while going through treatment was common for many traditional responders. Myra just handed everything over to her household helpers and let them cope. Carla did not have help, but she had similar feelings:

Looking back, it's as if it took over my life for the time being. . . . I realized after a year and a half, this thing has been controlling my life and telling me what to do. . . . I wanted my normal life back.

Like others, Carla found that she was able to feel she was regaining control by getting her life back to where it was before, rather than drastically changing anything. In her case, this was accomplished by going back to work. For Gabrielle, it was getting her hair back. As is discussed in chapter 7, hair loss was traumatic for women, because they associated it with deadly illness.

Carla made one important change, which harkened back to her guilt over neglecting her children. She told me that she became a more attentive mother after cancer, and she did this by making several changes in her life. She went out partying less often, and instead of returning to her office-based job, she performed similar data-entry work at home even though the pay was lower. She had made this change in order to be there when the children came home from school. She did not always find her resolve to focus on her children easy to sustain, noting that "sometimes I get upset with myself, because I forget these things I learned during cancer . . . with the girls—spending time with them."

Carla was able to make these changes because, toward the end of her treatment, she met a supportive man at a social evening for divorced persons. He had moved in with her, and they planned to marry. His financial help enabled her to work at home, and his companionship and emotional support lessened her desire to go out so frequently. Still, she struggled with her long-established self-doubt and feelings of unworthiness. As she put it,

> I can't say I live life to the fullest, because I don't. And I don't take advantage of every opportunity that's out there for me. I just don't have the energy. However, I have learned to sit back more. If it gets done, it gets done. If it doesn't, it doesn't.

Part of the reason for this inability to move forward even though her situation had changed was that Carla still found her cancer experience frightening and still worried about leaving her children motherless. Given her circumstances, these fears were not unreasonable. Carla constantly compared her situation to that of others:

> I know this is wrong of me, and I always say, "God forgive me," but when I find someone who had breast cancer, but they didn't have lymph node involvement—they just had the lumpectomy—I get jealous. And then on the other hand, I have friends, where they had the stem cell transplant,[26] and it went to a lot of their lymph nodes, so I'm like the opposite. I thank God that mine wasn't as bad.

Even though she was slowly moving forward with the help of the change in her life circumstances, Carla still felt buffeted by a life of powerlessness.

While Carla's big change was to try to become more involved with her children, some traditional responders changed by becoming more concerned about themselves as opposed to others. They used the opportunity their illness provided to lessen their lifetime commitment to women's historic responsibilities for nurturing and care.

Gabrielle is an example of such a woman. She noted that when she was ill, she learned for the first time in her adult life how to say no to requests for help:

> I was president of the band, and I was president of the association. I couldn't just be on a committee; I had to be the president. And I found out all those committees ran without me, and I learned to say "No" for the first time in my life. And I kind of pulled out of an awful lot of stuff to take time, and then I gave myself a year to kind of get better. And then I joined a painting class—I love to paint. . . . I could do something for myself that didn't deal with anybody else. . . . I don't

plan as much for the future. . . . I let myself have good night sleeps. . . . I got a cleaning lady.

Before breast cancer, Gabrielle had to be "super-mom, super-teacher, super-housewife." While her priorities had changed, she still struggled, telling me, "To this day, I still fight that person." Gabrielle's gendered responsibilities lessened as a result of the new rights a serious illness bestowed on her.

Many traditional responders worked hard after breast cancer to make changes in their outlook toward life and in their behavior. For many, this involved shaking off the victim role. Gina provides a good example of this:

> I have changed considerably. I had been depressed for a long time, for three years that I took care of my mother and for three years following her death. . . . I knew I was depressed, but I didn't know what to do about it. . . . Then this happened, and it changed me totally. . . . All of the things you hear people say, that life is precious and live every day as if it's your last. Well, it's all very true.

The desire Gina described, to see herself as transformed by breast cancer, is common among breast cancer survivors and appears frequently in the many personal accounts that writers have published about their breast cancer experiences.[27] Many traditional responders went so far as to say that they were better as a result of breast cancer and that they had a more positive outlook on life. This attitude was exemplified by Betty, an African American woman and traditional responder, whose husband had died shortly before her diagnosis. Even though we might expect her to focus on the sadness in her life, instead she insisted that her attitude toward life had changed for the better:

> I just knew I had to appreciate things. I would drive down the street and look at a tree and think, "God, how awesome you are to make a tree. . . ." I enjoy people. I enjoy family. I enjoy living. . . . It increased my appreciation. I've always had it, but I think it actually gives me a better appreciation.

Like most survivors of a serious illness, traditional responders wanted their illness to have meaning, and many found this in celebrating continuity and in reminding themselves of the good things in their lives. Of all the women in my study, traditional responders were most able to put cancer behind them and to continue their lives without making cancer into a career. Leaving medicine to the doctor enabled them to do this, and understanding this provides an alternative perspective to what at first appears to be a response to cancer based on fear and passivity. Like the other women in this study, traditional responders made choices constrained by life circumstances. Given their limited resources, their inability to confront doctors, and their family responsibilities, traditional responders chose to follow doctors' orders and to reassure themselves that their doctors had their interests at heart and the skill needed to cure them. When cancer was over, they were able to move on to other things.

The pattern described as typical of the relationships between women patients and their doctors—relying on doctors and believing in their authority and knowledge[28]—applied to traditional responders only. Others responded differently. The question then becomes one of why some women responded in this manner, while others did not. The class and status correlates of these patterns are not surprising. We might expect women who did not have college educations and lived on moderate incomes to be cognizant of tremendous status differences between themselves and doctors. No doubt doctors were aware of it too. The women in this response group fit the characteristics of the long-approved feminine character. In dealing with doctors, they presented themselves as too weak and too fragile to take care of themselves. Thus they were frightened by too much knowledge and were unable to make their own medical decisions. In spite of changes in women's status in the last several decades, many women still believe that self-assertive women will suffer.[29] And unless women have above-average resources to fall back on, they are often proved right.

In the following chapter, I turn my attention to a contrasting group. This group also believed in biomedicine, but they did not rely wholly on the doctor to cure them. Instead, they worked hard to create a partnership with their doctors and to direct their own recovery.

THREE

Patients and Doctors as Partners

When Joann, a thirty-four-year-old mother of three children under age seven, learned she had breast cancer, she was not surprised at being diagnosed so young. Her family had a history of breast cancer, including Joann's mother, her mother's sister, and her grandmother, and so she had long assumed she had inherited the risk.[1] At the time Joann discovered her lump, her mother was terminally ill with lung cancer, having survived breast cancer for twenty-one years. When her mother died a week later, Joann had told no one about her own lump; she waited until after the funeral. Joann was so confident that she had breast cancer that, prior to testing, she gave the surgeon her diagnosis. When he replied, with full medical authority, "You don't tell me you have breast cancer, I tell you," Joann responded, "I'm telling you. I know what cysts feel like, and I have never had anything like this."

Joann was unusual in her certainty that her lump was definite evidence of breast cancer. For most women, such a diagnosis is not legitimate until officially confirmed through a biopsy. Science, not feeling, determines whether or not they have breast cancer.[2] Dorothy Smith has argued that, in contemporary society, ways of knowing that formerly were grounded in everyday experience have become increasingly replaced by "objective," quantified facts and that social scientists have participated in creating this worldview.[3] Most women have no scientific knowledge about breast cancer in their everyday experience. Some have memories about the deaths of loved ones, but most have no experience in the diagnosis of the disease. Joann was unusual in that her everyday experience included some scientific training about breast cancer. She did not believe that she was just relying on intuitive opinion. Rather, she believed that she had the medical competence to distinguish a malignant lump from a cyst.

I talked to Joann in the conference room of the breast cancer support organization where she worked. A tiny and intense woman, whose life since her treatment ended had revolved around helping women get help and information throughout diagnosis, treatment, and post-treatment, Joann had heard about my work at a conference. She contacted me and asked to be in my study because she believed others would benefit from hearing her story. She wanted to testify to others about beating the odds so that they would learn how to help their doctors overcome cancer. Her narrative was similar to those of other women who looked for meaning in their illness experience. Presenting herself as someone who had not become a victim, in spite of life's raw deal, she was upbeat throughout her interview. Her heroic story of fight and courage was like that of many of the biomedical experts discussed in this chapter. These women believed in biomedicine, but they also believed they should be responsible for their health and their recovery from illness. Deborah Lupton, in her study of "consumerist" and "passive" patients, described consumerists as challenging the authority of doctors and becoming experts on their medical conditions. Such women were likely to be well-educated professionals, as were Joann and most of the other women in this group.[4]

Joann's mother had taught her to expect a breast cancer diagnosis at some time in her life. Beginning with Joann's sixteenth birthday, her mother had sent her to the gynecologist every six months to "learn to do a proper breast exam, when all my peers were going . . . to get a prescription for the pill for birth control." Instead of reacting to her diagnosis with shock and panic, as did many of the women described in the previous chapter, Joann was "kind of glad to hear it happen, because I was waiting for the anvil to drop." Prior to diagnosis, she had intended to undergo a prophylactic double mastectomy when her children were a little older, because she thought that this would lessen her chances of the disease.

Even though she was careful to present herself as in control of her treatment, looking back, Joann momentarily became somber. She had been prepared for the bad news, but the diagnosis was still "painful to see, knowing the reality of breast cancer and that I had the aggressive features of a typical young woman's breast cancer; every prognostic feature was poor." However, she comforted herself with the thought that coming from a "high-risk family" had "empowered" her to practice self-examinations and to stay "on top of myself so I could catch it early."

Unlike the women discussed in chapter 2, women such as Joann did not blame themselves for breast cancer. Joann's explanation was a family predisposition to cancer in general and specifically to breast cancer. Several biomedical experts had a similar family background; however, the majority had no history of breast cancer in their families. Still, they used scientific rather than self-blaming explanations for why they got the disease. Many of their explanations are similar to the "embodied risk" explanations given by some women in Anne Kavanagh and Dorothy Bloom's study of abnormal Pap smears.[5] In their study, such women had not anticipated a risk until they were told about their Pap smears, and at that point their bodies became the risk factor, rather than their lifestyle or something that was caused by the external environment.

In my interviews, most biomedical experts had not anticipated breast cancer until visited by it. Many women in this group had carefully followed the principles of good health promoted by the medical profession and had believed that these practices would prevent serious diseases like cancer. Prior to her diagnosis, Donna, a forty-eight-year-old lawyer, was typical in her view that breast cancer was "something that happened to someone else," principally because she expected that her healthy lifestyle precluded it. I interviewed Donna in the living room of the fashionable townhouse she shared with her husband and teenaged son, and she looked the picture of the successful, slender, career woman. So did Charlene, a forty-seven-year-old social worker and mother of two, living in a large modern home in an upper-middle-class suburb. Charlene understood that things may occur for no apparent reason:

> I just think bad things happen to good people. . . . I see so much of it in my work. . . . I didn't do anything to cause it. I'm not a religious person, so to me it just happens. . . . We want to explain everything . . . but, sometimes, I just don't think there's an explanation.

Even though she understood that cancer may occur by chance, Charlene's first reaction to diagnosis had been anger that her body had "betrayed" her, because, she said, "I took care of myself, I was pretty physically active."

These expectations, about the preventive powers of living healthily, illustrate an important aspect of biomedical experts' reasoning. Influenced by the health promotion movement in America, they thought that individuals should take responsibility for their own health and had imagined that they were avoiding serious illness by maintaining wellness.[6] When, like Joann, they had scientific reasons to think avoidance was impossible, they did what they saw as the next best thing and ensured the earliest diagnosis. But where those who had breast cancer in the family were knowledgeable about the disease even before diagnosis, the majority of biomedical experts only learned about the biology of breast cancer and its treatment afterward. This is because they had not imagined it to be in their futures. Robert Crawford has described the middle class as adopting self-control as a value and this stance as fundamental to the Western system of values. The women in this group typified this ideal.[7]

In their belief that women should take responsibility for their own health, biomedical experts were similar to traditional responders. However, when things went wrong, the two groups reacted differently. Where traditional responders saw themselves as victims and blamed a lack of control over their lives for their breast cancer, biomedical experts were firm in their faith that they had not failed at health promotion. Rather, they looked outside themselves and realized that, no matter what they did to promote health, breast cancer could still strike. When it did, they went into action to learn about their disease and not to be defeated by it. Thus they stayed faithful to the idea that they were in charge of what happened next. Their underlying assumption was one of personal control, and they maintained this stance throughout treatment.

The ability to control one's treatment in the face of illness results, in part, from the activism of the women's health movement. This movement was founded by women we might think of as biomedical experts. The best-known early breast cancer activist, Rose Kushner, was forty-four years old when she discovered a lump in her breast in 1974, and, from that moment on, she took charge every step of the way, from insisting that she be treated at a research hospital to visiting surgeon after surgeon until one agreed to sign a note saying that he would not use the standard one-step procedure of an immediate mastectomy, without waking her first, if the biopsy proved malignant.[8] She learned everything she could about her illness and the options available in different countries for its treatment.[9]

Kushner was a journalist who had written about medical issues, so she felt comfortable undertaking the research she needed for her arguments about breast cancer treatment in the United States. Like Kushner, many of the biomedical experts I interviewed had the background to undertake research on their treatment options. Eve was a fifty-three-year-old scientist with a Ph.D. in molecular biology. She knew little about breast cancer when diagnosed, and although she regularly performed breast exams, she "wasn't trained to do them right." After diagnosis, her scientific background served her well. Like other biomedical experts, Eve's explanation for her cancer relied on science rather than guilt:

> No one in my family gets cancer. . . . I might have increased risk factors in terms of starting menstruating at eight and not having my child until I was thirty-two, and some hormone stuff in connection with fertility and being on replacement therapy for a short while after menopause.

Eve's brief analysis raises five scientific theories—genetics, early menstruation, late childbearing, hormone-based fertility treatments, and hormone replacement therapy—common in the medical literature to explain breast cancer, four of which she applied to herself. Eve was one of the few seriously overweight women in the biomedical category and, to give a full list, she could have used her body weight in addition to the explanations she gave.[10] This is perhaps the only time she let sentiment—embarrassment about her weight—outweigh science.

Eve first realized something was wrong when, returning from an overseas conference, her "breast felt heavy." She "went to the washroom on the plane, felt around," and discovered that "either I had a rapidly growing cyst or I had a big problem, because it felt two by three inches." The quick appearance of such a large lump told her that this was serious, but Eve responded carefully and deliberately. On arriving home, she first called her family doctor, who confirmed her fears about the existence of the lump and got her in to see a surgeon within a couple of days. After a surgical biopsy confirmed the cancer, Eve took stock of her options before further action.

Biomedical experts, like traditional responders, believed the cultural messages about the supremacy of biomedicine. Both groups thought science could cure them or at least extend their lives for the foreseeable future. Yet biomedical experts differed from traditional responders in that they did not want to rely on the medical profession for their recovery. Instead, they saw it as their personal responsibility to manage their treatment, to select the right doctors rather than accept the first ones assigned, and to create a partnership with these doctors in deciding on treatment. Unlike traditional responders, these women were not especially deferential to doctors. Indeed, their faith in biomedicine did not lead them to think all doctors were knowledgeable or worthy of respect. Nor did they always agree with doctors' recommendations. They searched for the best possible care using the research skills that they, and many of those close to them, had.

A number of these women had medical backgrounds and were familiar with medical terminology, even if they had known little about breast cancer before diagnosis. Even those who did not have a medical background believed that they had enough education and professional experience to learn and to understand everything they needed in order to work with doctors, rather than simply defer to them. This is why I classify these women as biomedical experts: they believed in biomedicine and they thought they had or could gain the expertise to make decisions about treatment.

These women felt entitled in their relationships with their doctors, and this entitlement had its origins in their social locations. While their age distribution is similar to the total sample, although a little more concentrated in the middle categories, the other demographic differences are striking. As a group, these women lived privileged lives. They had higher than average incomes—over one-third had family incomes in excess of one hundred thousand dollars per year and frequently much higher. And although they had relatively high marriage rates—two-thirds of biomedical experts were currently married compared to just over half the traditional responders—they earned much of this income themselves. Two-thirds of the women had a college degree, and of these, the majority had graduate degrees. Most had either prestigious professional occupations or worked in a women's health profession such as nursing. Their affluence and their occupational histories provided them with the kind of medical insurance that entitled them to obtain second opinions and to consult their doctors of choice.

Biomedical experts were particularly overrepresented among Jewish women. About half the Jews I interviewed were in this group, and they were even more affluent and better educated than the group as a whole. Furthermore, almost all had professional occupations. These are the reasons I analyzed Jews separately; so many of them were comfortable dealing with the medical profession and felt entitled to issue challenges when necessary. Joann is a good example of such a woman. She had been doing routine breast exams since having her first child at age twenty-seven and occasionally before that, and she believed that her knowledge could match that of the doctor.

Most biomedical experts, particularly those with no family history of cancer, had been less rigorous about breast exams than Joann. Like traditional responders, if they did exams, they did them incompetently, as did

Table 3   Biomedical Experts by Selected Variables

	White (not Jewish)	Black	Jewish	Total
Age				
Less than 40	1	0	2	3
40–49	4	1	4	9
50–59	10	0	3	13
60 and over	6	1	0	7
Family income				
Less than $20,000	0	0	2	2
$20,000–$39,999	2	0	0	2
$40,000–$69,999	4	1	1	6
$70,000–$99,999	8	0	1	9
$100,000 and over	7	1	5	13
Education				
12 years and less	2	0	0	2
13–15	6	0	1	7
16–17	7	0	1	8
18 and over	5	2	7	14
Missing	1	0	0	1
Marital status				
Currently married	16	1	6	23
Divorced	3	1	0	4
Never married	2	0	3	5
Widowed	0	0	0	0
Total	21	2	9	32

Eve, or sporadically, as did Donna. However, the reasoning was different in the two groups. Where traditional responders thought they should do breast exams but often found it too hard to remember or too scary, many biomedical experts did not do them because of their assumptions that breast cancer happened to others. Women with no risk factors for breast cancer knew their odds of getting it were low, and they saw no reason for vigilance. Their health efforts were directed toward a lifestyle they hoped would protect against any and all illness. This is an argument found frequently in popular health books and articles.[11] And as is discussed in chapter 1, this is a message promoted by women's magazines and other media.

However, once diagnosed, biomedical experts went into action. Instead of panicking about death, a response that led traditional responders to rely unquestioningly on their doctors, they held on to an optimism that they could control their destinies. They quickly came to terms with the diagnosis and planned their next steps. Above all, they wanted to stay in control. These successful career women embraced liberal feminist attitudes about success. Susan Bordo has described such women as embodying "qualities—detachment, self-containment, self-mastery, control—that are highly valued in our culture."[12] Donna exemplified this attitude in reporting that, while she wondered how this could happen to someone who ate sensibly and exercised regularly, "I don't want to say that I took it in my stride . . . I was just trying to think, 'How am I going to get to one step from the next?'" She did not feel betrayed by her body as did some women in this group.

Because they wanted to ensure that they made the best decisions, biomedical experts tended to be less anxious than traditional responders to have surgery quickly. Their tolerance for a small delay before undergoing surgery is in accordance with most medical recommendations.[13] After her mother's funeral, Joann wanted treatment to start quickly, because her cancer was something she had anticipated and she had already waited several weeks. Still, she took steps to ensure that her medical care was the best. She called a family friend—a hematologist/oncologist—living some miles away and asked him to "be my second opinion, so I don't have to traipse around the city." When she met her surgeon to discuss her options, the friend "did a telephone consult while I was in the office. . . . My friend spoke to the surgeon, and then after they came to their conclusions . . . the surgeon handed me the phone, and [my friend] said, 'You're in good hands.'" Like many in this group, Joann had social networks that she could call into play to help her make medical decisions. Traditional responders had family and friends who tried to help, but the quality of their help differed, in part because they did not bring the same levels of expertise to the issue at hand. The marked class differences between the two groups had an impact on their ability to interact with the medical system.

Like other biomedical experts, Eve described her reaction to diagnosis in clinical terms. Although she did not know much about breast cancer yet, she knew women died of rapidly growing tumors like hers. To stave off anxiety, she "preoccupied" herself "with the most aggressive treatment possible." And she rationalized to herself, "Obviously you don't want to lose a breast, but you would rather lose a breast than life." Things moved fairly rapidly after diagnosis, but Eve remained in charge each step of the way and researched all proposals thoroughly before agreeing to anything. She underscored her newly found expertise by telling me her story using medical language to describe her type of cancer and what could be done about it. Her comfort with the terminology came not only from her years of working as a scientist, but also from her determination to be the equal of her doctors when discussing her case, and her confidence that she could learn what they knew. She did not have to tell herself not to defer to doctors. She took it for granted that she was a lot smarter than some of those who were treating her.

The surgeon performed an excisional biopsy,[14] removing a "tennis-ball" size lump but without obtaining "clean margins."[15] Eve needed further surgery so, like the majority of biomedical experts, she did two things. She got two second opinions about the best treatment, and, in choosing which opinion to follow, she educated herself on the medical protocol for her particular case. The first opinion came from the general surgeon who had performed the biopsy. She asked knowledgeable friends and members of her family where else she should go. They suggested a prominent community hospital several miles away in an affluent suburb, where the group of doctors she saw included a surgeon who specialized in breast cancer. Finally, she consulted the comprehensive cancer center at a prestigious university hospital.[16] In choosing among more than one opinion, biomedical experts tended to select hospitals and doctors on the basis of national prestige, but Eve relied on her scientific acumen to follow a different reasoning:

> The advice from the general surgeon was just to have a mastectomy right away. . . . The advice from [the community hospital] would be to have preliminary chemotherapy and shrink whatever was around and then do surgery. . . . [The university cancer center] . . . wanted to

resection and just kind of go by sets of approximations until they got plain [clean] margins. They were very unorganized. . . . I would get lost in the shuffle. The other thing was that they would do the lymph node biopsy right away, and then, maybe, I would qualify for the bone marrow transplant, which I did not want.[17] The people that I knew that did that were dead.

Eve decided to use the community hospital for several reasons. She wanted an experienced breast surgeon, which eliminated the first doctor. She did not like the experimental nature of the university cancer center recommendations, and she felt that, given this hospital's size, she would not get full attention.[18] Her final reason was the clincher. She went on the National Cancer Institute Web site and found that the community hospital's recommendation was "in accordance with the latest FDA protocol," and she wanted her treatment to be in accordance with evidence-based medicine.

The term "evidence-based medicine" describes the research methodologies used to distinguish reliable and valid results from other, suggestive findings.[19] They are applied by doctors to determine the correct protocols to use for treatment of disease. They have been controversial from time to time, for example among AIDS activists, who have argued that important treatments were being delayed by clinical trials that held too closely to this research ideal.[20] But biomedical experts appreciated understanding that their treatments had been subjected to what they saw as rigorous testing. Eve's training in science had led her to believe in scientific medicine and to believe that she could understand her treatment options and choose rationally among them.

For many biomedical experts, the search for expertise led them to the top of the medical hierarchy. Charlene used a comprehensive cancer center—a hospital for cancer patients only—because she reasoned that "If I live close enough to cancer centers, this is where I am going to go." She checked her surgeon's credentials and noted that he came "highly recommended at Sloan-Kettering," an important credential in her opinion.[21] For Charlene and other well-educated women who believed in biomedicine, the prestige of the institutions a doctor was associated with, or had trained at, told them whether or not he was the best, and the best was what they wanted. Traditional responders assumed that their doctors were the best because they wanted to think they were in good hands. Biomedical experts used prestige rankings of educational institutions and hospitals to assess who was best. Their belief in biomedicine led them to trust biomedical rankings. This faith, combined with their belief that they could and should take responsibility for their own treatment, led them to examine doctors' credentials, often with the help of the knowledgeable persons in their social networks.

A good example of this behavior was provided by Hedley, a forty-three-year-old anatomy professor, whom I interviewed in an older suburb near the city. Since she taught students who were training for the health professions, Hedley considered herself to have a fair amount of expertise. She knew nothing about cancer, but given her background, she believed she could learn. After much preliminary checking, she selected a team of doctors at a comprehensive cancer center. She then gave these names to a close friend—an oncologist at a national research center—for a more intense level of checking. This friend also examined all of her pathology reports and evaluated the recommendations of the doctors Hedley had already seen. He then approved Hedley's choices.

Because they believed that biomedicine is only as good as its practitioners, biomedical experts did not hesitate to challenge doctors' recommendations. This ability to treat doctors as consultants and colleagues, rather than as authority figures, set the women in this group apart from their more traditional, and generally less resource-rich, sisters, even though both groups put their faith for a recovery in biomedicine. After diagnosis, Joann decided to follow her original plan and have both breasts removed during her surgery. Although her second breast was cancer-free, she wanted to do this as a prophylactic measure. Her surgeon could not fathom why a young woman would willingly part with a healthy breast, and he told her that he would talk to her about the second breast after her cancer treatment was over, if she was still interested. Joann realized that he thought she was acting out of panic and that time would cure her "irrational" desire. The doctor was adamant that he would not perform the prophylactic mastectomy at the same time as the one on the cancerous breast.

Since Joann believed the surgeon was competent and did not want further delay, she was unsure how to proceed. She then turned to her hematologist/oncologist family friend to complain about the surgeon's intransigence and to ask for advice. The friend proposed that the surgeon proceed as planned, but that, in addition, he should check to see if there was cause for concern. The surgeon followed the friend's recommendation by performing a "mirror-image biopsy" of the second breast, while removing Joann's cancerous breast.[22] When the results of the biopsy of her second breast showed "atypical hyperplasia," Joann felt vindicated in her fears and, armed with this evidence, persuaded her surgeon to perform a prophylactic mastectomy eight months later.[23] She described her efforts to gain his understanding:

> Before I went to sleep [for the second breast surgery], I grabbed his hand, and I said, "Thank you so much for making this a reality. . . . You keep telling me I need a quality of life after this. I will have a quality of life, if I don't have to worry on a daily basis that this is going to happen at another time."

Joann's self-confidence that she could manage her surgeon and get him to go along with her plans in spite of his initial reluctance was a product of her class enlightenment.

In addition to managing doctors, biomedical experts were not afraid to criticize what they saw as medical incompetence or arrogance. Hedley described a run-in with her oncologist over his responses to her long list of questions:

> He was really taken aback by these questions. He said, "Maybe you do not know what an abstract is." I was gritting my teeth. . . . Then I asked him about menopause. . . . His eyes got really big. We were sitting at a table, and he leaned towards me and said, "Are you thinking about having kids or something like that?" I said, "No, I'm not thinking about having kids." Then he said, "Oh well, you may or may not [go into menopause]." I was just furious . . . shaking . . . livid.

Hedley's science training had led her to believe that early menopause could have negative health consequences for women, for example, a possible loss of bone density. She became angry at the oncologist's apparent indifference to her fears and his suggestion that the only cause for concern lay in the potential loss of reproductive ability. After consulting knowledgeable physician friends, Hedley decided not to tolerate such an unhelpful and patronizing attitude, and she found a new oncologist. Like Joann, she had discovered that, while she wanted to partner her doctors, some doctors would rather take charge and could be patronizing about what they apparently viewed as interference. The old standard of patriarchal doctors who wanted compliant female patients sometimes collided with biomedical experts' desires for involvement.

In line with this, some women, such as Charlene and Donna, who were affluent and well educated but not scientists or medical professionals, complained about physicians who responded to questions only briefly and did not volunteer information. They handled this by refusing to be intimidated by a doctor who was not as forthcoming as they wanted and by insisting on more detail. Donna noted that even this could be unsatisfactory. Although her surgeon answered all her questions, "The problem was finding the right question."

Eve's greater scientific knowledge led her to doubt her surgeon's competence in the middle of treatment:

> When he told me about the mastectomy, he said, "Well, based on your multiple tumor type, I think you should have a mastectomy." I don't have multiple tumors. I would like [him] to look at my chart sometime. And by then I was pretty committed and I really like the oncologist, and I figured, "Okay, his memory may be going, but his hands are still good."

While this made Eve "uneasy," she sorted through her options and decided to continue with the surgeon rather than start over. She also understood that oncology had already shrunk her tumor smaller than it was before. Her realization that the oncologist was more important to her than the surgeon is one that a woman with less knowledge would have been unlikely to make.

Yet, as we have seen in Hedley's story, even the most knowledgeable biomedical experts were not always able to obtain the desired treatment or responses, apparently because some doctors resisted patients' attempts to treat them as colleagues. As a result of this, where traditional responders could leave medicine to the doctors and concentrate on other aspects of their lives, biomedical experts never relaxed during their treatment. Instead of trusting their doctors, they felt a constant need for vigilance, and they worried continually about the quality of their treatment. This was because biomedical experts recognized that knowledge about breast cancer is unstable and imperfect. Treatment recommendations change constantly, and new procedures and protocols replace accepted ones.[24] Furthermore, as was the case with Eve, obtaining second and third opinions could mean that the complex information and contradictory recommendations gathered would have to be sorted through in coming to a decision. Eve was able to obtain several opinions because she had a comprehensive insurance plan that would pay for them, but this advantage did not come without problems.

Regardless of the group women belonged to, they could not escape the debilitating effects of breast cancer treatment. How did biomedical experts, who had generally placed great emphasis on feeling and looking healthy, cope with this? As a group, they worked hard to stay in control even when their side effects became severe. To do this, they informed themselves about what was happening, or was about to happen, at every step of the way. They did so by using the plethora of information available to cancer patients in books, on the Internet, through educational programs, and by consulting knowledgeable others.[25] These were not women who "did not want to know too much," as traditional responders often told me. They wanted to know everything, and they believed they could understand everything.

Much has been written about the medicalization of women's bodies. Writers such as Emily Martin have documented the ways in which formerly routine life events for women—menstruation, pregnancy, and menopause, for example—have become medical conditions in need of treatment.[26] While this expansion of medicine's domain has generally been seen as oppressive to women, biomedical experts embraced medicalization. They wanted their illness to be explained solely by science and medicine, and they liked believing in a rational system of information that could be justified on scientific grounds. This empowering aspect of medicalization has been described by Elianne Riska, who has noted that the Internet has enhanced women's capacity for active involvement in health decisions.[27] The Internet in recent years has become an important source of health information and has enabled patients to learn medical terminology and to understand medical practice. This in turn has demystified patients' encounters with doctors. Michael Hardy has argued that, because the Internet presents all material as equally credible, this "dissolves the boundaries around areas of expertise upon which the professions derived much of their power."[28] However, since much of the information is of a fairly technical nature, not every woman finds it equally helpful, as we saw in the case of traditional responders.

Joann was an example of someone who found medicalization liberating. She described herself as having been much more knowledgeable about cancer than anyone in her family, even before diagnosis. While she went through treatment, she explained what was happening to those around her. She had seventeen lymph nodes removed, and three were positive for breast cancer. However, she made sure she got a list of all the exercises needed for postoperative arm recovery, did them "religiously," and "eight days later I had my sutures removed and I drove my children to the shore."

Donna described a decision-making process that was typical of the majority of biomedical experts, that is, the ones with no family history of breast cancer and little knowledge about it before diagnosis. Donna said, "What I usually do is seek a lot of people's opinions first, and then I get all of those different opinions, and then I decide for myself." As she acknowledged, "It's a convoluted decision-making process." In Donna's statement, there is no doubt about who was in charge of the decision. Eve also talked things over with those around her. Her husband is a research scientist in a field close to hers, and she discussed everything with him. In fact, he "set up this whole thing of breast cancer sites that I could go to for information." She also talked things over with her boss, a medical doctor who could answer many of her questions. Eve had expertise in her social networks everywhere she looked.

In addition to consulting others, biomedical experts consumed masses of information. Where a low level of knowledge was sufficient for traditional responders, biomedical experts wanted to learn a great deal of scientific information in order to feel comfortable that they knew enough.[29] They all bought and read books about breast cancer intended for the general public, especially *Dr. Susan Love's Breast Book*, which is the best-known breast cancer book in America. This was typically the first book they read after diagnosis, and they referred to it and similar books every time they had a question.[30]

Many went further, seeking information not available in breast cancer books intended for lay audiences. For example, Charlene and her husband "spent a morning up at [their cancer hospital's library] . . . using the Internet and their research facilities, when we were deciding mostly about the chemo." They did this because Charlene "just wanted to read the studies about it myself, because the doctors will tell you one paragraph about it and I really wanted to know a little more." Even though she had no scientific background, Charlene was not intimidated by reading technical information intended for physicians. She was confident that she and her husband were the intellectual equals of her doctors.

Although many biomedical experts appreciated the Internet, it was not always satisfactory, for the reasons summarized by Hardy. Some women found the information overwhelming and could not tell which sources had the correct information. When biomedical experts used it, they tended, like Eve, to confine their use to sites they viewed as prestigious and reliable: the National Cancer Institute site and sites maintained by famous medical schools, such as Johns Hopkins, or by prominent cancer hospitals, such as Sloan-Kettering. They judged information to be "reliable" based on the standards of scientific medicine.

This desire to know was not based solely on a quest for understanding, although this was part of the motivation. The knowledge biomedical experts gained from books and the Web helped them deal with their doctors on an equal footing, especially when their doctors were not forthcoming. As Donna explained, "I wanted to get enough information, so I could ask the right questions and so that I knew the terminology the doctors were using." She reasoned that doctors would pay more attention to her questions if she appeared knowledgeable. It should be noted, how-

ever, that the biggest advantage that biomedical experts had over traditional responders was not in their willingness to learn so much but in
their connections to knowledgeable family and friends who helped them
navigate the medical system. This resulted from their class position,
which enhanced their comfort that they were the social equals of the doctors who treated them.

Biomedical experts were more inclined than others to insist on the
most aggressive medical treatment, even if it was more unpleasant. Joann
felt particularly strongly about this:

> I was told that AC,[31] at the time, was the gold standard of care for
> my diagnosis, and that there were no clinical trials, at that time, that
> I was eligible for. . . . [The oncologist] had already met me once before
> the pathology was known. . . . He said, "When we get your pathology,
> we'll talk about whether or not you need to see me for treatment."
> And I sat up in bed, and I said, "I don't care what the report says.
> You will administer chemotherapy to me. . . . If that's an insurance
> policy that my odds for metastasis will be less, then I want it. . . ."
> He was stunned.

Other biomedical experts also pushed for aggressive treatment, and,
when they did so, they used biomedical evidence to bolster their arguments. Charlene requested chemotherapy because of a study showing "a
small statistical advantage to women with no node involvement and
small tumors," even though the oncologist did not push it.

Biomedical experts reacted differently than others to unpleasant side
effects, because they understood their origins. In fact, some even commented that bad side effects meant the treatment was working. They
tried hard to keep a stiff upper lip throughout treatments. Joann reacted
to tiredness and depression by keeping busy with her "three little boys."
She added, "I got up every day. I got in the shower. I put my makeup on.
I went out. . . . I really tried not to play the victim." Donna said that when
the chemotherapy left her depressed and crying, "I had to remind myself,
this is chemical. . . . I could almost tell the days when the chemicals were
leaving my body." And in spite of symptoms including "mouth sores
[from a thrush infection] and painful patches," Eve resolutely avoided

the morphine she had been given for her difficulties, because she knew it was an addictive drug that could cause additional problems. Surviving treatment heroically was an important part of the narratives of biomedical experts and contrasts once again with the more victim-like reactions of traditional responders. We should not be surprised that heroism and privilege go hand in hand in breast cancer narratives. This is a society where individuals frequently take personal credit for the successes in their lives.

As part of managing treatment, biomedical experts were able to describe in detail both the potential side effects of the drugs they were treated with and the actual side effects they experienced. They also knew which were the best and latest palliatives, and they took them where needed as long as they viewed them as helpful rather than harmful. Compazine, a drug commonly used to treat nausea, did not work for Joann, but "it was right when Zofran was FDA-approved" so, at her request, her oncologist switched her to this costly new and effective drug. As a comparison, I found a Canadian pharmacy on the Internet selling discount drugs. Compazine tablets could be purchased for twenty-four cents a tablet, and Zofran tablets were nearly ten dollars a tablet.[32] Women with severe nausea might take two or three tablets a day, so it is easy to see why oncologists started everyone on Compazine. Changing to Zofran happened when women complained loudly about nausea and knew that a more effective treatment existed. It was more common for biomedical experts to receive Zofran than for traditional responders to do so. Some of the explanation for this was in the demands of the biomedical experts, but some was because they had prescription drug coverage, which paid most of the cost for the more expensive medicine.

Although biomedical experts did not always have an easier time with breast cancer treatment than other women, their greater devotion to postoperative exercises gave them a clear advantage in recovery. Because of their personal involvement in regaining their health as well as their histories of healthy living, biomedical experts learned and followed the prescribed exercise regimen to recover the use of their arms more diligently than did traditional responders. If the hospital did not teach them these exercises, they learned them elsewhere: from radiation oncologists, by making physical therapy appointments, or from Reach to Recovery volunteers who visited them in the hospital.[33] Traditional responders were also often taught the exercises but tended to do them sporadically, whereas biomedical experts did them conscientiously, at least in the beginning.

Biomedical experts were less likely to experience lymphedema than traditional responders, and there appear to be two reasons for this. First, the exercises helped them gain full, or close to full, mobility. In addition, they were more cautious about subsequent warning signs, such as insect bites that might swell or get infected.[34] Charlene—who reported that she was very good about doing the postoperative exercises for the first six months, but not later—had a pain in her arm one time:

> I just called my general doctor and said, "I don't know what this is, but I never had this before. It doesn't appear to be very swollen." He said, "We don't care. We are putting you on antibiotics."

Hedley had two episodes of insect bites on her arm after her surgery, and, each time, she took an antibiotic. Neither of these women was the least bit hesitant about calling the doctor about something that might or might not be a problem.

This combination of exercise and care allowed biomedical experts a high degree of comfort about the use of their arms on a day-to-day basis, and as a group, they tended to take only minimal precautions once their arms recovered. Joann's account was fairly typical. Although usually conscientious about not having shots or blood pressure taken in the affected arm, she reported:

> I had a memory lapse several years ago. I got a flu shot . . . in my affected arm and I realized it afterwards. . . . [The nurse] was beside herself. . . . Yeah, I protect it. . . . I carry [packages] all the time, and I think about it. . . . Oftentimes I'm carrying the heaviest packages with my [other] arm. . . . I'm better about [gardening]. There are times when I don't. [With insect bites] I kind of look at it and wonder, "Is this gonna be the thing to push me over the edge . . . ?" I just kind of blow it off.

Biomedical experts tended not to face the same burdens from family and friends as traditional responders, so they had more time and energy to devote to themselves. Their higher than average rates of marriage were part of the reason for this support. Husbands provided both emotional and practical support. Eve was typical in talking every decision over with "my best friend, my husband. . . . He went through everything with me." Eve felt safe having the person whose judgment she trusted most as her sounding board. In addition, those who were married frequently recruited their husbands for practical help in learning what they needed to know and in communicating with others. Donna's description was similar to many:

> I tend to be someone who learns by writing notes. And [my husband] really listens [to the doctors]. . . . He was really helpful . . . kind of a hub, I guess, for telling. So I didn't have to take all of the calls. . . . He did kind of group e-mails to a lot of people. And he was really good at the technical stuff, explaining to people who wanted to know what was going on all of the time. He was much more into that, as opposed to how I'm feeling.

For "feeling," Donna turned to friends, of whom she had so many that her husband helped her manage them by answering their questions and thanking them for their concerns.

Even when telling a family member was difficult, the recipient of the bad news often responded in a supportive manner. Joann drove about sixty miles to visit her father, one week after he buried her mother, to tell him she had breast cancer. She took her brother with her. They arrived without having told their father they were coming, because they did not know how to explain the visit in advance:

> He came out the front door. . . . He looked very startled. He wasn't expecting anyone. . . . [He said] "What's going on? Where is everybody . . . ?" We went in and sat down. And I said, "I want to tell you why I'm here. . . . The bad news is that I just learned two hours ago that I was diagnosed with breast cancer. But the good news is that it's out of me. It's been removed, and I'm here to tell you that I'm fine. And that I'm gonna be fine. No matter what my path is, I need you to hear that." And he stood up . . . and he gave me a hug. And he said . . . "If you get twenty-six years like your mother did after her breast cancer, then you're ahead of the game."

Of course, family members were not always so noble. Joann's in-laws did nothing to help and instead told her, "Don't dwell on it," as if ignoring it would make it go away. And while her husband increased the amount of time he spent with the children when Joann was in the hospital, when he came with her to chemotherapy, she made him stay in the waiting room because the first time, "I could turn and look and see him turn white."

Hedley also had mixed family support. She criticized her mother's response to the cancer, but her story told as much about Hedley's relationship with her mother as it did about maternal indifference. Her mother came to stay with her during one of the chemotherapy treatments:

> We don't have a very good relationship. . . . That was the first time I actually vomited, that I really got sick. . . . I came down at one point, and she was crying, and she started cooking dinner. . . . And I thought she was crying about me. And she said, "Hedley, you'll never know what it feels like to have your daughter go through this. . . ." So in retrospect, it felt like she was telling me how she was feeling, not anything about what I was feeling.

Hedley interpreted her mother's reaction as one of self-absorption, but her mother's statement can also be interpreted as one of fear of losing a beloved daughter. Hedley contrasted her mother with her sister, who traveled across the country to look after her in the days immediately following surgery.

Sometimes families created unintentional problems, particularly if there were elderly and infirm parents. At the time of the interview, Eve, at her husband's request, had not yet told her in-laws about her illness, because her father-in-law was struggling to cope with his wife's early-onset Alzheimer's. Eve understood that this silence was not a lack of support for her, but rather a way of coping with competing crises.

The high level of competence biomedical experts showed during treatment sometimes had the effect of shutting out those nearest and dearest. Joann's account of her relationship with her husband is not unique:

> There were times when he wanted to hold me or wanted to say something, and maybe it didn't come out the way it felt supportive. And I would yell. . . . He was trying, and I didn't perceive he was trying. So then he stopped trying. And we had our biggest arguments down

the road, with me saying, "You were great when I had my first chemo experience and then those last three treatments, I was like on my own and I don't understand that." I remember him blaming me and saying . . . "That's because of you. You didn't let anybody help you. You have this presence of, 'I can do it.'" I said, "I did it, but I was on my last legs. . . . I wanted to lie down." He said, "I couldn't read your mind. . . ." He was right. . . . How does a young woman with a family strike that balance of not wanting her children to worry more than they already are . . . ? I was looking for support, but I wasn't enabling him to give it in an easy way.

Loved ones in this situation felt guilty about drawing attention to themselves. Where traditional responders devoted time to supporting those around them, biomedical experts were too busy managing breast cancer to pay attention to the anxieties of others. They had well-educated and supportive families and friends who believed in putting the patient first, so this usually worked, but it sometimes left hurt feelings. After treatment was over and biomedical experts looked back on their behavior, they had enough self-confidence about their emotional intelligence to recognize their own culpability and to forgive themselves for it. The language used by biomedical experts is strikingly different from the language, especially of self-blame, traditional responders typically used and reflects not only the greater resources of biomedical experts but also their practice at dealing with problems by obtaining professional help and by engaging in self-examination.

Most biomedical experts had professional careers and knew women like themselves. It was to these women that they frequently turned for emotional support. Joann reported that her friends allowed her to say "whatever I wanted, and they listened, and they never made me feel that they couldn't handle it." Donna turned to those of her friends who had "personalities [that were] particularly helpful, and up, and supportive," while avoiding those who were "more gray and dour, and kind of looking for the worst." The mother of one of Charlene's closest friends had had breast cancer, and Charlene reported that her friend "identified very well with me. She and I had lots of talks and cries." This is in contrast to traditional responders, who were more likely to need friends to provide practical support, particularly for those who were single parents.

One thing the two groups had in common was sharing a concern for how their children would cope with their mothers' ordeals. Biomedical experts handled this by talking to their children openly and encouraging their questions, and by paying for professional assistance with their children. In other words, they felt that their children had the same right to an education about breast cancer as themselves, and they had the resources to provide this education and to get other kinds of help with their children. In her determination to get through breast cancer and stay in control, Joann hired a babysitter, over the phone from her hospital bed, to take care of her young children during treatment. She also sent the children to a psychologist. She was concerned that they would find her cancer terrifying because, "My mother died. They knew my mother had cancer. And they were babies. . . . It was very important to me . . . that they knew that not everyone died who had cancer." This is in marked contrast to Carla's story in chapter 2 about her desperate efforts to get her family to help with her children while she coped with treatment and her recognition that her children had been emotionally scarred in the process.

Charlene's son had lost a friend to cancer, so she made a point of sitting her children down and reassuring them that hers was a small treatable lump, caught early. "Then I looked at my son, and I said, 'Understand that this is curable. It is nothing like your friend.'" Donna also insisted on telling her son herself, so that she could reassure him. She monitored his reactions carefully, looking for signs of trouble, and applauding his growing ability to cope with the news. Her son was particularly upset when she had to go back for a second surgery, a mastectomy this time:

> He had two responses. One was, "Are you going to die . . . ?" And the other was, "Do we have to tell anybody?" He said, "You always tell everybody everything. Do the people at school have to know . . . ?" I said, "I am not going to announce it, but I am going to tell the people whom I care about. . . ." Over the months, he started bringing people over here, and I think it was important for them to see me, that I was up and around. And I tried to go to school functions, so that they would see me. And then he went to the Race for the Cure, and he actually put his number in his locker. . . . He really changed just in the few months, from not wanting anyone to know, to basically advertising it.

In telling her son that she retained the right to talk about her feelings, Donna did not put her concerns aside for his sake. Instead, she encouraged him to come to terms with his mother's illness, and she interpreted his changing response as psychologically healthy.

These descriptions of how biomedical experts coped with children contrast greatly with the difficulties traditional responders had in the same situation. First, biomedical experts were much more confident of their abilities to cope with their children's fears and to do so in a way that would not leave scars. Second, they did not report that dealing with their children's issues greatly increased their own stress. They were clear that their own survival was the most important issue, and they felt that, if they focused on that, their children would benefit. It is most likely the case that, because these women stayed calmer throughout their treatment, their children became less frightened. It is difficult to know how much this greater calm resulted from the social capital that education brings and how much was simply a result of greater resources. No doubt both these factors played a role. The result of this was that the women in this group did not keep things from their children. They simply faced the issues head-on and, with the aid of their greater financial resources, used therapy as a backup, when necessary.

What other kinds of support did biomedical experts resort to, in getting through treatment and in dealing with the aftermath of cancer? Like traditional responders, they did not find support groups helpful in general, but their reasoning was different. Traditional responders became depressed when they attended support groups because they had to deal with other women's breast cancer, including women with frightening symptoms that it was possible to imagine getting.

Biomedical experts did not find support groups scary, but neither did they find them especially useful. Charlene noted, "There are support groups at every place I went to," and the physicians and nurses who treated her had encouraged her to attend, telling her, "Some people like it now; some people don't want it now but later on will want it." So she had tried going "once or twice to [a friend's] support group, because she would tell me about interesting things that they were talking about." In the end, Charlene concluded this was not for her, and she repeated a biomedical mantra in explaining her reasoning, "I'm a strong believer in continuing the treatment, continuing follow-ups. . . . The most important thing is just to do the medical things. That helps me enough, and I don't need a lot of the support groups and things like that." Charlene put her faith in medical science, not in time-consuming talk with strangers, talk that had an unproven benefit.

An equally common reason for avoiding support groups was that biomedical experts were better informed than the average breast cancer patient and so found the information there redundant. Hedley attended one on the advice of her oncologist friend and found it helpful for the first three times, "then it became very repetitive." Another friend who had had breast cancer a decade earlier offered to be her support, so they met each week during Hedley's treatment. Hedley reported, "It was actually more informative than a real support group."

Some biomedical experts became so knowledgeable by the end of their treatment that they started support groups for others, often as a result of being asked repeatedly for advice by newly diagnosed women. Joann, who had tried support groups "only to walk away from each of them" because she knew too much already, was asked by

> [T]he rabbi at my synagogue . . . to co-facilitate a support group with him, which is very unique . . . a support group with a real spiritual component. . . . That was the only way I agreed to do it. I said, "If you can structure it differently from what women can get in the community, I will be happy to join forces with you." She provided the information, and the rabbi offered "relevant prayer."

A few biomedical experts did go to support groups, but their experiences differed from the usual pattern. Eve knew enough to find her large and rapidly growing tumor scary. The more she learned the scarier it got; her prognosis was frightening. While going through treatment, she did not join a support group because, "I was just managing my life and I didn't have the strength to do that and to talk about it." She knew she needed help, but the first group she tried "was all ladies who were older than me, with pictures of their grandchildren, and I really did not fit in." Eve was not looking for information—she had access to plenty—but she "hadn't really talked about it before." She attended a therapeutic support group.[35] The leader was a skilled clinical psychologist who required a ten-week commitment, unlike most support groups, which women attend as often and for as long as they want and which are not run strictly as group therapy. Eve's group discussed the issues she wanted:

> Communicating with others, a sense of loss at losing a breast, and ways of dealing with stress. . . . We all set little goals for ourselves, and they were short to mid-term goals. To me, they were steps to goals . . . a very supportive atmosphere and a lot on communication and learning to listen to others without interrupting. . . . We had eight people . . . completely different backgrounds and yet you felt a closeness to them because of shared experiences.

Eve told me that had she not been in such a "supportive atmosphere in which we could talk about it," then "I wouldn't have talked to you either." Her husband had assisted her through every step of her treatment, making time in his busy schedule to help her figure out the science and to second-guess her decisions with her, but she wanted a therapeutic intervention as well.

Most biomedical experts had family and friends to provide emotional support and care. When they went outside this group, it was for professional help such as Eve found in group therapy or for medical information presented in a way that allowed them to ask questions and to clear up misunderstandings. They were the largest consumers of the many educational programs offered by hospitals and by organizations such as Living Beyond Breast Cancer, the National Breast Cancer Coalition, and the American Cancer Society.[36] Joann was one of the most extreme examples of this, attending numerous programs, training for Reach to Recovery,[37] and finally getting a job doing educational outreach with a breast cancer organization. Even with a job that involved her with breast cancer throughout her day, she remained active with a number of other organizations and presented at both national and local conferences.

Donna's story is more typical of the ways in which biomedical experts used the educational and other resources available to women recovering from breast cancer:

I went to a few educational programs. . . . One was on cancer fatigue, one was a general day-long conference based on medical information, some social, some exercise stuff, and then I went to three Living Beyond Breast Cancer [conferences]. . . . They were extremely helpful, in just the little things . . . trying to hook me up with people who might have had a similar problem. . . . I saw a nutritionist at the University of Pennsylvania who was really helpful. I went to an acupuncturist also for pain and to boost my immune system. . . . I never wore makeup before, and I got all of that free makeup [at Look Good . . . Feel Better][38]—that was a very positive experience—and how to tie scarves. [Reach to Recovery] automatically came into your room. . . . I had somebody come twice. And actually, I didn't let her come after that. . . . She was asking all these questions. I had enough already. . . . I went to a program at the Wellness Community.[39]

The programs Donna chose stayed close to organized medical praxis, although she deviated somewhat when she went to an acupuncturist. Most biomedical experts avoided things they considered to be outside the realm of scientific medicine. Eve, for example, praised a presentation that she had attended by Larry Norton, a prominent oncologist at Memorial Sloan-Kettering Cancer Center in New York.[40] In fact, she liked him so much that she consulted him before she started taking Taxotere, a drug he helped develop. Yet, in the next breath, Eve described Norton's cospeaker on the panel, a physician who has pioneered the use of alternative medicine in one of the nation's top medical schools, as a "real loser." She viewed such medicine as unscientific.

This general unwillingness to try treatments that are outside the mainstream breast cancer regimen did not extend to every area. Biomedical experts had grown up with the women's health movement and its mandates about personal responsibility for health. They continued to believe that they must follow behavioral mandates for a healthy life even if these do not specifically guard against breast cancer, so most increased their vigilance in this regard. The two most common changes were in diet and exercise, even though few cancer physicians say much about either. In fact, the most common recommendation received about diet, for the women I interviewed, was not to lose weight, especially when they were undergoing radiation. This is because measurements taken as treatment commences are based on the patient's weight. As weight changes, so do the needed radiation angles. Furthermore, cancer doctors customarily tell women that their bodies are facing enough abuse from surgery and chemotherapy, without having to adjust to weight loss. And since many women become nauseous from chemotherapy, oncologists typically tell them to eat whatever they can. As a result, many women gain weight during chemotherapy.

This medical indifference to a healthy diet encouraged traditional responders to make few dietary changes and to eat what they wanted during treatment, but biomedical experts felt they were doing something by becoming more concerned about what they ate. Joann, for example, reported that she changed her diet significantly after diagnosis by cutting out red meat and substituting turkey. Here is her description of a typical day:

> There's a health food store right around the corner [from work]. We often get the macro-plate. So I'll get some steamed veggies and whatever. . . . Or I'll have some tuna fish or something like that. And dinner's typically chicken and turkey. . . . I make a lot of stir-fries. I'm doing shrimp or chicken with multiple vegetables, cooking it on top of the stove. It's not fried in anything, and I make a lot of rice. It's easy and everyone in the house likes it. I avoid a lot of sweets. I snack . . . pretzels, and I look for the no-fat things.

Charlene did not compromise on her diet for the sake of her children. She had an elaborate regimen, which she described as "pretty much the same" each day. It was similar in content to the post-cancer diet in *The Breast Cancer Prevention Diet* by Bob Arnot, the popular television doctor.[41]

> In the morning, I eat granola or oatmeal. Then I have raisins on it. I have flaxseed and wheat germ—usually another fruit like bananas, strawberries, blueberries, whatever—a large bowl of that and a juice. I am trying to stay away from citrus juices, or maybe a small citrus with something like pineapple-orange or mango. . . . Lunch is usually a whole-wheat pita with hummus and vegetables, maybe some pretzels. Dinner I eat pasta, usually half regular, half whole wheat, and I'll use vegetables. I'll use sun-dried tomatoes, usually that. Fish, I do eat fish, salmon especially. . . . Chicken, I do eat chicken. Once in a great while, I'll eat

some kind of meat, like a little bit of pork . . . beef hardly ever. Maybe fruit for dessert. Or, sometimes, I'll eat frozen yogurt, and occasionally I'll cheat a little too. I mean I'm not a total fanatic. . . . I do eat soy. My family, unfortunately, does not participate in this diet. . . . [The children] don't like anything that's good for them.

Like many biomedical experts, Charlene had followed a healthy diet before she had breast cancer, but the changes she made after diagnosis were specifically designed for breast cancer prevention. They included the following:

I eat a very large breakfast now. I have never eaten breakfast in my life. I eat whole grains, fruit, and yogurt. . . . I got rid of meat entirely. Not 100 percent, but pretty much so. . . . Oftentimes I would eat a sandwich with like a lunch meat and cheese kind of sandwich. . . . I cut that out too. I cut down on eggs. . . . I've tried different things, which I had not tried before. In winter, soups with kale and things I was not familiar with.

These food descriptions contrast markedly with those of traditional responders. Once again, they illustrate the lengths to which biomedical experts went to reassure themselves that they would not be victims of a life-threatening illness. In spite of their greater resources, biomedical experts seemed to find it more difficult to put cancer behind them than did traditional responders. Charlene, for example, had learned about the dietary recommendations she followed through the educational programs she attended and in the books she bought after diagnosis. And she was not unique. Eating a health-conscious diet was one of the most important distinguishing features of this group. The details differed; for example, some ate tofu, while others avoided it.[42] Most of the dietary rules they followed are those that doctors recommend as being good for people in general: low fat, low meat consumption, and lots of whole grains and fruits and vegetables. They did not usually take dietary supplements of the kind found in health food stores, since they considered these to be untested medically.

Why were biomedical experts so interested in diet as a way to control breast cancer, in spite of oncologists' indifference? We might have expected them to conclude from the scientific evidence that diet was not an issue in preventing a reoccurrence. The answer may lie in the discourse around breast cancer and health more generally. As Susan Yadlon found in her study of the rhetoric of breast cancer, diet has been one of its mainstays. There have been many studies on the link between diet, especially dietary fat, and breast cancer, and while there is still little evidence of a relationship, most studies conclude with the recommendation that women should lower their intake of fat if they wish to avoid getting the disease or having a reoccurrence.[43] It is not surprising that the biomedical experts were strongly influenced by the use of this language in biomedical discussions of breast cancer. It does, however, underscore Bruno Latour's observation that science is not simply based on an impartial reading of the evidence.[44]

Biomedical experts were equally concerned about exercise. This is another healthy lifestyle tenet that is not clearly related to breast cancer, although some evidence appears to exist that a lifetime of exercise may reduce the risk, possibly because it lessens the likelihood of obesity.[45] Joann, for example, walked three miles four times a week. She wanted to join a gym but could not fit it in between the job and the children. Donna also walked regularly and attended a gym four times a week, where she did both aerobic and weight-bearing exercises. She did the latter because a consequence of her treatment was early menopause, and she was now having some bone density problems.[46] Both aerobic and weight-bearing exercises help increase bone density and lessen the chance of osteoporosis.[47] Biomedical experts were determined to combat the difficulties they faced and, once again, portrayed themselves as heroes rather than victims.

Not surprisingly, some biomedical experts had been active athletes before breast cancer and remained so afterward. Hedley, who did not have the obligations of motherhood, played golf and tennis regularly, and she ran fast enough to come in second among survivors at the Race for the Cure.

Part of the reason biomedical experts placed so much emphasis on diet and exercise was because they wanted to maintain their active and in-charge stance. Attention to diet and exercise is approved of by the medical establishment, and following the rules of best practice in this area made them feel like they were keeping a reoccurrence at bay. Although there are few well-documented dietary or exercise recommendations for breast cancer, biomedical experts were used to including these things in their lives. They had come to breast cancer with a history of looking after their bodies through diet and exercise. Although this history had not prevented breast cancer, they saw no reason to give up healthy living in response to their diagnosis. Rather, they became even more vigilant.

This was probably exacerbated because the biomedical establishment has responded to increasing competition from alternative medical practitioners by incorporating some alternative offerings into their own educational programs. Almost every such program has sessions on diet and exercise. For example, when I asked him about the relationship between breast cancer and diet, my oncologist told me that there was little evidence diet helped, but he added that it was a good idea to eat a healthful diet. And hospital-based and other establishment educational programs, such as those of the American Cancer Society or Living Beyond Breast Cancer, almost always include a dietary component.

Susan Bordo has noted that women often become involved in extreme exercise as a way of maintaining absolute control over their bodies.[48] As an example of this, Charlene responded to my question about loss of control during treatment by describing how diet and exercise helped her:

> I'm a fairly in-control person. . . . I don't mean controlling others. It's a personal thing. I want to know what's going to happen . . . and this has been a lot of, you know, not knowing. . . . Even friends would come up to me and say, "We couldn't believe that happened to you. You take good care of yourself and everything." I said, "Well, unfortunately that's not good enough." You can't control any of these things. . . . I can control my diet. . . . It allows me to feel I am doing something. . . . My thing is exercise and diet.

Charlene did this in spite of understanding that one cannot prevent things like cancer, no matter how carefully one manages one's lifestyle, because, as she noted, "Bad things happen to good people." These well-educated women wanted to put their abilities to work preventing a reoccurrence of breast cancer, and undertaking a program of healthful diet and adequate exercise seemed like a good idea.

Control was a big issue for most of the biomedical experts, because unlike traditional responders, they had long prided themselves on being in control. Except for Joann, who had anticipated her cancer and viewed diagnosis as "an opportunity to take control because of my legacy," most women had not planned a life with breast cancer in their future. As Eve described it, "Here I was coming back from a successful meeting, and I think that things are going great in my life," and "all of a sudden, I have this big thing thrown at me to deal with." Where many women would have panicked at her prognosis, Eve reported that she "dealt with it in a controlled manner":

> I'm a project manager, so the way I coped was by making a project for survival and having my software for project management and making a Gantt chart with boxes.[49] We had all the appointments, and all this, all that, everything on it and managed it. . . . I don't know if it was just a diversion. . . . The thing about cancer is it makes you realize you are not in control of anything, so to compensate, to make yourself feel a little better, you pretend to be in control of something. . . . I still planned everything. And I planned activities for after each treatment, so I had something to look forward to. You try to put whatever control in that you think you can, and, if things don't work out, you change your plans.

Biomedical experts saw science and medicine as ways to make life's uncertainties more predictable, but they knew that science itself contains much uncertainty and that sooner or later one has to face this. Thus they kept faith in science as the supreme form of knowledge, even though they were unsure about their own futures and about how to prevent the worst. They tried "to hold on to some control," as Hedley put it, by talking to the doctors and taking charge of those things they could. Sometimes, they felt they were failing in this. Donna reported feeling a loss of control when her first chemotherapy made her feel "real shitty," so she regained a semblance of it by calling a therapist. Turning to an expert was her logical first response.

How did biomedical experts process their experiences and move forward after breast cancer? They reported two main changes in their perspectives on life, and each is related to the theme about control. First, they became acutely aware of life's fragility and concluded that they should not postpone its pleasures. Eve described both her husband and herself as "workaholics," but they had decided not "to wait until I retire to think about how easy to take things." As a result, "We're putting in time for ourselves and not postponing things." For Charlene, this translated into no longer taking life for granted. In discussing the changes in her life, Charlene returned to her theme of people's life chances:

> I've become more aware of the lack of control that we do have over things. And maybe my expectations of others are a little more realistic than they were. I was always able to look at that fairly well, with the kind of work that I do. I work with disabled, and aged, and low-income people who have many, many problems, far more than I do. I always try to say a lot of these people are in situations not of their own making, but because they had no control over things. So I have always been aware of that, but I guess this is personal.

Charlene had gone through life holding herself to different standards than others. Now, although she still strove for control, she also recognized the fallacy in her stance.

The second theme shared by biomedical experts was that breast cancer had made them more appreciative. Other women reported this, but biomedical experts took this position even while acknowledging that this might not really be true. Donna spoke for many when she said, "I try very much to figure out what's important and what's not important and not let little things get me down." So, "I do think it's kind of given me a new lease on life. And maybe, I've talked myself into that. . . . I think it's important to be optimistic, even if you do a number on yourself."

Hedley's realization that life can end at any moment had forced her to face her problems. One of her first acts upon diagnosis was to end a difficult affair she had been having with a married woman. She described the way in which she had consciously worked to change herself:

> I have learned to make a real decision, to search for healthy choices for me. . . . I guess that comes back to realizing that we are mortal and stopping and saying, "I don't know when my life is going to end, but I don't want to spend my life being unhappy. . . ." The most profound change has been to say . . . "I need to let go of those things that are making me unhappy, whether it's relationships, or work, or family, or whatever."

Easier said than done, but I think that is the most profound change, to really make conscious choices. . . . I'm really sorry it took a sledgehammer to get it in to me.

Hedley had moved into a more trusting and loving relationship than any she had had previously and saw this as resulting from the way her illness had forced her to change.

Joann saw cancer as helping her to "realize the important things in life and the things that are not that important." To illustrate this point, she told of a friend who called her all upset because "her daughter got a bad haircut." Joann replied, "Big deal. . . . Who cares? Be happy she's got [hair]." Joann was trying to teach her husband, as the children got older and more oppositional, that he needed to "Pick your battles" because the "annoying little things" were "not a big deal."

Because of their desire for control, biomedical experts had wanted to decide things for themselves and to go it alone to some degree. And in looking back, many of them saw this as a mistake. When asked how they would do things differently, if they had cancer treatment to do over again, the most common response was that they would have let others do more, even though they were not always sure they could have changed. We saw how Joann shut her husband out when he wanted to help. The only time she had let her brave front down was alone in the hospital for eight days with a clot in the catheter that had been implanted for chemotherapy. Joann noted that "In a perfect world, I should have let people do more for me. Maybe I should not have been such a tough cookie." Then she added, "But I think I did it for the right reasons." Even when I interviewed her, Joann still wanted to be the one to make decisions. She still kept a careful watch over herself, telling me she was "determined to find something before anyone else does." As a result of her conviction that she was "still in touch" with her own body and that "If I feel a change or a difference, I'm going to report it to one of my doctors," Joann found that whenever she went for a cancer checkup, "I just feel like it's this annual thing. . . . I never truly worry."

Hedley also felt she had been too stoical going through her treatment, but she was more adamant than Joann that this had been a mistake. She blamed her attitude on her upbringing:

> I grew up in a family where stoicism and bravery were values, and I was a good child if I didn't complain or get sick. If I got sick, I'd say, "I'm okay." And that is how I got through breast cancer. I wouldn't do it that way again.

Hedley described her new relationship in glowing terms, and she commented, "It's just wonderful to have a friend who holds my hand and recognizes that it's scary each time I go back." She added, "I just remember sitting there alone so many times."

Control could also be achieved if women could find an ironclad scientific explanation of the cause of their breast cancer. Most of the women from families with a breast cancer history did not want to know for certain if their illness had a genetic explanation because such knowledge would be frightening for their offspring. But the biomedical experts who had breast cancer in the family wanted to know because they wanted to plan for every eventuality. And some had genetic testing, even without a particular family history. Donna reported that the only time she cried was with relief when she was told she did not have a genetic marker for breast cancer. Again Joann differed from others:

> I did have the *BRCA1* and 2 [genetic] testing done way back as part of the clinical trial . . . in women diagnosed under forty. I got a letter back saying I didn't test positive, but they refined the lab technique and I should be retested because it may not have been accurate. . . . I will do it again . . . so my kids know it's part of their genetic background when they're older. I wouldn't share it with them now. It's for cousins of mine who are female, who want to know. . . . I asked them, "When I get this information, do you want me to share it with you?" And they said, "Yes."

Where traditional responders continued with their day-to-day lives as much as possible by handing breast cancer over to their doctors, biomedical experts put other things in their lives on hold. Breast cancer was their priority. They became more knowledgeable about the disease than other women and took a greater part in treatment decisions. This does not mean that they coped with their cancer better than more traditional women. In his book on the history of breast cancer research, Barron Lerner observes that the complexities of breast cancer treatment and the current emphasis on patients' rights to make a decision can create problems for women who feel the need to decide on complex issues they barely understand.[50] Many biomedical experts became obsessed with their cancer experience, staying immersed in it by eating right, by exercising, and by keeping informed about the latest cancer discoveries and treatment techniques. For some, this became a full-time job, and, for almost all of them, it created a vigilance they rarely escaped. Many continued this vigilance even after their treatment ended. Traditional responders were more easily able to turn their backs on cancer and to carry on with their lives as they had lived them previously.

Biomedical experts, until their diagnoses, seemed to have achieved the enviable status of "having it all." They had interesting careers, the majority had loving husbands and families, they had lots of friends, and they believed that they could achieve whatever they wanted. These were the women who had benefited from affirmative action programs to achieve their educational and occupational goals, and they were confident that they had their lives in order. Breast cancer was a blow to this confidence, but they used the skills they had developed and the resources of their education and income to manage this new problem. Their education and affluence and their personal connections enabled them to get all the medical services available. Yet, in their pursuit of everything out there for breast cancer, they may have become consumers of more than they needed and allowed their bodies to become needlessly medicalized. To this point, we have considered only those women who viewed scientific medicine as the basis for a cancer cure and who followed the tenets of biomedicine either by doing what the doctor told them to or by creating a partnership with their doctors. We now turn our attention to women who had less faith in biomedicine as the ultimate source of a cancer cure.

FOUR

Faith in the Ultimate Authority

Bella, an African American woman in her sixties, looked much younger with a spectacular figure and lovely face. She had worked with cancer patients, so she knew that breast cancer could happen to anyone, and she checked herself "at least once a week." She reported that the lump leading to her own diagnosis "just stuck right out of nowhere." She attributed this early warning to God; she reasoned that God "had to be there. I mean it just stuck right out of nowhere." Even so, she was stunned when the subsequent biopsy revealed breast cancer. Her immediate reaction was that death was imminent. She no longer looked with pride at her beautiful breasts; instead, "I looked at my breast . . . and it reminded me, 'I got cancer.'"

I interviewed Bella, who lived alone, in her immaculate living room in a public housing project in the outer suburbs. She is representative of a small group of respondents, about one-tenth of those I interviewed, who were like traditional patients in that they turned the responsibility for a cure for breast cancer over to a higher power. But, where traditional responders relied on doctors and medicine to place them on the path to recovery, women like Bella relied on faith rather than science. Many women in the study prayed to God for endurance and emotional support during cancer treatment, but most of these saw prayer as a supplement to their medical treatment. The women discussed in this chapter reversed this procedure. They followed doctors' orders for the most part, but they believed that only God could bring about a recovery. Indeed, they assumed that God had a purpose in putting them through this trial, and that this purpose would become known to them in time. I call these women "religious responders." They chose not to take personal control over the course of their illness, and they relied on faith as the basis of their recovery. Furthermore, they had religious explanations for their disease.

Most, but not all, of the women in this group were African American, and their religious faith had long supported them in all aspects of their lives. As noted in chapter 1, had I not made a point of interviewing a large number of African Americans, I would have missed this group in my analysis. It is possible that other racial or ethnic groups with a history of religious conviction and church attendance, such as Latinos, would have given a religious response also, but I had only one Latina in my sample. There is an extensive literature showing that African Americans are typically more religious than whites.[1]

Religious responders also had lower than average incomes and less education than any other group. This is related to race—the two white women in this group were affluent and college graduates. Members of this group were almost all currently married, even though they were somewhat older than average. So the group consisted largely of African American women who were economically and educationally disadvantaged even though married. For these working-class women, the church was the mainstay of their lives, providing them with resources and social support otherwise lacking.

The importance of the church to the black community has long been

Table 4   Religious Responders by Selected Variables

	White (not Jewish)*	Black	Total
Age			
Less than 40	0	0	0
40–49	2	2	4
50–59	0	2	2
60 and over	0	4	4
Family income			
Less than $20,000	0	2	2
$20,000–$39,999	0	3	3
$40,000–$69,999	0	2	2
$70,000–$99,999	0	0	0
$100,000 and over	2	1	3
Education			
12 years and less	0	6	6
13–15	0	2	2
16–17	2	0	2
18 and over	0	0	0
Marital status			
Currently married	2	6	8
Divorced	0	1	1
Never married	0	0	0
Widowed	0	1	1
Total	2	8	10

*No Jewish respondents were religious responders.

recognized.[2] In a national survey of black Americans, 70 percent identified themselves as church members and 71 percent attended on a regular basis.[3] Political scientist Cathy Cohen has called the black church "the glue and motor of the community."[4] The church has served as a social support system and refuge from a hostile world.[5] In a survey of the seven major historically black denominations, C. Eric Lincoln and Lawrence Mamiya found that 70 percent of the ministers they interviewed cooperated with social service agencies in solving community problems.[6] For generations, access to health care and other social services has been problematic for African Americans. Many have written about racial disparities in health care.[7] In general, blacks receive later diagnoses and fewer procedures for the same illnesses, compared to whites. As a result, the church in the black community has a long history of providing for the health needs of church members. This has been accomplished through a variety of programs, including free health clinics.[8]

Black women have relied on the church as a support system to a greater extent than have black men.[9] In a study of African American women's approach to health care, Mary Abrums argued that religion was the basis for how the poor and working-class women in her study faced illness and dealt with the health care system.[10] No doubt the preponderance of African Americans among religious responders in my study is a result, in part, of the lack of good quality care received by many minority women.[11] Black women have less reason than whites to believe that biomedicine has their interests at heart.

These differences exist for cancer treatment. In a study published in 1989 of over 7,500 women treated for breast cancer at more than 100 hospitals, Paula Diehr et al. reported that African Americans were less likely than whites to have health insurance or to be treated by a board-certified physician and were more likely to be treated in large public hospitals. Yet, even when the authors controlled for these differences and for demographic factors, whites received better care and more follow-up services.[12] While it is difficult to document the impact of discrimination against minority patients, in one study, one-third of African Americans reported having been discriminated against by the health care system. In another study, African American patients were four times as likely as whites to state that they believed racial discrimination was common in doctors' offices.[13] Part of the explanation for their poorer health care lies in the higher percentage of African Americans who are uninsured, even when they are employed.[14] Jean Hardisty and Ellen Leopold found that whereas 13 percent of whites were without health insurance, 30 percent of blacks were.[15] One of the consequences of this lack of medical insurance is that black women are diagnosed at later stages on average than whites and thus have higher mortality rates for breast cancer.[16] For all these reasons, it is not surprising that African Americans look to God for support in dealing with illness rather than relying solely on biomedicine.

Women who lacked the education and resources to make decisions for themselves typically turned their illnesses over to their doctors. Yet African American women in this situation often had other reasons to mistrust biomedicine. So they frequently turned to religion to see them through breast cancer, just as they no doubt turned to religion in other times of crisis and in dealing with hostile social institutions.

Caroline, age seventy-one, was a retired factory worker who lived with her husband in a small, sparsely furnished older house in the outer suburbs. Like Bella, she reported that God had helped her obtain an early diagnosis of her illness:

> They had hurt me so bad [at the previous mammogram] . . . I decided I was not going to get it. . . . Diahann Carroll came on the television, and she was saying if you had not had a mammogram recently, within the past year, "Please, please, please." And it looked like she was pleading with me. . . . I thought, "Lord, she must be talking just to me." And I made the appointment that very day.

Shantal also saw God's hand in her diagnosis. Shantal was fifty-one years old and a longtime city employee with a high school diploma, living in one of the city's historically black neighborhoods. When she had her annual mammogram, the radiologist noted calcifications but told her that they were nothing to worry about, and her gynecologist agreed with this assessment. Although Shantal was normally stoical and private about health concerns, she felt compelled to insist on a biopsy, and was proved correct in being fearful.

This belief that God was instrumental in ensuring a diagnosis, so that a woman of faith would be cured, is similar to that reported by Holly Matthews and colleagues in a study of black women with advanced breast cancer in North Carolina. While the women in that study were more fatalistic and had been resistant to having cancer treatment, many of them changed their minds, and, when they did, they used God as the reason.[17]

Religious responders did not fit Anne Kavanagh and Dorothy Broom's typology about how women explain their illnesses.[18] This group did not blame lifestyle, as did the traditional responders, nor did they see their cancer as emanating from the body itself, like the biomedical experts. Nor did religious responders refer to the third category of most-likely blame—environmental risk. The illness narratives of religious responders make them a group that Kavanagh and Broom did not find in their data. While only some of them described God as causing the cancer, all thought that he had helped them face the diagnosis and survive the treatment. They also believed that, in letting them have cancer, God had a specific goal for them. Shantal reported that as soon as her fears were realized, she prayed:

> I got down on my knees and I just prayed . . . I said, "This is too big for me Lord, you have to take care of it and take care of me." And when I came up from that prayer, I haven't been the same person.

Although they were like traditional responders in some ways, religious responders differed in not using self-blaming reasons for breast cancer. They knew that their cancer was caused by forces outside themselves and that they had been chosen for some reason to bear this burden.

Religious faith and a personal relationship with God strengthened some women's resolve in dealing with biomedicine from the beginning of their cancer experience. Rosamund, a forty-five-year-old business executive, insisted on a mammogram that her gynecologist thought unnecessary. When her fears that she had breast cancer were realized, she, too, found support in her religious beliefs:

> I thought about scripture. They always say the Lord doesn't give us more than we can bear, and I thought and believed that. So I thought I must be able to get through this, because, if I couldn't, it wouldn't be happening.

The themes that religious responders used in their narratives of breast cancer did not resonate with the cultural messages found in the media to the same extent as did the narratives of those women who believed that biomedicine was the route to recovery. In his influential work, Bryan

Turner argued that medicine has replaced religion as the dominant moral guardian of Western society.[19] While this has been challenged, most notably by Malcolm Bull in his study of Seventh-Day Adventists, the argument appears to hold for most residents of Western societies and it is certainly the message to be found in media discussions of breast cancer.[20] The media may make mention of religion in breast cancer stories, but they do so in a secular manner; they position religion as one of a number of supports. Religious responders were in the minority in viewing God as their central support.

Another way in which religious responders differed is that their stories were neither of victims nor of heroes. Instead, they were stories of redemption. These women told of getting sick and recovering by leaning on a God who took a personal and palpable interest in them. Although doctors were visited and treatments were followed—as might be expected in a culture where biomedicine is accorded such great authority and esteem—doctors were viewed as being under God's rule, just like the rest of his children. Religious responders had a close relationship with God, and they considered this relationship to be their main anchor in all aspects of life. In their interviews, they talked about God as an intimate, and they were most comfortable in the fellowship of those who felt as they did. Through their reliance on faith, religious responders tended to reject the pressure toward medicalization found in our culture. Scientific truths were not paramount in their worldview, in the way they were for the groups discussed in chapters 2 and 3.

It is hard for less religious persons to comprehend the emotional strength religious responders gained from their faith. Physicians, for example, are not always sympathetic to such beliefs. In a study of cancer patients and the decision-making process, Tovia Freedman described how an African American patient chose to follow the surgeon's rather than the radiation oncologist's advice, because the latter showed disrespect to her mother who had sat in the examination room reading a prayer book.[21] African American patients, who could not always rely on the sympathetic understanding of doctors, found comfort in believing that doctors were subject to God's authority also.

Among religious responders, family members could be skeptical about religious conviction. Shantal's husband asked her a question that many less religious persons might ask: "How can you serve a God who would let you have cancer?" Shantal replied, "I don't know if He's responsible." In telling me this story, she added that she never felt angry with God, and her statement was echoed by most of the women in the group. When Rosamund's friend gave her a book about dealing with anger at God, Rosamund's reaction upon reading it was, "This is not how I feel."

Some religious responders did not deal with the diagnosis as calmly as Shantal or Rosamund. Bella described feeling stunned and being "in denial for a long time." Even so, she coped with her fears through prayer and through her church. She continued to feel fearful from time to time, but, when this happened, she knew where to turn. Like Bella, Jenna, age forty-five at diagnosis and one of the two white women among the religious responders, did not face the diagnosis calmly at first. Jenna was an upper-middle-class homemaker married to an executive. Like Bella, she found the diagnosis emotionally traumatic, reporting that she "couldn't even say that word. . . . I kept thinking 'Call it anything but cancer.'" She added:

> I guess the first thing that really came into my mind was my mortality. . . .
> It all of a sudden hit me very strongly that that was a possibility, and I
> was going to have to travel a path that I did not want to travel. . . . I didn't
> want to do chemo. I didn't want to do the radiation. I didn't want to go
> through the surgery. I just didn't want to do it, but I knew I had to.

The above quote is reminiscent of traditional responders. Both groups found it difficult to make decisions about their treatment and needed outside support. The difference between the two groups lay in the source of this support. In addition to the racial differences between traditional and religious responders, there were many more young women in the group of traditional responders. These women had child-care responsibilities and sometimes no husbands and did not have the time or energy to turn to a nonmedical source of support. In contrast, the religious responders were in a better position to give time to church and religion because they were less burdened by family responsibilities. Their children were grown and their marriages long-lasting and secure.

Jenna was one of the few women in the group to report anger at God when she was diagnosed, but she immediately "felt that it was inappropriate for me." However, a friend who shared her strong beliefs asked her, "Jenna, don't you feel God's shoulders are strong enough to handle your feelings?" Realizing that a loving God would turn the other cheek, she allowed herself to feel "angry that I had to go through it," without feeling guilty about her anger.

Some religious responders overcame their anger when they began to understand God's purpose. Bella, who had suffered an abusive childhood, was angry because "On top of that, he allowed me to have this." However, she ultimately felt "bad that I felt that way about God, because through all this he was disciplining me." Bella's comment helps in understanding why religious responders did not lose faith when diagnosed. Where traditional responders most frequently blamed themselves for their cancer and biomedical experts looked for scientific explanations, religious responders viewed their illness as part of God's larger plan. The women in Abrums's study viewed Jesus as being in charge of their bodies and believed that they had to surrender their illness to God.[22]

Some religious responders saw God's purpose as one of promoting their personal salvation; they saw God as wanting them to become better Christians or to overcome earlier difficulties. This was particularly true of those who reported that their first response had been anger at God. Bella believed that God caused the cancer to help her finally overcome the pains she still carried from her childhood:

> My background is horrible. . . . As a child, I mean, it was a nightmare. Then why give this to me now? I think, up until then, I was a very angry person, from my childhood on. But today, I could tell you, I am not angry. . . . I enjoy life now. . . . Life has so much meaning now. . . . It's like God gave me a second chance.

A belief like this is a comfort in an unkind world. Bella had had, and continued to have, a hard life. There was no comfort to be found in science for her pains, but in religion, with its promise of salvation, illness could be seen as a good thing, not as a final blow.

Jenna thought that there might be a genetic explanation for her breast cancer because her mother had been similarly diagnosed at approximately the same age. Even so, Jenna's primary explanation was that God used cancer to strengthen her faith:

> My faith was tested, like it never was before, through this process. I really look at this thing as a real refiner's fire I had to go through. And I feel I'm a better, stronger, wiser, more trusting Christian because of this. . . . I cannot say, "Thank you, Lord, for giving me this cancer or for allowing it to happen. . . ." I haven't yet got to that point in my life. . . . I certainly have seen his hand in the entire process. . . . My faith was very immature and very baby-like before the cancer. I think I considered God a miracle worker or just kind of like a Santa Claus. . . . When I prayed, he would do it.

In contrast to these individualistic explanations for cancer, other religious responders saw their cancer as a sign that God intended a larger ministry for them. This was particularly true of those who reported no anger at God for giving them cancer or at least for not preventing it; as Shantal's and Jenna's comments demonstrate, religious responders may not always be clear about this point. Both Rosamund and Shantal became active in the breast cancer movement after completing treatment, and each believed that God had called her to this task. Rosamund prayed to God to "Let me know what to do and let me be strong enough to do what I need to do." Later in the interview, she added:

> I read this book once. . . . It was talking about pain and suffering, and it really stuck with me. It said, "Sometimes, I need for me to suffer. . . ." I look at what I went through, and I think I went through it because I would do something with it. . . . He knew that I would get through it, and I would do something that would help other people.

Rosamund followed up as she believed God intended. She recounted several examples of how she had improved the lives of other breast cancer sufferers. For example, after she did a radio interview about her experience, the interviewer called and told her that he had gone to his barber's a week later:

> The barber said his wife had breast cancer, was real down, depressed, you know, not dealing well with it. They were on their way to chemo, when they heard me on the air. He said they pulled over and listened to

the broadcast. He said she changed her whole attitude and said, "That's it. I'm getting through this. . . ."

Rosamund added, "I don't have a clue who this woman is." But, inspired by experiences like this, Rosamund continued to feel God's hand upon her shoulder as she worked for a myriad of breast cancer support programs. Like Shantal, she saw herself as a conduit for God's plan. She was not doing this alone or even getting most of the credit. In this way, religious responders differed greatly from biomedical experts. The stories of religious responders did not portray heroines but rather faithful vessels for God's larger plan.

The most remarkable story about faith and activism is that of Shantal. She described her whole breast cancer experience as culminating in a mission to help underserved African American women learn about breast cancer, to get them diagnosed early, and to cope with the treatment. Among the explanations offered for the higher breast cancer mortality rates among black women, in addition to a lack of access to medical care, is a continuation in the black community of silence and shame about the disease.[23] Many health providers and others in the breast cancer community believe that this mortality differential cannot be lessened without more education and support geared specifically toward African American women, and groups like the American Cancer Society have struggled to accomplish this.

Immediately after hearing the bad news, Shantal called her pastor to ask him to pray for her. Like others in this group, she first thought about her religious faith as a way of obtaining personal support as she went through her treatment. The minister, who was newly appointed to Shantal's church and was still getting to know his congregation, responded, "Come in and meet me." When she did so, he told her, "There's a need for a woman to do this." Shantal understood that he was passing on a call from God that she should minister to others in need. Another sign that she had been called was that, where before she had been extremely private about medical problems, this time, "I told everyone straight away. . . ." Shantal added, "Knowing me, my husband said, first thing . . . 'What do I tell people?'" Her reply was, "Tell them I have breast cancer."

Shantal quickly became inundated with requests for help from other African American women with breast cancer. Then her pastor, who had not forgotten his earlier comment, asked her to run a program for women at the church about the disease. In this way, a breast cancer educational program for African American women was born to provide a number of services, including a well-attended support group that combines religious faith with breast cancer education. The group provides scientific information to the women who attend, but the help is packaged in the message that faith is paramount. Shantal attributed to God her decision to become involved in this, saying, "I believe spiritually that this is something God has assigned me to do." And as is discussed in chapter 8, on activism, her ministry has had a great impact on many women of color and others in need of help.

Religious responders' faith that God would be by their side as they went through treatment did not stop them from obeying their doctors. It did, however, lessen the emotional impact of dealing with the medical system. Almost all religious responders wanted surgery and treatment over with quickly. This was not because of family demands as in the case of traditional responders. Rather, they wanted to devote their time to God's agenda, instead of spending it around doctors and hospitals or in learning lots of medical information. Almost none of the religious responders went for second opinions. Jenna came closest; she did not go for second opinions but she had an oncologist cousin through whom she passed all of the doctors' recommendations. Many religious responders did not have sufficient health insurance or the financial resources to pay for second opinions. Jenna was one of the few exceptions—a woman who had medical experts in her social networks.

Religious responders also reported liking their doctors in the main. Like traditional responders, they tended to stay with the doctors they were first assigned. Some had insurance issues that made it difficult to be picky about doctors, but most reported confidence that God would ensure they were in the right hands. Caroline spoke for many in this group in stating that she did not want to become too involved with the medical side of things, "because the Lord will take care of me." This fatalism that the future was out of their hands led religious responders to say little about their doctors, including whether they found them satisfactory or not. Once again, this illustrates the ways religious responders sought miracles at the hand of God and not in the medical system. These mostly African American women did not need to rely on a system they had not always found to be friendly.

Religious responders' attitudes about doctors and treatment extended to learning about treatment recommendations. Noting that she "did not read anything that had anything to do with cancer," Jenna "did exactly what I was told by my husband and by my doctors." As she put it, "I wasn't the type that went home and looked it up and read about it and wanted to know what the diagnosis was or anything like that." Shantal did call the American Cancer Society, and she read the information they sent her, but she learned little about breast cancer while undergoing treatment. Rosamund also called the American Cancer Society, but she preferred to read books about successful survivors rather than learning the details of the disease. Many religious responders had a strong sense of service to others, so it is not surprising that they were especially interested in the experiential aspects of breast cancer. When Shantal and Rosamund became active in the breast cancer movement, they learned about the disease in order to minister to others, but even then, their focus was on providing emotional support. In this way, they were similar to traditional responders, except that they were not so focused on family demands.

Where biomedical experts coped with treatment side effects by learning about them and by asking for aggressive countermeasures, religious responders took a different route. Their narratives were about the healing power of the Savior; in them, illness took second place to faith. Shantal gave the following account:

> I've had surgery before, and I've been very sick after the anesthesia, sleeping for hours and upchucking. This time I had none of that. When I was wheeled to my room, I could see all of my family members standing there, waiting for me. And their faces were concerned, sad, anxious. And they said, the smile on my face, it was a wonder. . . . And I asked for dinner. Before, I would never eat until two days after because of upchucking. . . . I ate it all. . . . And I feel that, within my soul, it was the power of God.

Even Jenna, who found after chemotherapy that "I couldn't look at vegetables in the grocery store, I couldn't drink coffee, and those are things that I normally love," added, "It was livable, and I wasn't miserable." She had similar contradictory descriptions of her experience with radiation. Although she got burned and her skin peeled, she "was just incredibly amazed at how well I felt and how well I did."

Caroline, who reported few side effects, explained her philosophy and, in doing so, spoke for many in this group:

> I'm a person who accepts things as they come. You know, I don't try to make problems. . . . Life is too short for that. You accept every day as it comes and enjoy the goodness of the Lord, and you have no problems.

Caroline's stoicism in the face of pain speaks of a lifetime of accepting what cannot be altered and of leaning on God for support in doing this.

And for Rosamund, whose treatment side effects were quite serious, the Lord stepped in to help:

> There was a woman at church who said, "I've never known anyone have this difficult of a time. But there is someone I think who went through similar experiences, and she's in Virginia. . . ." I called her, and she just started talking to me and sharing that she knew what I was feeling and going through. She could relate to the spiritual side. . . . I talked to her regularly. She would just wake me up some mornings and say ". . . You were in my heart today. . . ." And she arranged a prayer circle for me. . . . If I was having a difficult day, she called up all the prayer partners that she had lined up for me and said, "We need to pray for Rosamund today."

In this account, we see that the support provided by church members gives religious responders further evidence of God's loving intervention. For many black women, used to an indifferent medical system, believing this was so comforting that they felt they could survive whatever difficulties treatment wrought.

Like traditional responders, family members gave religious responders mixed help. Often these women worried about grown children or husbands who were extremely upset when the family's main caregiver faced a life-threatening illness. Rosamund reported, "My daughter wanted to drop out of school. So I had to reassure people that I would be okay." Her husband was even more difficult:

> One of the issues I had was that he was making it so about him, you know, with all the crying and everything. And I remember once, he said, in the very beginning, of all the things that he had to go through in life, he never thought he would have to go through this. And I was just so amazed that he would feel that he was going through this. And I got real tired of people saying how fortunate I was . . . that he's there and what he does. . . . I wanted to say, "This is me. What about me?" So I got upset with him, and once I told him, "I'm so tired of hearing what you did, when I have breast cancer."

Other religious responders, such as Caroline and Bella, had daughters whose education exceeded their mothers', and these daughters took on the role of family expert. Jenna's mother, who had herself been diagnosed with breast cancer, also took on the role of expert. However, all three of these religious responders were less interested in medical expertise than they were in sustaining their faith that they would be fine. For this, they turned elsewhere.

Family members who became upset at a breast cancer diagnosis did not always respond as did Rosamund's husband. Some tried hard to keep their grief away from the patient. Shantal's family followed her example and kept up brave appearances when they were around her. They said nothing to her about how they were feeling, but they "fell apart" when she was not there. They dealt with their fears away from Shantal, and they told her later that, "They couldn't fall apart around me, because I was so strong; I never showed any signs of crying or falling apart myself." Shantal's husband, in particular, struggled to be brave:

> The day we left the hospital from the biopsy, he said he had to go to the store. . . . He cried, walking . . . just walking down the street crying . . . visibly. And people were, you know, looking and moving out of his way.

Shantal did not hear this story until months after her treatment was over. She was asked to give a speech about her experience and asked her husband for input. Shantal attributed her family's stoicism in her presence to God's intention. God, she believed, wanted her to survive her ordeal with the least possible trauma, so she would have the strength to follow his mandate. Her religious beliefs helped her when she was sick and provided her with an obligation that she is still repaying.

Perhaps the most important distinction between the experiences of religious responders and those in other groups lies in the support they got from their churches and from prayer groups. Shantal, for example, talked to many people in her church and in the prayer group she belonged to at work. She described the spiritual counselor who worked with the prayer group as a continuing support.

Rosamund's ambivalence about her family was in marked contrast to her feelings about her church family. The church gave both practical and emotional help:

> They had a schedule for preparing meals, when I needed that. One woman took responsibility for lining up my rides. . . . I wore different wigs to church before I lost my hair, and everybody gave their opinion on that. . . . My minister shaved his head . . . to support me with that. They prayed for me all the time. I was always in the weekly bulletin. . . . They called all the time. . . . I explained to them, "When I have chemo, don't call me for three days," so people respected that.

Bella described her minister as a "godsend," adding, "He already got his crown." She also noted that, if she ever missed church even up to the time of the interview, "Members would start calling." Religious responders used their churches as support systems to survive their treatments, which further placed biomedicine in the background. Most of the women went to historically black churches, which have long taken on the role of providing help in times of personal crisis.

Since they tended to be older than other groups of responders, most religious responders had grown children and did not, therefore, have to explain their illness to little ones. However, they still worried about how their children would respond to their diagnosis. Bella, for example, found it difficult to tell her daughter, because she "feels like I'm gonna be here forever, and I always protect my daughter." Caroline did not tell her daughters until she knew for sure, because "I wasn't going to tell them, and then it's not true; I wanted to spare them that." In both cases, daughters provided their mothers with educational guidance and information.

However, Bella and Caroline felt the need to protect their daughters as long as possible.

Those who told their children right away used faith to gain the courage to break the news. Shantal had never told her children about previous surgeries, but this time, after she prayed, she told her daughters immediately. Jenna told her children along with her friends, because she "knew they would be praying" for her.

Like other women with breast cancer, religious responders worried about daughters who might be at risk, and they went to lengths to minimize these risks. This was a rare place where they did not rely on religion. Jenna's daughter was going to participate in a clinical trial of a drug that might prevent breast cancer in high-risk women, and Caroline's daughters had started going for regular mammograms at her urging. Shantal went one step further. Given her own mother's death from breast cancer, she reasoned that her programs for women of color should include the women in her family, and she provided all kinds of information to them. She found her younger daughter's resistance particularly frustrating:

> I don't think the youngest one has been screened. I've been constantly talking to her about it. [The older one] attends my sessions, so she's been educated. The youngest one, she's been invited, but she hasn't attended any.

And she fretted that the rest of the women in her family might not be doing enough:

> They're not old enough to get the mammogram, but did say they're having Pap smears on a regular basis. So I just hope they're not giving lip service to me. . . . We have a family reunion. . . . And I always supply breast cancer literature and prostate cancer literature. . . . Whether they heed it and adhere to it, that's another thing.

Hospital-based support groups are another possible source of support for women with breast cancer, but religious responders did not use them. Some women in this group had thought about going to support groups but had not gone to them unless they were faith-based. Most reasoned that they did not need support groups because they received emotional support from their church and their own prayers bolstered them even further. Several, like Shantal and Jenna, belonged to prayer groups that provided spiritually based emotional support. Jenna described the difference between a prayer group and a support group by telling me she did not want to go to a support group because she did not want "to sit and talk about it." Instead, she added:

> I'm very involved in a [Bible] group. And those women, those thirty or so women, were an incredible support to me, both spiritually because they prayed for me and they prayed with me, and that was invaluable; and they were practically helping me, because they brought meals, and meals, and meals, and I think I went for six months without getting meals.

Most religious responders did go to other kinds of programs. A few went to educational programs dealing with biomedical aspects of cancer but most went to programs describing alternatives to biomedicine. Rosamund liked the programs run by Living Beyond Breast Cancer (LBBC), an organization founded by a radiation oncologist, Marisa Weiss, to address women's ongoing need for support after treatment.[24] LBBC runs twice-yearly conferences on a variety of topics, and, although the emphasis is on biomedical information, Rosamund always chose "the ones on holistic approaches . . . about vitamin therapies and everything." Many of these—meditation, visualization, or yoga, for example—have a spiritual or mystical component, which might be expected to appeal to religious persons. Most of these types of treatment require faith in their efficacy, because hard evidence is lacking. Religious responders are comfortable with this. Furthermore, since they do not privilege biomedicine, they are willing to try other things. Rosamund made the connection clear:

> [I learned about visualization] in one of Dr. Chopra's[25] books, talking about if you can picture what is going on with you and come up with a visual image of it, and then what you want to do to take care of it. So I decided that my tumor was a lump of coal, and that the chemo was snow. And it was falling on it. And it was freezing, and it was melting the way in, it was dissolving. . . . The spirituality part of it was very key to me.

Religious responders modified their diets a little or not at all. The following description from Shantal is a good example of the type of diet most religious responders followed after diagnosis. It is similar to the diet many Americans follow, when they are trying to eat healthfully without too many complications:

> Cereal in the morning. At noon, I may eat soup, grilled cheese. I try to eat vegetables, a meat, three pieces of fruit a day. . . . For dinner, I may have a small piece of meat, like a noodle starch, and then that vegetable—string beans, corn, peas, or something like that. . . . I love sweets. . . . Chocolate candy bars I don't do any more. Maybe a jellybean. I'll count them now, where before, I would, maybe, take a handful. Instead of the whole Tastycake, maybe just a piece of the Tastycake. . . . [Before] I would eat a steak hoagie, no big deal for lunch, every day. And now if I have that, it's a treat.

Shantal was extremely busy helping others and had no time for the more complex diets biomedical experts often embrace. And she was less inclined to take medical decisions into her own hands anyway.

The other religious responders gave descriptions similar to Shantal's, sometimes adding statements such as "Anything that's not nailed down" (Bella), or "I eat a lot of stuff I shouldn't" (Caroline). While most made a concerted effort to change their diets, they still differed from biomedical experts, most of whom ate less fat and more fruits, vegetables, and whole grains than the diet described above. Since religious responders did not feel pressure to steer the course of their medical destiny, they did not feel the need to make drastic dietary changes. On the other hand, their religion did place moral injunctions on them not to be too self-indulgent about food or other pleasures.

Exercise is a similar story. Some religious responders did a limited amount of formal exercise; for example, Rosamund went to the gym for about thirty minutes three times a week, and Jenna tried to walk a mile every night. Many were like Bella, who reasoned, "Every day I do housework, so I consider that my exercise," or Caroline, who reported, "I walk around the block a couple of times, whenever I get the chance," but added, "There is usually so much work to be done in the house that I can't get out and do it as often as I would like." None followed the kind of rigorous exercise program commonly undertaken by the biomedical experts. The religious responders had similar intentions about diet and exercise as the biomedical experts but did not follow these intentions to the same degree. This is not surprising, given that they believed that God was in charge of their recovery and that they were reluctant to focus on themselves. These factors limited the extent of their independent actions in pursuit of a cure.

Most religious responders reported that they did not feel a loss of control during treatment. A few, like Jenna, felt like "a walking zombie for months," but Shantal's comments were more typical. Shantal did not "have that feeling" of losing control, because of "my faith in God again— no—no problem." And Rosamund said that she never felt that she had lost control; instead, breast cancer helped her increase her sense of control because, "It continues to help me refocus and prioritize."

After her treatment was over, Jenna came around to a similar point of view:

> I had a change, maybe a year or two after the whole process was over . . . when all of a sudden I realized I wasn't thinking about cancer every day. . . . I guess a lot of my confidence was taken away from me when I had cancer. . . . [If I could do it over] I would probably have been a little more knowledgeable and less trusting of every doctor I looked at. . . . I felt that I had very good care. . . . I really believe it was more through God's guidance than anything.

Jenna believed that she should have challenged the doctors more when she believed they were wrong, because God was on the sidelines influencing her judgments. She did not always do this, because of a lifetime of gendered deference to authority, and afterward she regretted it. Other religious responders remained somewhat independent of doctors because of their belief in a higher authority guiding them through cancer treatment. The African American women in this group were more independent of their doctors than the white women, no doubt because they had more reason to distrust the medical profession and because in the main they had fewer resources. Both the white women in this group were stay-at-home wives and mothers with husbands in well-remunerated and prestigious occupations. These two women belonged to the same prayer group, which was composed of women like themselves. They had a lot of free time on their hands with grown children and husbands who were away from home much of the time, and religion may well have filled a void in their lives.

After treatment was over, most religious responders stated that their experience had transformed them. This is not surprising since they believed that the purpose of having cancer was for a transformation of some kind to occur. Shantal put this point of view very clearly:

> [My life] changed tremendously. . . . Life is precious. Each day is fulfill-ing. And what happens each day is important, and I review it, and I digest it, and what I can't do anything about, I get rid of. And what I can, I do, in a positive way . . . concern for other people, other women, especially in reference to breast cancer. Closer ties to my family. I thought it was close before, but now it's closer. But the concern for people, in reference to breast cancer, drives me now.

Where many women claimed to be different as a result of cancer, Shantal was able to show, quite convincingly, just how she had changed.

We return to the issue of activism in chapter 8. It is sufficient here to note that religious responders believed that, since God had a purpose in letting them suffer from breast cancer, they should change their lives to live up to his expectations of them. Some, who were less active in the fight against breast cancer than Shantal, saw God's hand in a more per-sonal way. Caroline reported, for example, that her main change had been an increase in her "faith in the Lord." Jenna, who had always "had a very positive attitude towards life," said that now, "I certainly appreci-ate life more than I did before, because I feel very blessed." But others—like Shantal and Rosamund—stated that following God's intention had led to a greater involvement in social causes.

Religious responders took their faith with them into the doctors' offices after breast cancer treatment ended. Many said that they had no fear when they went back for checkups, because God would look after them. Some who were fearful put their fears in the hands of God. Caroline was not fearful because, "If you have that faith, that the Lord has done this for you, you're not going to doubt it." Shantal took care of any fears she might have by praying "more, harder, longer, that this hasn't come back in any way." And Rosamund said that she dealt with her fears by "coming to grips with 'There's a reason.'" She added that this reason is what "everyone wants to know." And she concluded that if she did not know she had God's support, "I'd be stuck with 'Why?'" Given the higher rates of mortality among black women diagnosed with breast cancer than among white women, religious responders had more to fear when they returned to doctors. Yet they were able to minimize this fear by using the faith that had helped them through a lifetime of the daily grind.

The mind-set of women who see God as a personal savior, helping them every step of the way in life, made religious responders face each day differently than did those in other groups. Some of the ways they operated throughout their treatment reflected their higher than average age and lower than average education. They were not used to challenging doctors or even to receiving fulsome explanations. The fact that so many of them were African American reflects their long-standing use of the church for social support in all manner of situations. Religious responders were already active in their churches and in prayer groups long before they were diagnosed. And no doubt many of them had had bad experiences with doctors in previous contacts with the medical establishment. They were more comfortable in the familiar, welcoming, and accepting churches they went to than the alien and sterile medical institutions that treat breast cancer.

But the demographic explanation for these women's lack of fear provides only a partial understanding. Many traditional responders were likewise older and less well educated, and yet they had many fears about their disease. The difference between the two groups lies in the intense religious convictions of religious responders, which led to much of the calm they evinced in the face of a life-threatening disease. They simply did not believe they were going through the experience alone. Traditional responders, who placed great faith in the power of their doctors to cure them, and biomedical responders, who had extensive support from family and friends, were essentially alone in the end. This is why so many women were fearful even after their treatment finished. Some of those who believed in biomedicine became even more fearful once medication stopped, because taking medicine had given them a feeling of security that that they were fighting the cancer. In contrast, the knowledge that they were not alone gave religious responders what Caroline described as "a sort of calmness." Caroline added that her faith is stronger after breast cancer:

> We went to church twice yesterday. In the afternoon, I just felt like I was, you know, close to the Lord. And, I just felt He was right there. I just felt that He was telling me, "I brought you through this. . . ." And, I just felt so emotionally filled up about that, that He would do this for me. And I know if He would do this for me, He would do it for somebody else as well.

With this kind of belief, doctors and their practices were merely human interventions and paled in comparison to divine intervention.

The faith that religious responders relied on was not blind. They believed that God wanted them to follow doctors' orders, and they did so for the most part. However, their core belief system told them that prayer would be the key to getting them through their illness and that, without prayer, their chances would not be as good, no matter how expert their doctors. In some sense, this is fatalistic—a belief that they could not influence their health by themselves but must rely on God for a cure. Yet they also believed they could influences their chances of a cure through prayer, and their churches responded to their needs by providing all manner of help. Furthermore, some of the women in this group felt called upon to become active on behalf of others.

This way of responding to a serious illness such as breast cancer has been largely ignored in the medical sociology literature. Writers note the ways in which biomedicine is reified in our culture and in the pressure individual women feel to take responsibility for their illness. They are especially interested in the activists, who discuss breast cancer from a social perspective rather than an individual perspective. However, few have discussed the role of religion in helping women make sense of the disease and in coping with treatment. The women in this group did not reify medicine, but they still took an individualistic approach. Each woman saw herself as having a personal explanation for cancer.[26]

In the following chapter, we turn to the final group of women. This is a group that shared with the religious responders a belief that biomedicine alone was not sufficient, and as well, most of them were suspicious of the claims of biomedicine. However, like the biomedical experts, they did not rely on a higher power to see them through their illness. This was a ship they needed to steer themselves, and, frequently, they steered it into uncharted waters. At the same time, their explanations for breast cancer tended to be more social than those of other groups.

FIVE Opposing the Mainstream

Before her breast cancer diagnosis, Violet, a fifty-year-old American writer living in Greece, had little confidence in the medical profession. However, since her mother's death from breast cancer some years earlier, she had become anxious about her breasts and had started having regular mammograms. A self-described hypochondriac, Violet reported that her self-exams were not consistent or thorough. Instead, she said, "I would just go grabbing at myself, anytime I was having a panic attack." She noted that she did these exams "more in a sense of coming out of fear than just as a routine," because "I knew it was going to get me at some point." And Violet had assumed that, when it did, she "would be powerless" in the "grip" of cancer.

Yet once she was diagnosed, Violet did not act like a powerless person. She took immediate charge, and she made her own decisions about which treatments she would agree to. She took, as she put it, "responsi-bility for my own healing," but she did so in a manner that differed from that of biomedical experts. Violet represents a group of women who made their own decisions about treatment but who did not really trust conventional medical science. Indeed, they were frequently hostile to doctors and hospitals, viewing them as part of the problem rather than the solution. As James Olson has noted, "Cancer has always spawned a counterculture." Olson added that from the beginning some women look to alternatives to standard biomedical protocols.[1] The women discussed in this chapter fall in this group. I call them "alternative experts" because they had a profound distrust of biomedicine even when they succumbed to its directives, and they wanted to make decisions for themselves rather than rely on the expertise of others.

Selecting a few representative women proved to be more difficult with alternative experts than with the other three groups. Women in this group were often angry about the increased medicalization of American society and particularly about the medicalization of women's bodies.[2] They had colorful things to say about their experiences with doctors, and their responses to diagnosis were often idiosyncratic. Furthermore, their responses showed two types of motivations for these reactions. One motivation was that earlier negative experiences with doctors and hos-pitals had caused them to lose faith in medical solutions to illness. They trusted themselves more than they trusted others, and they explained their cancers, at least partly, in personal terms. They often combined bio-medical treatments with more radical, alternative ones, because they wanted to do everything they could to effect a cure even while they mis-trusted biomedicine. Yet they also had political explanations for their dis-ease. They viewed cancer as resulting from a flawed and toxic society where women's health, in particular, was sacrificed in the unregulated quest for corporate profit.[3] Most alternative experts incorporated both of these perspectives to varying degrees.

It is not surprising that women with a political viewpoint about breast cancer should also explain it in intensely personal ways. They viewed themselves as living in a dysfunctional society that had negative conse-quences for individuals. And, as many activists have noted, the cancer experience is personal, even if shared with others. After all, political activism cannot substitute for treatment when one is diagnosed. As Zillah Eisenstein wrote, "Bodies are always personal in that each of us lives in one in a particularly individual way." But, she added, "They're also always political in that they have meanings that are more powerful than any one of us can determine."[4] In an analysis of feminist autobiographical accounts of breast cancer, Laura Potts underscored Eisenstein's point by saying that "Women's experience of breast cancer is both personal and private, and collective and connective."[5] This combination of the personal and the political is also found in accounts by Sharon Batt, Audre Lorde, and Jo Spence.[6] It is also unsurprising that women with a critical viewpoint of American society would be skeptical about the claims of conventional medicine and would look to alternatives.

In his book on the history of the health promotion movement in the United States, Michael Goldstein noted that, although this movement began in the nineteenth century, the late twentieth century saw a great increase in adherence to the cause.[7] Goldstein identified a number of factors that helped further the ideas that individuals are responsible for their health and that medical intervention may not be the best path to wellness. In particular, he described those involved in this movement as questioning science and technology and as critical of what Peter Conrad and Joseph Schneider have described as the medicalization of increasing aspects of the culture.[8] Several writers have noted that women are more attracted to alternative medicine than are men, in part because they perceive biomedical practitioners to be paternalistic to women patients.[9] The women described in this chapter meet these criteria. They defined health holistically—as a positive state rather than an absence of disease—and they believed that this could be achieved through self-help and self-healing, rather than solely through reliance on evidence-based medicine. They did seek outside help in their quest for a breast cancer cure, but they chose this help selectively from both outside and inside the medical profession. Finally, many of them had experience with the women's movement and were inclined to view American society, including its medical institutions, as patriarchal.

As a result, many of them had what Christy Simpson described as a social ideology about illness.[10] They viewed disease as the result of societal and environmental conditions, which meant they were concerned with the experiences and responses of groups, rather than those of individuals. A number of breast cancer survivors have written accounts from the societal perspective. For example, Judy Brady explained her breast cancer as resulting from exposure to radiation, because she grew up in California near a number of nuclear plants.[11] Batt blamed hers on environmental contaminants, as did Eisenstein, even though Eisenstein acknowledged the likelihood of a genetic component, since her mother, aunt, and two of her sisters had breast cancer also.[12] Still, this is a minority viewpoint in our culture. Susan Sherwin has argued that, in Western societies, cancer is usually addressed as a disease of individuals, even though evidence exists that many cancers are preventable at the societal level.[13]

In background, alternative experts were similar to biomedical experts, although a little younger and less successful. They were mostly middle aged—almost all were between 40 and 59—so they had few small children to worry about. While not quite as affluent and educated as biomedical experts, almost half had family incomes in excess of one hundred thousand dollars at diagnosis and over half had graduate degrees. Where they differed from biomedical experts is that they were much less likely to be married at the time of diagnosis—only one-third were married, a proportion lower than any other group. About one-third were divorced and one-third had never married. Part of the reason for this was that all but one of the seven lesbians I interviewed were in this group. This put them at the margins of the conventional social world to a greater degree than any other group. Violet is a good example of this. Many of those who were not lesbians had been involved with radical movements before diagnosis, so they came to breast cancer with a well-thought-out political ideology.

So even before diagnosis, the alternative experts I interviewed had, as a group, been more critical than any other group of what they saw as corporate medicine. Religious responders turned their backs on medicine for positive reasons—they did not dislike doctors; rather, they saw God as the ultimate healer. Alternative experts, however, looked outside biomedicine for help and information, because they trusted neither the medical profession nor the larger establishment supporting it. Their reasons

Table 5   Alternative Experts by Selected Variables

	White (not Jewish)	Black	Jewish	Total
Age				
Less than 40	1	0	0	1
40–49	4	1	3	8
50–59	4	1	2	7
60 and over	1	0	0	1
Family income				
Less than $20,000	1	0	0	1
$20,000–$39,999	0	1	1	2
$40,000–$69,999	1	1	0	2
$70,000–$99,999	2	0	1	3
$100,000 and over	5	0	2	7
Missing	1	0	1	2
Education				
12 years and less	1	0	0	1
13–15	1	2	0	3
16–17	1	0	2	3
18 and over	6	0	3	9
Missing	1	0	0	1
Marital status				
Currently married	5	0	1	6
Divorced	3	0	2	5
Never married	2	2	2	6
Widowed	0	0	0	0
Total	10	2	5	17

for seeking other treatments were negative rather than positive. Like religious responders, however, their narratives did not follow messages appearing in the media, which tend to emphasize biomedicine. Instead, they were critical of the media, viewing them as part of a corrupt and profit-hungry corporate America.

John McKinlay and Linda Marceau have listed a number of reasons why late capitalism has seen the erosion of the status of doctors and of patient trust. In the current study, only one group, traditional responders, treated doctors as they had been treated during what these authors call "the golden age of doctoring."[14] And no group was more critical of doctors than alternative experts. They saw them as part of corporate America rather than as the authoritative and esteemed guardians of the nation's health.

Like Violet, Hannah, a divorced mother of one child living in a middle-class suburb just outside the city limits, had seen her mother die a terrible death from breast cancer. And, like Violet, she "thought it was in my future," but she did not expect it to happen "until I was in my sixties." Hannah, who worked for a women's health organization, started to pay more attention to her health after both her mother and her aunt died of breast cancer. Like Violet, she came to her diagnosis with an existing critical stance toward the medical establishment, which she had long believed exploited women. In Hannah's case, this was not the result of bad personal experiences with doctors but of occupational experiences with poor women who struggled to get access to biomedicine and then to get respect once they had obtained access.

When Hannah's mother died, Hannah started to do everything she could to prevent her own diagnosis and, in the event she could not, to ensure an early diagnosis. She became careful about diet, stopped taking birth control pills, had annual mammograms, and performed monthly breast exams. When Hannah was diagnosed at age forty-four, she "felt my body betrayed me." Alternative experts were more pessimistic than biomedical experts about their ability to control their personal environment, but they still believed in trying and were upset when they failed. After diagnosis, Hannah wanted to remain in charge, and she immediately went "into control mode." Like biomedical experts, alternative experts tended to take personal control when illness struck.

Both Hannah and Violet had political ideologies to explain breast cancer, although the personal played a role also. In contrast, Janet's explanation was mainly personal but was backed by political arguments. A successful investment analyst living with her husband in an upper-middle-class condominium in the outer suburbs, Janet appeared the face of conventionality. It was not until we talked that her unconventional beliefs and practices surfaced. She had had no thoughts of breast cancer before diagnosis, because there was "no profile for breast cancer in my family," but when she found a lump, she made sure she had it checked during her annual gynecological exam. At age fifty, she had never had a mammogram until the doctor sent her for one to aid in diagnosing the lump. When I interviewed her, she stated, "I knew for a year that I had been sick, but I could not put my finger on it." In hindsight, she decided, "It was the cancer." Janet viewed her cancer as invidious and felt sure that it had attacked every part of her being. She also believed that routing it out was not just a matter of following the prescribed medical treatment. Janet was militant about which treatments she would have and what she would not agree to. After diagnosis, she permanently altered her entire life to respond to what she believed was her continued threat of cancer. It is hard to explain how a successful corporate woman such as Janet became an alternative expert rather than a biomedical one, but sociologists recognize that personal biography has importance in addition to social location, and Janet had had previous bad experiences with doctors. Her own personality no doubt played a part also.

Alternative experts were similar to biomedical experts in that, except in the minority of cases where their mothers had been diagnosed previously, most had not worried about cancer. But they differed from biomedical experts in the explanations they gave for their diagnoses and in the treatment choices they made. For example, Sarah, a fifty-four-year-old psychotherapist living in a historically liberal, racially diverse, and upper-middle-class area of the city, had not thought of cancer as something that would ever happen to her. She too "had a primitive kind of infantile construct, that since I was doing mammograms every year, I was safe." When diagnosed, however, Sarah's first explanation for her disease was social in nature and illustrates the marked distinction between alternative and biomedical experts:

> It's an epidemic. So I don't need a reason. I just need to be in this population, in this environment. ["Do you mean physical toxins?"] Yes, and I think maybe even on a deeper level—maybe on a spiritual or cultural level—this is one of the diseases of our time . . . just kind of the social milieu we live in.

In addition, Sarah had personal explanations, although she put them in a social context:

Number one, I think I'm in that group—I had a lot of acceptance about it. . . . I'm not above the rest of the women in this world. . . . I smoked for a very long time, so I had internalized a lot of toxins in my body. . . . I've had a lot of heartache . . . female pain and suffering in terms of my sister's death at thirty-seven and being so intimately involved with her dying so young. . . . My youngest daughter had a lot of difficulties. . . . There were years when she was very alienated, and I found that very difficult and painful. All of which I associate with kind of being a woman in the heart.

Janet also explained her breast cancer as a result of the weight of the world, but she saw this in terms of its personal effects on her, even when her explanation was political:

I was working a full-time heavy-responsibility corporate job, plus volunteering for this and that, and this and that. And not just volunteering, but taking on responsibilities like treasurer. . . . From dawn to midnight, my time was committed, because that's just the kind of person I am. . . . I think the growth hormones in the beef were one of the things that helped cause the cancer, because of the time frame of when they started putting growth hormones in beef. . . . And, you know, I drank a lot of milk too. There's the growth hormones in milk.

To these external causes, Janet added individual factors:

Eventually, as I figured out what made me well, I understood what made me ill. The beginning of the whole thing is the fact that the pancreas doesn't work right and process sugar properly. So that puts a stress on the body. . . . I had made a major dietary change almost ten years ago, before I was diagnosed with cancer, which had put an extra stress on my body. That extra stress plus dietary inherited stress, plus the job stress; that was all a very, very stressful thing.

In these quotes, Janet's explanations illustrate the ways that alternative experts think about health. They emphasize wellness, which they see as more than the mere absence of illness; in their view, in order to understand illness, one must first understand what one needs to do to be well. They also see themselves as victimized by an indifferent society, which permits growth hormones in animal diets to extract extra profit in disregard of human safety. These are the kinds of arguments to be found in many best-selling books about health. They inform the educated, middle-class women who read them that taking a critical stance toward medicine is the best way to promote one's own health.

Regardless of group, women with breast cancer in their families saw genetic explanations for their diagnosis. However, when such women were alternative experts, they blamed the system also. Hannah's story illustrates this:

> I certainly have, I'm sure, a genetic predisposition—my mother, her sister, my grandmother had cancer. . . . I think that we all grew up in an area I know of, since then; other women who are my age whose mothers have died of breast cancer all in that same neighborhood. . . . We lived near a creek. . . . There were factories there. . . . I don't know how awful the water was. Basically, growing up, I ate totally unhealthy. My mother had no concept of healthy food. We never had fresh vegetables. . . . And the other thing, I think, is emotional. I'm sure losing my mother was a major blow to my immune system, and then losing my aunt . . . I'm not pointing my finger at any one thing, but there are enough factors that don't surprise me.

Violet's explanation for her breast cancer provides, perhaps, the best example of the way alternative experts combined the personal and the political to explain why they and others were succumbing to breast cancer, in what they assumed were epidemic proportions. First, Violet looked to larger social issues:

> My commitment to understanding and research became very powerful in relation to the environment and the environmental sources for this disease.[15] I knew that pollution could have an effect when my mother died. . . . She lived on Staten Island. . . . Her friend across the road had another kind of cancer. . . . There's definitely something going on out there. And it's definitely not about what kind of drug is gonna save me. I was much more interested in what caused this. And I was not accepting the explanations that were being given. I know that this is part of an international corporate cover-up, basically about what is happening to us.

To corporate conspiracy, she added personal pathology:

I accepted responsibility for being a hospitable host for the disease through my fear of it, through the stresses that were existing in my life. It was a wake-up call for me. There was stuff that wasn't working, and I wasn't paying enough attention, and it finally erupted into this— including my own basic stance towards fear of life.

Although most alternative experts disliked conventional medical practitioners and feared medical treatment, it is a testament to the power of biomedicine that, faced with cancer, no woman among those I interviewed rejected it entirely. Alternative experts were educated and had long taken a critical stance toward biomedicine, often based on experience, but they found it hard to turn their backs on its promise of a cure when the alternative might be death.

Regardless of their stance on doctors, all the women had surgery. This does not mean, however, that they all liked their surgeons or that they followed all their surgeons' recommendations. After going for a second opinion, Janet returned to her original surgeon for a mastectomy. She described him as "straightforward," by which she meant that he answered her questions but did not volunteer any information she did not ask about. Instead, "He emphasized that he was an excellent surgeon" and "He crowed about his work in the follow-up." Things did not deteriorate between Janet and her surgeon until she told him she had decided not to have chemotherapy. Upon hearing this, Janet reported, "He blew up at me. He said, 'You're gonna die of breast cancer' and stormed out of the room."

Sarah's "philosophy about those doctors" was "I do not need them to be any more than courteous. I want them to do their job. I can get what I need from other people." Sarah's statement contrasts with both the desire biomedical experts had for a partnership with doctors and the admiration for their doctors held by traditional responders. No one in the other groups spoke about doctors in such disdainful terms. Women in the other groups might dislike or discount a particular doctor, but not the whole profession. Part of the reason Sarah took this position was that, as a lesbian, she had to decide whether or not to come out to each of her doctors. She told me that her surgeon knew she was a lesbian, "but our relationship was professional," by which she meant that her lesbianism did not affect her treatment. She approved of the fact that her surgeon acted conservatively, by performing a succession of wide-excision biopsies until the margins were clear and the surgeon was confident that the cancer was completely removed. The surgeon based this decision on her "philosophy . . . that you can always go in and scoop a little more, but you can't put any back." Sarah appreciated this, but she still saw her relationship with her doctor as formal.

Some alternative experts developed a warm relationship with at least some of their doctors. Hannah, who disliked her oncologist so much that she never went back for checkups once treatment was over, loved her surgeon. However, this feeling resulted not from his expertise, but from the emotional attention he provided. Saying, "He and I really formed a bond right away," she spoke approvingly of the emphasis he placed on attitude:

> I said, "Can you tell me what my chances are?" He said, "I never, never, never tell people percentages, because everybody's different. . . . But I can tell you one thing—I've worked on enough people that, based on people's attitudes, I can tell you who's going to be successful in terms of dealing with this. You will definitely do great handling this. . . ." And that was like the boost I needed. I don't know why doctors don't tell people positive things.

Hannah disliked the way medicine often ignores the human element, and she contrasted this with the way her surgeon treated her:

> I had a very amazing experience with my surgeon. . . . He knew that I was a single parent. . . . And, when I called to go to his office to have the bandage removed and the tube taken out, he said that he'd come to my house, because he lives near me and he thought it would be easier for me. . . . So he came by with his own small child, who my child entertained and played with while he took my bandages off.

Hannah's professional experience in dealing with women's issues was the basis for her determination to manage her own illness and to do so in a way that did not privilege doctors. When she made an exception, it was for a doctor who treated her as a real person.

Violet had an especially hostile relationship both with doctors and with biomedicine in general. The following is typical of her many state-ments on this theme. In this case, she was discussing the lymphedema that she developed after surgery:

> They don't even tell you that you're gonna hurt. That you're gonna have to work at getting your arm back again. They don't tell you that more painful than the actual surgery is lymph nodes, and that that's a lifetime experience. . . . That you're gonna be numb in here for the rest of your life. . . . What happens is like you're in an emergency mode with red lights flashing, and it's like they're gonna do things to take care of this emergency. And they say absolutely nothing to you beyond that.

Given their attitudes, what kinds of treatment decisions did alterna-tive experts make in the days following diagnosis? As noted above, all had surgery. However, they were ambivalent about other treatments such as radiation and chemotherapy, and they were even more ambiva-lent about tamoxifen. Their fears were fueled by books warning that chemotherapy and tamoxifen are more toxic and less effective than con-ventional doctors acknowledge.[16] These arguments from critics of the medical establishment made alternative experts hesitant to continue with treatment. After her surgery, Sarah, for example, "took a break—a long period of investigation—because I was not going to do radiation at first." Her description of her decision process is instructive:

> Doctor [X] at [Y] hospital said, "You know, this is what we do." I said, "Well, it's not what I do . . ." and initially I decided not to do radiation. But then I decided I needed to do some real research. You couldn't make this decision on what I felt. . . . I decided to do it, because I kept thinking about it. I'd say, "Put it to rest. You're not going to do it." And then three days later, it would be coming up in my mind. So I really honored that as a way—that was my own wisdom.

Again, we see alternative experts resorting to feelings as a guide to action, in spite of their denial of this mode of decision-making. With their antagonism toward biomedical evidence, alternative experts often let their feelings substitute for data.

Sometimes alternative experts were torn between doctors' recommen-dations for treatment and their own suspicions of medicine, so they compromised somewhere in the middle. Hannah described this in reference to tamoxifen, which is typically prescribed for five years:

> I read a lot of research, not a lot that was here in this country. . . . It really elaborated on the dangers and the side effects. I was very angry. . . . I would talk about the side effects. They'd say, "No serious side effects." I'd say, "The literature is quoting liver cancer. I don't want liver cancer." . . . I did it for a year, figured I got my benefit. . . . Made a lot of people uncomfortable when I went off.

As is discussed in chapter 8, on activism, tamoxifen is considered one of the most controversial treatments by the more radical activists. They particularly disapprove of the drug because its maker, AstraZeneca, has massively promoted tamoxifen, and it is a very profitable drug. AstraZeneca is also the company that owns the rights to the newer hormone therapy, Arimidex. AstraZeneca also made pesticides and herbicides until 2000, when it sold the business to a new merged company, Syngenta. Alternative experts never lost the political analysis they had incorporated into their daily lives, a result of both their education and the experience of living in opposition to society. AstraZeneca was an easy target.

Violet was even more hostile to tamoxifen than Hannah:

> All my friends are . . . "You have to take that." "No, I'm not taking that, because . . . studies show that tamoxifen can also cause uterine cancer. . . ." I totally resisted the tamoxifen thing, and I'm very glad that I did. . . . I think it's a treatment which is promoted for economic interests. I think it can be dangerous. And I think anything that's continuing the myth that we're just gonna give the drug right here—you have to be careful. . . . They give you one thing but then you've got to take another thing to take care of the effects of the thing they gave you.

Violet had already decided that if chemotherapy were recommended to her—it was not—she would refuse, because it had caused her mother so much pain and sickness.

Janet's hostility to biomedicine was so strong that she refused both chemotherapy and tamoxifen, even in the face of strong pressure from her doctors. Yet her hostility to medical expertise did not prevent her from using biomedical arguments to support this decision:

I did go, at the behest of the surgeon, to the oncologist. . . . And I listened to him and then politely told him that I take two aspirins a year and that's the extent of my taking drugs. . . . With the lymph nodes having been part of the cancer, it was standard procedure to do chemotherapy. . . . I was already prepared with knowledge of how the whole thing works. . . . The most telling thing—besides the fact that I just don't do drugs . . . the downside is worse than what they do—was the statistic about chemotherapy, where 75 to 80 percent of women who have breast cancer end up with metastasized breast cancer or breast cancer come back again in the other side. . . . That said to me, well, did those 20 percent of women, were they not even gonna have it anyway, if they had not had the chemotherapy?

When asked for the source of her data, Janet replied:

It's a common statistic. And if you ask any chemotherapist about it, they'll say that. . . . It also depresses the immune system tremendously. The immune system is already depressed, or the cancer couldn't have gotten hold. So you depress the immune system further and get well? No logic there.

I was not able to find the statistics Janet quoted, and available studies show much lower rates of reoccurrence and metastases than Janet reported.[17]

In their arguments, Janet and Violet made all the points used by alternative experts to justify their decisions to reject doctors' recommendations about drug therapy. These included that the treatment is toxic, that it depresses the immune system, that it is ineffective, that it is sold only to increase drug company profits, and that it causes more illness than it cures. All of these arguments indicate a profound distrust of doctors and their pharmaceutical allies. This opposition to medicalization contrasts with the attitude of biomedical experts. Alternative experts saw medicalization as rendering women as victims, rather than empowering them to control their illnesses.[18] Although the two groups had a lot in common in terms of class and race/ethnicity, they had very different views about society. Both groups saw themselves as in control and viewed the others as passive dupes.

Like biomedical experts, those who relied on alternative methods read and absorbed lots of information to inform their decisions and to cope with treatment, a not-surprising finding given their class backgrounds. But where the former obtained their information from Dr. Susan Love's critically acclaimed book and from hospital-based Web sites, the latter looked elsewhere. A number of best-selling books make the argument that traditional medicine falls short in treating patients. Alternative experts used these books by well-known healers to learn about nontraditional treatment.[19] Hannah, for example, did not find Love helpful. Instead, she read *Quantum Healing* by Deepak Chopra, a medically trained doctor who markets spiritual guidance and Eastern religion as ways to health.[20] He has written numerous books on health and healing, and he lectures all over the country. Violet read the best-known alternative practitioner, Bernie Siegel. Siegel is the source for much of the language that appears in the alternative medical literature. For example, he emphasizes wellness rather than curing disease: "Don't do things to not die but do things to enhance the quality of your life and you may be surprised by how long you do live."[21]

This is how Violet described the differences between traditional medical knowledge and that of alternative practitioners:

> There are two kinds of information. One is the left-brain information, which is really about the disease, diseases in general, healing, alternatives, stuff like that. Then there's the right-brain information, which is information about what is the nature of the disease and what is the meaning of healing.

Violet acknowledged that she benefited from "factual" information, but she liked to obtain it in a context that did not simply provide a biomedical perspective:

> At my daughter's house, she had *Our Bodies, Ourselves,* and they had a section on breast cancer. . . . I was really comfortable and enjoyed looking at it alternatively or from a spiritual perspective. But as soon as I started getting down on the raw basic data and statistics . . . they were saying there's really no certainty that surgery, or radiation, or chemotherapy would make a bit of difference in terms of the outcome. . . . You have cancer and you've got it forever. . . . Whatever illusions I may have had, "Oh well, I've just done something, and now it's okay . . ." at some

level [the book's statistics] really disrupted that. And I think that's a good thing.

Janet was especially hostile to biomedical sources of information. After telling me that she "did a lot of extensive reading on alternative treatments," she added, "Most of the stuff on the Web is self-serving, even Oncolink," which is the Web site of the University of Pennsylvania's comprehensive cancer center, and one of the best-known cancer Web sites in the country. This hostility to science has been noted in other studies of those who question biomedicine and its assumptions, including not only breast cancer patients but AIDS activists and community activists working on toxic waste and leukemia.[22]

Since they used lesser invasive medical procedures than other women, alternative experts had fewer than average side effects. When they did undergo medical treatments, they counterbalanced them with alternative medications, as Sarah's radiation experience illustrates: [23]

> I was doing a lot of ointments from a Chinese herbalist. And so, though I was doing this treatment, I was also bringing to it other things. . . . I took what they gave me, and then I added.

As Sarah noted, this did not always work:

> I would say the first four weeks, my breast was just as pink as could be and fine. And the techies were going, "Oh my God, I can't believe this." Then all of a sudden, shhh, you know it just turned gray. In fact, one of my good friends who's a body worker would look at it, and she'd say, "Nothing's going to grow in there. Don't even worry about it."

This joke by her friend that radiation had killed both the cancer and the breast underscored Sarah's earlier hesitancy to undergo the treatment. Alternative experts simply did not trust what they viewed as heavy-handed evidence-based medicine. This is in part because of their more generalized hostility to the biomedical-industrial establishment, in which they saw physicians, drug companies, and major cancer centers as critical components.

While both biomedical experts and alternative experts considered their own personal authority to be most important, one of the main differences between the two groups was that where the former received lots of help from family and friends, the latter did not. This is partly because most alternative experts lived alone and their family contacts were few. It is hard to know whether their iconoclastic viewpoints resulted from or caused their greater social isolation, but it is likely that the causal direction went both ways. Violet had one daughter in her late teens and living elsewhere at the time of diagnosis. She chose not to tell her daughter at first, and when she finally did tell her, the daughter was upset:

> [She] was terribly upset that I had not told her immediately. . . . Then offering to come, and then my telling her, "I think it'd be best that you not come. . . ." There were times we'd be together and first it'd be okay, but then the days go by and all that yucky stuff comes up, and I guess, at some level, I didn't want to deal with that. . . . As soon as I got back to the States, I went to her house. . . . She was not emotionally there. And when I tried to pursue it, she said that she was pissed that I told her not to come. . . . I ended up leaving and getting on a bus and coming up to New York to stay with my friend.

The rest of Violet's family "had passed away already," except for one brother whom she described as a drug addict. He did not come to see her in spite of promises. Violet did have a partner at the time of diagnosis, with whom she shared everything "at the emotional level." However, the relationship did not survive her treatment, because their inadequate sex life became even less satisfying during radiation.

Hannah's surviving family was small, and, as a single parent with a young child, she had few relatives to fall back on. Sarah had family, including two daughters, but they lived in distant places and confined their support to an occasional phone call. At diagnosis, she too was in a relationship that did not survive treatment, although Sarah described that as a coincidence. In addition, Sarah decided not to tell her mother:

> I felt it would cause me additional emotional stress . . . for her to know. She has a histrionic personality. And it would have been all about her and her upset. . . . I discussed it with my daughters and my nieces, and we all decided it would be the best thing. . . . That meant I couldn't tell my brother too. . . . My mother's nickname for me is Mrs. Fine, because

I'm always, "Everything is fine in my life." I had, of course, growing up, in earlier years, tried to share and tried to have a real relationship. But the price of it was so high, and upsetting, and anxiety producing. And my mother and brother have that relationship.

Janet was married, and she described her husband as "totally supportive," but she made it clear that all decisions were hers. She reported that she "tackled it clinically, so there wasn't much of an emotional component to it." She did not tell her daughter at first. She did so eventually, because her husband planned a trip to California, including a visit to their daughter. He told Janet to tell their daughter because otherwise, "It's going to be kind of odd when we start talking about you, and I have to avoid the subject."

We might expect women with so little in the way of family support to have lots of friends, and it is true that alternative experts relied on friends more than family. However, even here, they did not usually have the large circle of supportive friends that the biomedical experts had. Violet was involved in an international women's group, and she described the women in this group as "kind of family." They cared about her and went with her to radiation but gave relatively minimal support because most of them knew little about breast cancer and were busy dealing with their own lives. Janet also described her friends as having "their own lives," and she said that most of the time she "ended up being the support of others."

Even Hannah—whose friends created a schedule for her and came around with food—found them a burden:

> I couldn't stand them coming around and kept them all away. . . . I actually found it difficult to have everyone underfoot and treating me like I was incapacitated. . . . There was one friend . . . we had a major fight during my treatment. . . . People in her family were doctors, so she wanted me to get more medical opinions . . . and she was appalled I was doing things the way I was. . . . A surprise party we were planning for another friend—she and I had a major blowup over it, because I was supposed to do something with the invitations, and she said I didn't do it right. "I know you are going through all these treatments, and you probably can't think clearly." Like I didn't do it her way, so therefore I did it wrong.

This story underscores the desire alternative experts had to stay in control of their lives—a desire exacerbated by their sense of living in a world run amok.

Alternative experts' lack of personal social ties contrasts with the experiences of each of the other response groups: less family demands than traditional responders, fewer friends and a less supportive family than biomedical experts, and no church community like the religious responders. This illustrates their outsider status and helps explain an ideology of alienation from American society. It is this ideology that allowed them to be so critical of the biomedical culture faced in dealing with cancer.

Given their limited support from family and friends and their suspicion of organized medicine, where did women in this group go for support? First and foremost, they were the biggest consumers of the myriad of programs and alternative medical treatments both for breast cancer per se and for health in general. In particular and more than any other group, alternative experts went to support groups. In a time of stress, they found strangers easier to cope with than friends. Contrast Hannah's experience in a support group with her previous description of problems with friends:

> It was fabulous. . . . I was just about to start treatment, and I remember getting to the group early . . . and sitting there and watching the women as they came in and being amazed at how healthy and vibrant they looked. . . . I sat there at the first meeting deciding whether it was a group I was going to be in, because if they weren't going to facilitate the group tightly, I wasn't going to stay. They were very skilled. . . . People dealt with major issues, but it wasn't a group of women who spent time feeling sorry for themselves. . . . We talked about healing issues . . . emotional support issues . . . treatment issues. . . . How much people knew about alternative therapies. . . . How to deal with the other people in your life.

Alternative experts found the "other people in their life" a burden that the strangers in the support group helped them with. In a therapeutic culture, this should not be surprising.

The women in her support group became Hannah's friends as a result of their shared experiences. It was common for alternative experts to develop friendships as a result of their dealings with the alternative health system. When asked about support from friends, Sarah, for example, replied that, "My acupuncturist is a good friend of mine, and one of the healers I go to is one of my closest friends, so they have a lot of knowledge." Expert knowledge seemed a good thing to have in a friend.

Like biomedical experts, alternative experts spent many hours learning how to manage their illness and to get the best attention possible. The difference between the two groups lay in the types of expertise sought. Where biomedical experts looked for the latest medical science, alternative experts tried many different treatments and services, ranging from alternative programs within the medical system to things that were out of the mainstream altogether.[24] We have already noted that the two groups read different material, but the differences were far greater than this. Hannah provides a good illustration of these differences, not only in the variety of programs she tried, but also in her focus on emotional support. One of her goals had been to avoid replicating her mother's experience of breast cancer. She described her mother as "having had a great deal of difficulty with it emotionally," adding that "she kept it to herself." Hannah wanted to be like her aunt, who had "decided to be a fighter." So, like her aunt, she "looked to alternative treatments." The first thing Hannah did was to go to a "gifted therapist" who "did Gestalt work with me" by putting "my mother in one chair and my aunt in another chair" and having "me talk to them." As a result of this encounter, Hannah decided "that I didn't have to go down the path my mother went down." Hannah viewed her resistance to conventional medicine as a way of staying in control.

Since her aunt had "put herself on a macrobiotic diet," Hannah also decided to change the way she ate. Her changes were quite different from the dietary changes made by biomedical experts. Instead of switching to a generally healthy and low-fat diet full of the antioxidants that some argue can prevent cancer, Hannah tried something more radical. She went to visit Susan Silberstein, who runs an organization called the Center for Advancement in Cancer Education (CACE).

CACE describes itself as bridging "the gap between the shortcomings of conventional cancer therapies and those of the nonconventional world." The center takes issue with conventional treatment, which it views as "tumor-oriented" rather than "host-oriented," because "the failure of radiation and chemotherapy to cure most cancers has become more apparent in recent years." As a result, "Dozens of alternative cancer therapies have commanded increasing attention." The center functions as a clearinghouse for alternative treatments, many of which it describes as no better than conventional medicine. Its Web site states, "The programs which have produced the most consistent results are those which recognize the body as a self-healing mechanism by giving it the essential tools for immunocompetence and self-repair."[25] This is what CACE means by host-oriented. While "there are dozens of unconventional approaches to cancer treatment, such as diet, nutritional supplements, traditional Chinese medicine, Western herbs, immunotherapies, meditation and yoga, that have been helpful to many patients," Silberstein views diet as especially important in effecting a recovery, because by strengthening the body's immune system, diet focuses on the host not the tumor.

The CACE approach, including its hostility toward conventional biomedicine, is similar to the viewpoint of many alternative experts. Hannah, for example, used the information she found at CACE to develop a holistic eating regimen to help her through treatment:

> When I was doing my treatment, I had somebody . . . who came to my home and made deliveries once a week. And he brought me all organic produce—meat, chicken, vegetables. So I was pretty vigilant initially, didn't eat any meat out, didn't eat any chicken out at all. Now it's relaxed, so, when people see me eat red meat, they're surprised.

When I interviewed her, Hannah was still buying "only organic milk, yogurt, and organic produce when I can get my hands on it," and she also bought organic meat and chicken. She was not eating a lot of meat, instead eating "primarily carbohydrates and fruits and vegetables."[26] And she took supplements in waves. When she went to the acupuncturist during treatment, she got "all kinds of dreadful-tasting Chinese herbs." By the interview, she was taking "a B-complex, an antioxidant complex, and then anything else I can throw in, like coenzyme-Q10." As she noted, she tended to "make up rules as I go along." As an example, she "decided that beer may be less dangerous than wine because grapes have all the toxins," adding "I like it better anyway."

In addition to changing diet and adding supplements, Hannah went to numerous programs run by well-known alternative practitioners. These included one by "a very well-known healer, Belleruth Naparsteck," who is an expert on visualization, a meditation technique in which patients visualize the cancer leaving their bodies.[27] Naparsteck runs an organization called Health Journeys, which sells visualization tapes that patients often use during chemotherapy.[28] Hannah was thrilled when Naparsteck "came over to me and said she had a real sense of my energy and that I was on a healing road." She bought Naparsteck's tapes and "used them every night before I went to sleep," as well as listening to them during treatment. She also went to hear Joan Borysenko, a Harvard-trained clinical psychologist, who teaches meditation and holistic healing on her Web site and at spiritual retreats throughout the country. Borysenko's techniques combine biofeedback mechanisms with small doses of Buddhist philosophy.[29] She is particularly focused on women's health issues, and Hannah went to hear her give a "wonderful" workshop on diet.

The above list represents only some of Hannah's activities in aid of her recovery. She also did yoga, had a monthly massage during treatment, did acupuncture "to deal with the side effects," and took a course in meditation—although she reported that she found it difficult to sit still for long periods. She also became more involved in organized religion than she had been previously, but whereas religious responders relied on religion as their main route to a cure, for Hannah spirituality was only one among a number of techniques she practiced in her quest for healing. She had previously been a not-very-active member of a synagogue but now found "that being in a spiritual environment helps me connect with my own healing." This description of the healing benefit of religion is similar in tone to Hannah's description of Naparsteck's comments above—yet another tool.

Alternative experts' attitude toward exercise was similar to their handling of diet. Hannah, who was slender in build and fit in appearance, described herself as not doing enough exercise. She went to classes "in waves." She biked, walked, and was an avid member of a women's dragon boat crew composed of breast cancer survivors. In addition, she became involved in other activities, mostly political in nature, which are discussed in chapter 8.

Hannah was by no means unique among alternative experts in the number of treatments she tried. Her story shows the lengths that alternative experts went to in their efforts to fight what they saw as a malignancy of body and spirit. Why did alternative experts go to such lengths and try so many things? Given their oppositional ideology, they had long been antagonistic to the conventional power structure and they viewed biomedicine as part of that structure. Now they were faced with the possibility of death, so it was too frightening to turn their backs entirely on doctors and their treatments. However, they had the resources, both educational and financial, both to follow conventional medical treatments and to counteract them by compromising in their use of biomedicine and by doing lots of other things that allowed them to feel they were personally running the show and following their own beliefs. And they did not have significant others with the power to fight their decisions.

Alternative experts viewed conventional treatments as "toxic," and they used alternative treatments to combat these toxic effects. Many of them took some type of alternative therapy with them when they went for conventional treatment; witness, for example, Hannah's use of visualization tapes during chemotherapy. Likewise, Violet took a book by the psychic Jane Roberts to all her radiation sessions. Roberts "channeled this entity Seth," and the book consisted of "what came through her from Seth."[30] Violet added that "There was a whole lot of stuff that made sense to me in terms of how I could perceive what was happening to me. . . . It was really about how we co-create reality."

Violet approached her treatment believing that her vision of reality would affect the outcome. For example, here is her description of how she approached radiation:

> I was very much engaged in accepting responsibility for . . . the ways in which all of the treatments that were being applied would affect me. . . . Because I had responsibility for [giving myself the disease], that means I could also accept responsibility for my own healing. . . . The first time they did it, I was having a visualization where I was just going to let the radiation come in and go through me and make everything better.

During her treatment, Violet had an epiphany about the meaning of illness in her life. In the following quote, she describes her resignation to what she saw as the inevitable. This enabled her to move from panic to acceptance:

> Stephen Levine,[31] who is a Buddhist . . . had a paradigm that I would live with in relation to disease. . . . To truly accept that I am only a temporary visitor here, and that I am going to die, and so is everyone else. . . . Healing is a lifelong process. . . . We are born as isolated, broken beings whose journey in life is to become healed. . . . A life-threatening illness is really an opportunity to take a quantum leap in healing. . . . Healing is distinct from the cure. . . . Sometimes in healing you live, miraculously. And sometimes in healing, when you heal, you die.

Like Hannah, Violet also supplemented the conventional treatments with other alternatives. In her case, these included support groups, the self-healing practices of tai chi and qi gong, meditation, massages, deep breathing, and visits to a holistic practitioner to understand "how to release pain."[32]

Alternative experts used these techniques and others like them in abundance and saw them as changing their lives. More than any other group, these women described breast cancer as a completely transformative experience. Religious responders reported that they were transformed by faith but most did not change to the extent reported by alternative experts. The latter had been concerned about the world and their place in it before. Now they took on a new level of concern. For Sarah, breast cancer was an opportunity to put theory into practice:

> I think this really gave me a chance to try out some of my philosophical and ideological thinking about illness and aging and death. Ideas that I had thought about but never had to face myself. . . . Accepting the situation for what it is, and allowing, and walking in it, and seeing what is there for me to learn from this. And if this path would go to illness and death, really giving it a lot of thought and being real practical and clear about it for myself.

Violet described her changes in similar terms.

Hannah, who was an activist before diagnosis, described her feelings after cancer as "absolutely, dramatically different," adding that she approached her life "with a lot more urgency." This is in contrast to many women in other groups who reported getting less stressed and being calmer. The reason for this was that she wanted to "have an impact on the world," and now, she realized, she had "a limited clock, where other people don't think they have." As a result, she said, "I am not going to put off for twenty years what I could do now. . . . I get into many struggles with people, because I never spend any time on bullshit."

Janet's transformation was even more dramatic. When I interviewed her, she was practicing both qi gong and feng shui. Qi gong is a technique of traditional Chinese medicine that restores the balance in the vital energy or "qi." This vital energy comes into the body from the outside world and enables the body to heal itself. Feng shui involves the placement of objects in correct positions in the living spaces of those who wish to avoid "geopathic stress" from the earth. This is how Janet described her approach to healing:

> I'd always been very Western oriented. But all my readings said I need to turn to Asian medicine and Asian thinking. . . . I decided that qi gong, which is exercise, meditation, energy flow, would be one thing that I could start with. . . . I took classes for about a year . . . making sure the energy flows in the body, it all flowed properly. . . . Then, in their theory, you shouldn't have the disease. . . . I have recently moved with this thought of energy and Eastern into feng shui. That's not a personal body thing. That is a whole environment thing . . . [involving] some of the renovation in the house [being done] and the rearranging of things.

Janet's house was in disarray because she was in the process of having everything redecorated and rearranged according to feng shui principles. And this is only one aspect of the changes she made. Others were similar to the ones already discussed: diet, supplements, exercise, and a host of other treatments.

Janet's most radical change, though, was in giving up a comfortable income for a more marginal one:

> How I changed—it was no more corporate job—in fact no more full-time job. . . . Now I do anything that is interesting or fun. I work as a vision therapist, which is an alternative medical therapy. . . . Two days a week, I work for a nonprofit organization. . . . For plain old fun, I work as ground crew for a hot air balloon company. . . . It's part of the lifestyle changes.

Since she described her husband as someone who never really held down a serious job but instead "wandered through life," this meant that their family income had declined from well over 120 thousand dollars to between twenty-five and forty thousand dollars since Janet was diagnosed. Most of their income now came from investments Janet had made when she was earning a handsome living.

Alternative experts had a complex relationship with the issue of control during and after breast cancer. Control was important to them. Janet, for example, said, "The diagnosis did not make me feel I had lost control—the fact that I had it at all meant I had lost control." She regained it "with the reading, informing myself of what it was I was facing and had, and my options, and all the changes I made." Similarly, Hannah "fell apart when I went to get moled[33] for radiation," because, "I was in this dark room with all these machines coming down" and, "It was like the whole medical establishment had control of everything." Subsequent to this, Hannah "suddenly looked at my life as something I could manage and have control over" by taking "control of my mental health, my healing, how I handle things emotionally." Hannah concluded, "The control was mine, not the medical community's."

Violet also had a complicated relationship with control:

> I felt like I had lost control . . . that my body was somehow the betrayer and the enemy, and that I was helpless. I think what it put me in touch with was the ways in which, in fact, we are not in control of our lives or anything. . . . I think that's a healthy thing . . . I don't know if anybody else is actually in control, or anything else, although I think there is an order, a natural order that we are a part of. . . . In many ways, I got more control, because I wasn't as afraid. It put me through the terror and the fear and the anxiety that I had been living out and gave me another level of freedom that finally is another level of control—not to be mistaken for the larger control.

For women who had a critical analysis of what they saw as the oppressive nature of social control, the idea that there really is less control than they had imagined was a comfort.

In spite of the fact that both Hannah and Violet had mothers who died of breast cancer, neither seemed particularly concerned about the risk to their own daughters, and in this, they were similar to other alternative experts. Hannah said she did not really focus on this danger, even though her daughter was probably predisposed to breast cancer, because there were so many other issues for her to worry about. Violet had talked to her daughter, explaining that three generations had now had breast cancer, but her daughter followed her mother's beliefs. She was not happy with biomedicine and refused to have a mammogram. Violet added, approvingly, that "she mostly follows alternative ways of health care whenever possible."

In a similar fashion, Sarah said that her daughters did not worry about breast cancer because they had other, more prominent worries. And Sarah had not talked to them about any possible risks. Janet took a similar position. Acknowledging that her daughter was at risk, Janet added that she was not too concerned, because her daughter "has been basically a vegetarian and exercised a lot." The lack of concern alternative experts showed about daughters' chances of getting breast cancer reflected not only their weak family ties, but also their desire to place cancer risk at the social rather than the individual level. They also continued to view alternative health practices as the way to health, rather than the early diagnostic techniques of biomedicine. Given the high prestige of biomedicine in this culture, only well-educated women would have had the self-confidence to decide to follow a different way—at least in part.

As a group, alternative experts believed that they had handled their experience with breast cancer well. As Hannah said, "I was actually pretty proud of myself. I thought that I did a great job." When her treatment was over, she held a party for everyone who had helped her and then "closed the door" on the experience. In saying that she closed the door, Hannah meant that she was no longer focusing on her own health but instead was working on larger social issues. At the time of the interview, she still experienced times when she worried about cancer. For example, she said, "I wonder if I have to worry about long-term things . . . if I have to worry about my retirement."

Janet also said she would not have done anything differently. She felt that she took charge throughout the experience and handled it in a "thoughtful" manner rather than panicking, as she assumed others did.

And she continued to be vigilant. Sarah, who described herself as "thoughtful, but not nervous" when she went for subsequent checkups, believed that she handled breast cancer well by using Buddhist principles.

The last word on this goes to Violet. She described herself as "radiant" during her treatment, adding:

> That period is one of the best periods in my life in terms of my connectedness with myself, with life, and the sensation of being in relation to the world around me. . . . I was given permission not to do anything else . . . to just be and to heal. So I really entered into a spiritual, psychological experience that was truly extraordinary and had a lasting effect on me.

Alternative experts opposed scientific medicine because they believed that medicalization fragmented women's bodies and subjected them to patriarchal medical control.[34] This could cause women to feel estranged from their physical selves. Violet's quote above is in direct contrast to this, and yet she attributed it to her resistance to standard medical treatment.

Furthermore, while Violet had decided "not to have regrets over what I had done," she also stated, "I would probably never do that again." Unfortunately, she was apparently having the opportunity to put her radical position into practice:

> The [physician] I see here in Philadelphia was doing the feely thing, and she felt something in the breast that had had surgery, and she was trying to get me to feel it too. And it's a small thing. It's not clear if it's a lump, or a cyst, or a scar tissue, or whatever. . . . She said, "You also can go and have it checked." I finally decided I don't want to do any more of this constant running to some doctor to tell me if I'm okay. . . . I don't know what's gonna happen, but I'm not so willing to go rushing into the system anymore, after my experience. 'Cause once they've got you . . . the next thing you know, you're in this whole stream of, "You're gonna get the CT scan, we're gonna biopsy you. We're gonna put the needle in. Then you're gonna sit on a little platform. Then we're gonna stick your breast through a little hole. . . ." Even if it were cancer, I don't want to go to them anymore. . . . I'm on another track now, and it was the experience of cancer that put me there.

Violet's quote is a powerful statement of the antimedicalization position that appears often in the narratives of alternative experts. She did not want some impersonal expert to treat her breast as a part unconnected to her body. Instead she wanted the kind of healing that would make her feel whole.[35]

Before breast cancer diagnosis, alternative experts had believed that they were responsible for staying well. In this way they were similar to biomedical experts, whom they mirrored in education and income.[36] Where they differed is that alternative experts saw wellness in both physical and emotional terms and they did not assume that biomedicine was the path to this state. In fact, they saw the medical establishment as an impediment to staying healthy. Alternative experts were the only group to move explanations of breast cancer away from individualistic blaming, at least to some extent. This is difficult to do in a world where personal responsibility for health has become a mantra, echoed by the media.[37] But in describing breast cancer as resulting from societal pathology, this group took the responsibility for cancer away from the individual woman.[38]

Where biomedical experts had assumed that those who maintained wellness could not be diagnosed with a life-threatening illness, alternative experts saw their diagnosis as resulting from more than their own personal histories. This was true even for those with cancer in their families. A diagnosis of breast cancer had personal causes but also resulted from societal failure to create an environment conducive to wellness. When they were diagnosed with breast cancer, women who believed this felt the need to drastically change who they were and how they did things, in order to heal both their bodies and their minds. It is their mistrusting worldview that sets alternative experts apart from the other groups, and this worldview can be explained in large part by their social locations.

In the following chapters, we turn to the experiences of women after they finished treatment. Given the tremendous differences in their approaches to diagnosis, the similarities in the ways the four groups responded to the physical ravages of their illness are striking. This issue is explored in more detail in the next chapter. Women, regardless of their response group, found the loss of a breast or increases in weight traumatic, which is a testament to the power over American women of these body-image issues. All women faced similar issues around the topics of body and sexuality. Those women who had lumpectomies often had to come to terms with a malformed breast. Those who had mastectomies had to decide whether or not to have reconstruction. Those who had reconstruction had to decide what type and sometimes had to accept a less than perfect surgical outcome. And regardless of type of surgery, all women had to deal with changes in, for example, weight and sexual response. Chapter 6 discusses the physical and emotional consequences of breast surgery, and chapter 7 deals with changes in body and sexuality.

SIX The Assault on the Breast

Amanda, the youngest woman in my study, was diagnosed with breast cancer at age twenty-six. Amanda, who worked in information technology, responded to her diagnosis as a biomedical expert. She first worried about her chances of survival, and then, to reassure herself, she learned everything about her disease. Since she was single, she also worried that breast cancer would make it difficult for her to marry and to have children. Because her type of tumor had a high probability of a reoccurrence in the same breast, Amanda's physician gave her no choice about the surgical technique; he performed a mastectomy. Amanda "didn't even spend a second pondering" whether or not to have reconstruction; she considered it a given. She did spend time, however, researching the various options. She was especially interested in the effects each type of procedure might have on her body and her appearance.

For many plastic surgeons, the tramflap, which involves bringing muscle from another part of the torso—most commonly the stomach—into the chest and using it to reconstitute a breast, is the surgery of choice.[1] It does not involve introducing foreign objects into the body, it feels natural, and it changes in size with weight changes. In addition, many surgeons assume that women would like their stomachs to be flatter, and, often, they are right.[2] Cynics might add that it is a more complex procedure than implants and, therefore, more lucrative for plastic surgeons.[3]

Although appearance was important to Amanda, she had other considerations. She decided against a stomach tramflap. Reasoning, "You really need that [stomach] muscle there for when you get pregnant," she next considered having a tramflap with muscle taken from her back. She decided against this, when she "found out that it's really a lot of rehab to get the strength back" and that she could "mess up" her back.

This left a breast implant as her only option. Amanda had a saline implant.[4] The plastic surgeon inserted the implant immediately following the mastectomy, and for three months Amanda paid weekly visits to have it expanded. Because her new breast looked "gravity defying," she also had the healthy breast lifted to make her chest look even, and the surgeon used the extra skin taken from the second breast to create a new nipple for the reconstructed breast. This is how Amanda, an attractive, slim, woman who had really liked her breasts before surgery, described the end result:

> The whole breast is basically an implant now. It doesn't move. It just stays there. I call them my new improved models . . . and kind of like, "Wow, this is nice. . . ." I really don't like having this big hard implant in me, but I think I look a little better. It's like I really don't need to have those big push-up bras any more. . . . However, there's certain clothing I wouldn't wear. A lot of the styles now . . . tube tops, halter tops, in the past, maybe, I wouldn't have shied away . . . but now it's like, I really don't want my scars to show . . . they are kind of bad. I'm the type of person who tends to keloid [thickened scar].[5]

In spite of these concerns, when she woke from the mastectomy, Amanda felt grateful that she had still "had a little mound there." And she had no regrets about reconstruction. Once treatment ended, she started dating again, and, although she still felt that cancer created a barrier between her and potential partners, at least she had two complete breasts.[6] Although Amanda as a biomedical expert approached the issues of reconstruction as she had approached everything else about her illness, first engaging in extensive research and then taking personal responsibility for decision-making, her outcome is strikingly similar to that of women from the other three groups. No matter how they responded to breast cancer diagnosis or how much authority they gave doctors, women found the reality of a deformed or absent breast traumatic. The major variable in determining how well they coped was age, for breast loss or deformity was particularly difficult for young women. For this reason, I made the decision to deal with breast and body issues for the sample as a whole rather than group by group. To do the latter would have been repetitive. Differences by group are noted; in most cases, these differences were confined to the process of decision-making rather than the outcome.

In a culture so focused on the breast,[7] a missing or damaged one is a hard thing for a young, unmarried woman to face, regardless of class or race.[8] Philosopher Marion Young has written that women rarely feel neutral about their breasts; they are inextricably intertwined with their self-images.[9] Young added that rather than simply being objects of male desire, breasts represent female desire as well. They are seen by women as a source of power and pleasure. Yet, in spite of the truth of this claim about desire, how breasts look takes precedence over how they feel. In Daphna Ayalah and Isaac J. Weinstock's series of interviews with women who agreed to have their breasts photographed, no one was indifferent about her breasts. Although the women came from all walks of life and from every race, class, and age group, each woman had strong opinions about the look of her breasts, and many were unhappy with them. Most women had an idealized vision of breasts, and their real breasts usually provided a disappointing contrast, particularly as they aged.[10] Although breasts in this culture are a major source of erotic pleasure for women, the frequency with which this pleasure is sacrificed in the service of breast enhancement shows that the breast's appearance is the most important thing to women. Breasts as power apparently take precedence over breasts as pleasure, which is not surprising in a culture where women's looks count for so much.

In the early days of the mastectomy, most American surgeons did not attempt any type of reconstruction, because William Stewart Halsted, the inventor of the first breast surgery, was opposed to it on the grounds that it made detection of a reoccurrence more difficult. Although some doctors experimented with various types of tissue transplant, it was not until the 1950s and the invention of synthetic implants that the surgery became more feasible.[11] Since then, plastic surgeons have used breast cancer to argue for the continued availability of breast implants for use in breast enhancement as well as in reconstruction. They have used the language of the women's health movement to make the case that women have a "right to normal breasts."[12]

Most women with breast cancer are older than Amanda at diagnosis, and not all of them have a mastectomy. Women have the right to a choice between a lumpectomy with radiation or a mastectomy, where this choice makes medical sense.[13] This right has been a major triumph of the women's health movement.[14] However, the United States still has much higher mastectomy rates than western Europe.[15] A report at the 2002 San Antonio Breast Cancer Symposium on the ATAC trial, which compared the effectiveness of combinations of hormone treatments for women diagnosed with breast cancer in the United States and the United Kingdom, noted that 51 percent of the U.S. women had had a mastectomy compared to 42 percent of the U.K. women.[16] The U.S. rate varied by region, with the highest mastectomy rates in the South. It also varied by surgeon. A study reported at the annual meeting of the Radiological Society of North America in December 2000 found surgeon-by-surgeon rates ranging from a low of 19 percent of women receiving a mastectomy to a high of 81 percent.[17] Some variation in these rates may be expected because low-income women tend to be diagnosed at a more advanced stage and to be more likely to need a mastectomy, but the range is too great for type of patient to be the sole explanation.

Not surprisingly, mastectomy rates varied among the four types of response groups. Over half the traditional patients (55 percent) had a mastectomy. Of the biomedical experts, 42 percent underwent mastectomies, a lower rate than the U.S. national average and the same as the U.K. rate. Biomedical experts were more likely to agree with doctors than those less supportive of evidence-based medicine, but also more likely to question the need for a mastectomy than traditional responders. Rates were lower for those who did not put their faith in biomedicine (36 percent of religious responders and 37 percent of alternative experts). However, age is also a predictor of mastectomy, in that premenopausal women are more likely to need one than postmenopausal women, because young women's cancers grow more rapidly. Thus, it is likely that the low rates for religious responders can be explained by their greater age. Nor is it surprising that alternative experts would want the least invasive surgery, given their attitudes toward biomedicine.

Regardless of surgical procedure, all women who undergo breast cancer surgery must cope with an assault on the part of their body most frequently associated with womanliness and desirability.[18] Any malformation of the breast, including missing breast tissue, is viewed negatively by Americans.[19] In an analysis of the interviews with the women whose breasts were photographed, Raymond Schmitt concluded that women's breasts were an important part of their identities. These identities varied from woman to woman and changed as women aged. Breasts constantly reminded women that they were getting older—even twenty-six-year-old Amanda noticed how much younger her breasts looked after reconstruction. Most women had detailed opinions about various aspects of their appearance, but for many, breasts were the badge of womanhood.[20] In a series of interviews with plastic surgeons, Diana Dull and Candace West found that surgeons believed that women's concern over their appearance was an intrinsic part of being a woman.[21] Many women in the current study felt this way about their breasts, regardless of response group.

A number of writers have taken the position that women's responses to breast cancer and to its effects on their breasts are varied in both experience and meaning. For example, Kristin Langellier and Claire Sullivan, in analyzing interviews with seventeen women who had undergone breast cancer treatment, explained that the breast has a number of meanings for women. They described the medicalized breast as the result of frequent breast exams and of the common experience of lumpy fibrocystic breast tissue, which many women regard as a disease. Then they described the functional breast as the one that feeds and nurtures. However, they noted that, in Western culture, the gendered breast outweighs either of these meanings, because breasts are associated so closely with femininity.[22] It should come as no surprise, therefore, when a woman diagnosed with breast cancer experiences the disease as an attack on her identity as a woman. Most women I interviewed were farther along in their life's course than Amanda and were, or had been, in an established relationship. Most did not have to fear explaining to a potential life partner why their reconstructed breast felt unnatural to the touch. Even so, most mourned the disfigurement or loss of a breast. The fact that this was almost universally experienced testifies to the strength of our cultural expectations about women's breasts.

Even women who had lumpectomies were disturbed by the appearance of their breasts. Many lost a fair amount of breast tissue, either from surgery or because radiation caused physical changes, often shrinkage. Kimberly, a divorced mother of two adolescent sons and a biomedical expert, described these changes in detail. She viewed herself as someone who had not been overly concerned about her appearance before her diagnosis. She had thought her breasts "kind of nice" even though "They were not nearly so perky as they had been" before she breast-fed her children. This is how Kimberly viewed her cancerous breast at the time of the interview:

> It's quite a bit smaller. The scar is real. . . . There is a lump there. It is very, very hard. . . . And the nipple is kind of tucked in and points to the soap dish now, when I'm in the shower. . . . I have one going straight ahead, and one saying, "Right turn. . . ." I feel comfortable with it. . . . ["Are you willing to let others see you with no clothes on?"] Yes if they can stand it. Who cares . . . ? Nobody has thrown up yet. . . . I went to Filene's basement . . . and I was trying something on because I was going to be putting myself in a bathing suit. And I went like this, "Whew!" The scar, where the lymph nodes had been, was so vividly red. . . . That was upsetting.

Breasts are such an important part of women's identity that even a woman who claimed not to care about her appearance could not help feeling stressed in viewing the damage caused by the surgeon's knife.

Sophia was a traditional responder who was thirty-three years old and single. An attractive, slender woman, she had spent several months before her diagnosis recovering from a bad intimate relationship, but then her life had improved dramatically. She had started a new relationship and was living in her own small house in the Italian neighborhood where she was raised. Having recently received a master's degree, she was working as a university administrator. Although conscious that her body was beginning to age and, especially, that her breasts had "started to sag a little," she felt good about her appearance. Cancer changed that, at least temporarily. After surgery, Sophia underwent radiation, which caused burning:

> I used to joke that I had this Frankenstein breast. They saved the breast, but why? It looked terrible. . . . I spent a lot of time looking in the mirror at it, when it was black and blue. And the burns were terrible. . . . There were some days when I thought my body was going to look terrible forever, because it looked so terrible in the beginning.

The appearance of her breast gradually improved, and Sophia noted that the radiation burn had ended up "minimizing the scar, because it peeled so much." Still, her detailed description of the remaining problems— problems that appear minimal to an outsider—reflected the importance that the appearance of her breasts held for her:

> I'm embarrassed that you can still see—you know when you lie on the table you have to put your arm up. And then when you put your arm down, the area which was radiated has an odd shape to it, more of a diamond shape, and people imagine it is just your breast. In certain shirts, you can see that diamond come up, and it's brown now.

Even women who were no longer so young and who were more resigned to bodily changes could give intricate descriptions of the damage done to their breasts by lumpectomies and radiation. Sonia, age forty-five at diagnosis, was a religious responder who worked as a teacher's assistant. She had been unhappy about her excess weight, but she had loved her breasts:

> I always liked them. I liked to showcase them. You know—you see larger women—they usually wear low-cut stuff. ["Now?"] This one hangs down wrong . . . and the other one sits up a little bit more. . . . They're here and they're healthy. And they still give me pleasure, you know, so they're great, and I'm glad I still have them.

Sonia was one of the few women who mentioned her breasts as a source of personal pleasure. Most women focused only on the changed appearance.

If women who had lumpectomies experienced unhappiness over changes in the appearance of a breast, what then of women who lost a breast completely? As others have noted, mastectomies are viewed as a violation of femininity in our culture.[23] Beth Meyerowitz found that women experience great conflict when they need a mastectomy.[24] They feel pressure to focus on the disease and to discount breast loss as a small price to pay for recovery, but this contradicts the high value placed on breasts in this culture. As a result of such cross-pressures, women accept the need for a mastectomy, but they also feel ashamed of breast loss and generally hide it from view.[25] Images of mastectomies are rarely shown in pictures accompanying breast cancer stories, and when they are shown, they are shocking. When the model Matushka appeared on the front cover of the *New York Times Sunday Magazine* in 1993, revealing a chest with one breast missing, there was an immediate outcry, especially from survivors.[26] When Ayalah and Weinstock photographed women's breasts, they included four women who had had mastectomies. All had been disturbed by the mastectomy, at least at first.[27] In her autobiography, Betty Ford recounted how worried she had been, after her mastectomy, that she would no longer be able to wear low-cut dresses.[28]

Women in my study echoed this shame about breast loss.[29] No one responded as did Audre Lorde after her mastectomy:

> Ten days after having my breast removed, I went to my doctor's office to have the stitches taken out. This was my first journey since coming home from the hospital, and I was truly looking forward to it. A friend had washed my hair for me and it was black and shining, with my new gray hairs glistening in the sun. Color was starting to come back into my face and around my eyes. I wore the most opalescent of my moonstones and a single floating bird dangling from my right ear in the name of grand asymmetry. With an African kente cloth and new leather boots, I knew I looked fine, with that brave security of a beautiful woman having come through a very hard time and being very glad to be alive. [30]

What happened next is more typical. On walking into the doctor's office, one of the first things Lorde was told was, "You're not wearing a prosthesis." When Lorde explained that it did not feel right to wear one, the nurse replied, "You will really feel much better with it on." The staff, the nurse added, liked patients to wear them when coming for a visit, because, "Otherwise, it's bad for the morale of the office." This hostile response to Lorde's public and political statement about her missing breast is striking. In general, as other writers have noted, women with breast cancer are expected to hide from public view any damage to their breasts.[31]

It should be no surprise, therefore, that over two-thirds of those who had a mastectomy opted for reconstruction, although as with mastectomies, this choice varied by response group. The religious responders had the lowest rate, with only one woman in this group opting for reconstruction. Many religious responders had minimal health insurance that would not have paid for a new breast. In addition, the average age of the group helps explain the low rates. Only a few premenopausal women opted not to have reconstruction after a mastectomy, and when they chose this route, they did so in the face of strong opposition from their doctors. In contrast, a number of the older women did not have reconstruction. Not surprisingly, the traditional responders were the group most likely to have reconstruction after a mastectomy, with over four-fifths opting for the procedure. Surgeons generally put pressure on women to have reconstruction, and traditional responders listened to their doctors. Also, this group contained many of the youngest women. Half of the biomedical experts had reconstruction after a mastectomy, and two-thirds of the alternative experts did. While these rates cannot be generalized to the population, given the nonrandom nature of the sample, they are in line with what might be expected. Indeed, many women colluded with their surgeons and made hasty decisions to have reconstruction because of their own fears about not being whole.

In her book on plastic surgery, Kathy Davis argued that we should not view women who undergo surgical procedures to improve their bodies as "cultural dopes."[32] First, women often feel conflicted about cosmetic surgery, wanting to improve a perceived deficiency even as they have critical views about such surgery. They implicitly recognize that their feminine beauty may be used to equalize the power imbalance of the sexes and that breasts are one of their central tools. Diana Dull and Candace West found that women who had plastic surgery considered it to be correcting something that they found abnormal and disfiguring about their appearance.[33] Furthermore, most media coverage of reconstruction emphasizes its positive rather than negative aspects.[34] In my research, many women decided to fight the devastation breast cancer caused to their self-image by having surgical reconstruction in an effort to recapture, and even improve, what they had lost. These women came from different social locations with a variety of political perspectives.

What happened to women who resisted this cultural imperative for a full and even chest? Pearl, a fifty-year-old biomedical expert, was a physician's assistant and was comfortable dealing with doctors. She told me that she had always liked her breasts and had "never been so thankful that they are small" as she was at diagnosis. Pearl was one of the few respondents who realized that she did not have to act hastily after diagnosis. She took her time by going to four different breast surgeons for their opinions. She also considered breast reconstruction:

> It was first recommended by the surgeon who did the biopsy. Although I was not sure this was something I wanted, I trusted their opinions, and I didn't know how I'd feel about myself after the surgery. . . . When they explained to me what was involved in the surgery . . . I could not consider it. . . . They explained that psychologically it could be very beneficial to your health, but I trusted that psychologically I would be fine. . . . It was more involved than a mastectomy, and I thought, "This is insane."

When Pearl told the surgeon what she had decided, he responded, "Please, please go and see another plastic surgeon," because, he said, she had obviously spoken to the wrong one. She complied with his request but still decided not to have reconstruction. When she went for a second and third opinion about the cancer surgery, each surgeon she talked to pushed reconstruction. Realizing that she had seen three male surgeons, she thought that perhaps they were pushing reconstruction because of their gender. She went to a female surgeon "in one of the best teaching hospitals in the area," for a fourth opinion because she expected a woman to be empathetic about her stance on plastic surgery:

> To my surprise, she was shocked that I wasn't considering reconstruction and asked me why. And I told her that having gone to two plastic surgeons and found out what's involved . . . I would wonder why any

woman would go through that. . . . It was just not worth the health risk. And she responded back with, "Why? The reason why is to be whole."

Pearl was horrified by this statement, and it confirmed her stance against reconstruction.

Most of the women in the study who had mastectomies were encouraged by their breast surgeons to have reconstruction, or at least to have a consultation with a plastic surgeon. In her book on breast surgery, Nora Jacobson has recounted how this close relationship came about.[35] At one time, because of Halsted's opposition, surgeons who performed mastectomies did not encourage reconstruction. Plastic surgeons organized to change these attitudes by arguing that losing a breast after cancer was psychologically devastating and that reconstruction was the surest way for a woman to regain her lost femininity. They also argued that patients would be more appreciative of surgeons if they were able to have reconstruction after the mutilation of mastectomy.[36] Their arguments were so successful that nowadays surgeons routinely turn the patient over to the plastic surgeon while the patient is still under anesthesia.

However, as if this medical pressure was not enough, Pearl's "well-meaning friends" who "could not imagine living without a breast" were also upset with her for not seriously considering reconstruction. One friend even came up with the phone number of yet another plastic surgeon who "could persuade anyone." When Pearl finally prevailed, however, her husband and family told her they were happy that she was going to avoid unnecessary surgery. The pressure Pearl experienced is reminiscent of Lorde's story. However, Pearl did not want a constant visual reminder of her asymmetrical body, so she bought a self-adhering prosthesis that, except for sleeping, she wore constantly. She was satisfied with this solution because the prosthesis enabled her to feel whole when she looked in the mirror. As a biomedical expert, she was happy that she had come up with her own solution to presumed loss of femininity.

I visited a corset shop as part of my research and found a booming business in prostheses, accounting for about one-third of the store's business. The kind of prosthesis Pearl bought was not typically covered by insurance, because it cost over four hundred dollars and was more expensive than others. The owner of the store, who did all of the prosthesis fittings, estimated that she did about two hundred fittings a year. She did them not only for women who had mastectomies without reconstruction but also for women whose reconstructions had gone wrong, and for lumpectomies that had left a shrunken or misshapen breast.[37]

We should not be surprised that women face much pressure to have breast reconstruction. In this culture, even small breasts are seen as a liability.[38] Many women told me how unhappy they had been as late-developing or tiny-breasted teens. Women who undergo breast enhancement do so as a result of the social pressure for large breasts, which is how we imagine real breasts should look.[39] Breast reconstruction and enhancement are about gendered expectations and not about pleasure. Sometimes, physicians will tell women that their reconstructed breasts will feel normal, because they are thinking about how the breast will feel to a man and not to the owner of the breast.[40] The owner of a reconstructed breast does not experience the pleasures of a real one. Nor does it look like an actual breast. Even the most successful reconstruction looks like a self-supporting plastic breast that does not require a bra to hold it up. As Naomi Wolf has argued, our culture represents breasts in a particular way, rarely showing those that are soft, asymmetrical, or mature, which leads many women to become fixated on a so-called ideal breast that is perky and firm.[41] Thus, women may experience their breasts as separate from themselves, as objects to be assessed in comparison to the idealized image of breasts. The irony is that what looks sexy is no longer erogenous for the owner.

A woman without a breast makes others uncomfortable. A woman who chooses not to have breast reconstruction, especially if she is young, seems to be devaluing an important aspect of women's bodies. Often women who had chosen not to have reconstruction after a mastectomy reported that the pressure to "normalize" their bodies continued long after surgery. One woman reported, "My surgeon asks me every time I go for a check-up." Breast reconstruction is complicated surgery and carries serious risks, no matter which procedure is used, but, as Ellen Leopold noted in her book on the history of women and breast cancer, cosmetic concerns quickly overshadow medical ones. Breast reconstruction, she stated, can easily become synonymous in women's minds with recovery.[42] And many women in my study confirmed this, with statements indicating that they wanted reconstruction so that they would not be reminded they had breast cancer every time they looked in a mirror. These cultural pressures are so strong that they affected women in every group. Most of the time, the women were unaware of the social pressure; they simply knew they wanted breasts, and they took reconstruction for granted.

One of the largest and best known-breast cancer support programs is the American Cancer Society's Reach to Recovery.[43] This program specializes in providing advice and help to mastectomy patients about using prostheses and having reconstruction. The organization's goal is for every mastectomy patient to receive a visit from a Reach to Recovery volunteer while still in the hospital, and many do. This volunteer will also have had a mastectomy. The emphasis in the program is on helping women look and feel whole again by possessing two matching breasts. One of the American Cancer Society's other programs, Look Good . . . Feel Better, is complementary to Reach to Recovery. It provides women with free makeup, gives tips on how to use it, and shows them how to tie scarves to cover bald heads. In this program, "recovery" appears to be about regaining femininity.

This belief resonates deeply in our culture and is a message widely represented in the media. Perfect breasts are used to sell everything, and images of women's breasts—the kind that have no sag or blemishes—are ubiquitous. Regardless of group and of race and class, most of the women I interviewed believed that two matching breasts would aid their recovery. When mastectomy patients chose not have reconstruction, they did not attack the desire for femininity. Instead, like Pearl, they sacrificed femininity for the greater good of health. This argument was particularly common among biomedical experts. Some of these women worried about the length of extra time under anesthesia, especially with the tramflap, while others did not want unnecessary surgery at a time when their bodies were already weakened. Yet others decided to postpone the decision until they had finished treatment and were stronger. Some of the poorest and oldest women in the group did not have health insurance to cover plastic surgery and thought they were too old to worry. Only a few saw the lopsided chest as a remembrance of what they had been through and exulted in it, like Lorde.

For the majority of women, evenness was a worthwhile goal; unfortunately it was difficult to achieve. Women with lumpectomies often ended up with the cancerous breast smaller and/or less droopy than the healthy one. Women who chose to wear prostheses also had problems. First, the prosthesis does not alter in size with weight gain or loss, so breasts often became uneven over time. And even without weight change, women often found that they could not get a perfect match unless they were willing and able to pay for expensive prostheses not covered by insurance. It is a comment on the influence of surgeons and the cultural assumptions about femininity that insurance companies would not pay about four hundred dollars for prostheses that are molded to match the other breast and to adhere to the chest, but would pay thousands of dollars for reconstruction. And some insurance programs will pay for only one prosthesis, no matter what problems develop. The cheaper one the companies paid for frequently fell apart in time, especially if the woman was physically active.

In one of the more bizarre examples of this, Jenna, the religious responder discussed in chapter 4, was fitted with a prosthesis after surgery. At that time, she did not want implants, was nervous about the surgery involved in a tramflap, and was still figuring out God's intentions for her. When she needed a new prosthesis, her insurance company refused to pay for it. They would, however, still pay for reconstruction. She had been thinking she would like reconstruction anyway, and, when a friend told her about "a great plastic surgeon," she made an appointment. The surgeon performed a tramflap as well as a breast reduction on her other breast, which was larger than the tramflap breast. As was true in many cases, evenness was achieved only by surgery on both breasts. This is how Jenna described the result:

> I love it that I did the reconstruction. . . . I feel so good about it. . . . It's a wonderful gift, and I don't know if I'd be as thrilled about it if I had done it right away. . . . My stomach is wonderful. It is flat, I feel like I wear a girdle all the time. . . . I still have the scars. I have scars on this new breast where, you know, he had to fit it together like a puzzle. And I have a scar here from the reduction. I feel like a walking advertisement. I'll show anybody.

Jenna did indeed show me the reconstructed breast.

Women often showed me the results of breast reconstruction during the interview. As one woman said, it did not really feel like her breast. I assume this is the reason so many otherwise modest women were anxious to show me, when I was never shown lumpectomy scars. In their study, Langellier and Sullivan found that women with breast prostheses had a lack of modesty about them, which suggested that these women did not see them as real breasts.[44] This separation of the self from the body is an extreme example of anthropologist Emily Martin's argument that women see their bodies as something to manage rather than as something that is part of them.[45] It is an example of the medicalization of women's bodies that Jenna had surgery on both breasts because her real breast seemed wrong. This surgery on the second breast is a measure of the power of plastic surgeons, who have been able to convince insurance companies that it is medically necessary for women to have surgery on breasts that are healthy.[46]

Dana, age thirty-seven at diagnosis, was also pleased with her reconstruction, and she too had surgery on both breasts. Dana was a traditional responder who turned her treatment decisions over to her doctors in order to pay attention to her two young daughters. Dana had reconstruction because "No one suggested I shouldn't; no one gave me any bad talk about it." She described herself as having always been unhappy with her breasts. When she first developed breasts, she would "pray every night, 'Please wake me up with more,'" because she felt "insecure" and not "quite womanly enough." She was devastated at the thought of losing one and being even more flat-chested. As she did throughout her treatment, Dana followed her doctor's advice on reconstruction:

> I wanted the reconstruction right away, and, as far as not doing the tramflap or anything like that, the doctor said I didn't have enough fat to do it anyway. . . . A year later, after everything was done, this [reconstructed] one was a little bigger than that one. And he said, "Look, the insurance is going to cover it anyway; however you want to do it." And I said, "Well, I've always liked to be a bit of something instead of flat." So he ended up changing the first implant . . . and then [putting] one in here. . . . I'm glad I have the reconstruction. . . . I don't like how it's full up here. . . . And now this one is bigger than this one. . . . I just have to kind of leave it at that, I think. . . . I'm still not big. . . . I can joke about it and say, "Well, I guess I got something

out of it. . . ." I couldn't have got implants without having the cancer first because the insurance paid for it.

Like most of the other women who underwent reconstruction, this was not something Dana's husband pushed her into. "It didn't bother him to look at it at any stage," she said, adding, "My husband is very support-ive of the way I look." Her belief that small breasts made her less of a woman and that the loss of a breast would be even worse was something Dana had internalized while she was still a girl.[47]

Every woman who had a mastectomy told me that her husband put no pressure on her for reconstruction. Those women who decided against reconstruction described husbands who opposed plastic surgery because of the risks. To these husbands, breasts paled in importance when com-pared to the health of wives who faced a life-threatening illness. Women who had reconstruction reported that they did it for themselves and not for their husbands. There is truth, I think, in this—women had internal-ized the belief that breasts made them into women, and most husbands did not want wives to have additional unnecessary surgery. However, this point was not made in a response to a question; it was volunteered. Perhaps women found it necessary to describe husbands who loved and supported them no matter what they looked like. To say anything less would reflect badly on the husband. Women who had undergone recon-struction wanted me to understand that this did not mean their husbands wanted their wives to suffer in order to gain the two breasts every hus-band is entitled to.[48] These gendered beliefs about body and about love are widespread in this culture and affected women in my study regard-less of response group.

Since breast symmetry and perfection are so important to women, it was not uncommon for respondents to "fix" the other breast while under-going a breast reconstruction. As happened with Dana, plastic surgeons would frequently market a breast enhancement or reduction on the non-affected breast, since insurance companies would pay for this as part of the cancer treatment.[49] As we have seen, surgeons and plastic surgeons aggressively pushed reconstruction, and it was a rare surgeon who simply acceded to a woman's wishes not to have a plastic surgery consultation.

Almost all women with mastectomies, therefore, were sent to plastic surgeons, who gave them a hard sell.

Sometimes women found this use of commercial sales techniques offensive. Eve, the woman we met in chapter 3, on biomedical experts, visited a plastic surgeon on the recommendation of her breast surgeon, even though she "hadn't really thought about that" before. This entailed "driving over to some plastic surgeon whom I didn't really want to talk to" and who "showed me somebody else's picture book. Like why," Eve added, "would I ever go to a surgeon who shows me somebody else's picture book?" Eve had "been overweight since I was born," and she found it offensive to look at other women's bodies and breasts as an advertisement for reconstruction. Doctors who marketed breast reconstruction by showing pictures of other women's breasts did not suit Eve's idea of evidence-based medicine. Like the other women in her group, Eve was managing her own treatment and did not succumb to marketing pressure. She had had a very rapidly growing tumor and her health was now paramount, so she resisted breast reconstruction. Her management of breast loss was different than for more deferential patients, but her sadness at losing a breast was not.

Sometimes a second breast had to be created also, because women had both breasts removed. Most of the time, the second breast was removed for prophylactic reasons. Biomedical experts were particularly susceptible to this, because they made this choice more often than women from other groups. Although they were more reluctant than other groups to have breast reconstruction, since it was not going to prevent cancer, they were more likely to believe that they could prevent future medical problems through surgical interventions. Sharon was a nurse and a biomedical expert; she had the second breast removed about six months after her mastectomy. The biopsy of the first breast had shown the small precancers known as DCIS and LCIS,[50] in addition to invasive cancer.[51] She asked to have her other breast removed because she thought it likely that these precancers were not confined to one breast. She did not have reconstruction immediately after the original mastectomy because she needed time to decide about removing the second breast and she was not sure which kind of reconstruction she wanted. When she decided to have the prophylactic surgery, she did not "have enough muscle to reconstruct two breasts," so she had saline implants, which made her somewhat nervous because she had read the negative publicity about implants and knew that they could break.

Sharon was typical of the biomedical expert who knew a little too much and traded one fear for another. Although she had been unsure about whether or not to have implant surgery, when I talked to her Sharon was generally satisfied with the result. Even so, she worried somewhat about her appearance, and she mourned her old breast:

> I like them. I'm very happy with the reconstruction. . . . In fact, I show a lot of people. . . . I know I look at myself in the mirror a lot now. I look at my breasts in relation to my stomach and saying, "Hmm, do they look too high? I wonder if people can tell. No, I don't think they can tell. . . ." There are still some issues about not having real breasts. I mean I like how they look, but I think I would like to have my own breasts back.

In describing the old ones as her "own" and in showing the new ones to everyone, Sharon demonstrates the general attitude that reconstructed breasts were somehow not part of a woman's body. This was echoed by Sharon's husband. Sharon reported, "He really likes them a lot." Where he had no name for her previous breasts, Sharon's husband named the new breasts "the girls" in reference to their youthful, perky appearance. Sharon underscored this sense that the new breasts were objects she owned by adding, "We really enjoy them."

For every woman who liked her reconstruction, another was unhappy, and often extremely unhappy.[52] Ella, age thirty-four, was African American and a lawyer with a husband and baby when she was diagnosed. A traditional responder who had barely thought about breast cancer before diagnosis, her prior knowledge of the disease was confined to a scary experience she had had as a teenager visiting an aunt. Ella discovered to her shock that the aunt had had a mastectomy. Ella learned this when she was dressing up for church alongside her aunt and "saw that she had one breast, and the other side was flat." As soon as she was diagnosed, Ella "knew" that she "was going to have breast reconstruction" because she "wasn't going to be able to bear having that flat thing that I saw my aunt had all those years ago." When Ella visited the plastic surgeon she received a hard sell, but she noted that she had been anxious to have something done quickly:

> She explained to me about my different options. She said I could get an implant or I could have this tramflap . . . that they would use my own tissue. And she made it sound good, and she made the implant sound not good. And I can tell she was favoring the tramflap . . . how I would get the tummy tuck. . . . And I agreed to it.

However, things did not turn out the way Ella had hoped:

> I still have pain and itching from the tramflap . . . in my stomach. . . .
> Even in the breast . . . I have itching and discomfort because of the tissue being moved there. . . . The way the plastic surgery was explained to me, I knew it was not going to look like the other one, but I didn't think it was going to look the way mine looks. To me, if I was to go topless, I would make people scream. They didn't have a tattoo that was dark enough, and it didn't take. . . . It doesn't look like a nipple; it's just this thing that sticks out. [My stomach] feels tight, and I have no feeling. . . .
> I didn't need to be cut on my stomach. . . . It looks horrible . . . like a big laughing mouth.

Ella showed me her reconstructed breast. It did indeed look misshapen, although not as badly as she imagined. In retrospect, Ella believed that she would have been happier with an implant, but her cancer had been high on the breast and had necessitated taking part of the chest wall, so it is doubtful that an implant would have looked better.

Ella's unhappiness over her breast's appearance was related to her still-fresh grief at having breast cancer and belied the oft-stated reason for reconstruction, that it helps women feel whole and put their cancer behind them. However, others had horror stories also, and in each case, they had faced aggressive and sometimes unsympathetic doctors. Trish, age thirty-six at diagnosis, was an occupational therapist and an alternative expert. After the plastic surgeon showed her photographs of a mastectomy without reconstruction and then ones of reconstructed breasts, she thought that the latter looked "pretty good" compared to the former. The plastic surgeon gave her choices:

He offered me the tram . . . a tissue expander, the implant, or you could wait. . . . I was in a rush. . . . One of the things I would have to do if I was going to get the tram was to go that day and donate some blood in case I needed a transfusion. . . . I don't want to deal with that. I just wanted it off, but, definitely, I made a hasty decision.

Unfortunately, Trish's complicity in rushing into a decision designed to bring back wholeness led to an unpleasant but not uncommon result. Most women who have mastectomies do not need radiation, but, where the cancer has already spread to the lymph nodes, surgeons often suggest radiation of both lymph nodes and breast as an added precaution. In this case, it is advisable to wait for an implant until after the radiation.[53] However, some plastic surgeons are less conservative. Trish had implants put in before her radiation:

Nobody told me I might need radiation, and that if I needed radiation it might ruin the implant. And that is exactly what happened. . . . The implant just got hot, and it shrank up, and it just formed a capsule around it. . . . I've been having it out with my plastic surgeon. I just saw him yesterday. And he told me from his point of view he just sees the patient. He doesn't get the pathology report. He relies on the surgeon to clue him in. . . . It was mostly the breast surgeon's responsibility. . . . I wrote her a letter, you know, telling her what I was upset about. And she never responded.

When asked if the plastic surgeon would have waited had he known she needed radiation, Trish said, "No, he would have told me what the possible consequences would be." She added that the plastic surgeon did not think it was a "big deal," because problems do not always develop.

Trish had had her implant removed and was wearing a prosthesis when I interviewed her. She believed that her problems could have been avoided with a tramflap instead of implants. Here is how Trish felt about her breasts at the time of the interview:

I'm not real happy with the way this looks. You know, it actually looks worse than if I had just had a mastectomy, 'cause the implant kind of pushed down on the ribs and made a dent. I don't have a silicone prosthesis yet; I'm wearing a light one. . . . After I went for my treatments and the implant started to shrink up . . . I ended up getting a silicone prosthesis, but it was a partial one because I still had the implant in there. But the implant started to get so painful and tight that I really wanted it out. So the prosthesis that I had didn't fit, after they removed the implant. . . . I haven't gotten around to finding out if my insurance company will pay for another one.

As we saw in Carla's case in chapter 2, there is also controversy about whether or not implants are advisable after radiation because the radiated breast does not always take well to an implant.[54]

The problems with breast reconstruction appear to result from a combination of plastic surgeons who are overoptimistic about results and women, especially young women, who feel the need to have breasts so strongly that they push blindly ahead. Trish had been careful about other medical decisions she made, but she wanted breasts badly and she pushed blindly ahead. The surgeons are able to market their wares because they understand the desire women have for an appropriately gendered body. These women buy the argument that they need breasts to be whole. Evidence that desire clouds judgment can be seen by the fact that when things went wrong, women often decided they chose the wrong surgery, instead of questioning the whole process. Thus, Trish believed that she would have had a better result had she had the tramflap instead of implants, while Ella wished she had had implants instead of a tramflap. In both cases, they blamed the specific technology rather than questioning reconstruction in general.

A few women did come to understand that reconstructed breasts could create their own set of problems. Often these women were older and more resigned to bodily change and decay; aging represents its own loss of femininity. Jeanne, an alternative expert, had been fifty-five years old at diagnosis. A self-professed exercise devotee, she had discovered a lump on a morning when she was to run a half-marathon with friends, one of whom was an oncologist. The oncologist examined the lump and told Jeanne they needed to get her to a surgeon right away. After performing a lumpectomy, the surgeon told her she needed to go back and do a full mastectomy, so Jeanne decided to have the other breast removed as a precaution. She described herself as not thinking about having reconstruction. In retrospect, she could not really explain why she did it, except to say that she "thought it was automatic." She decided to have implants, because the surgery was quicker and less complex than tramflap surgery. The process turned into an ordeal. Jeanne "had to go back and forth for the implants," then she had to have expanders, and eventually she had the final implants inserted. She chose not to have the nipples reconstructed, because she had had enough surgery. She finally felt her life was returning to normal. Four years later, she faced another ordeal:

> About a month and a half ago . . . one of the implants just collapsed, and I was very upset. . . . The doctors were very casual. The plastic surgeon had since retired. So the new one said, "Oh, it's not a big deal; they're only supposed to last ten years." I said, "Ten years! If I had known, I would never have had them. . . . Why do this? It might not be safe." And the doctor said, "Oh, it's just saline. It's perfectly safe. . . . It's a silicone/saline mix."[55]

Until this crisis occurred, Jeanne had been unaware that her saline implants were encased in silicone. An environmental activist who blamed her cancer in large part on her father's extensive use of pesticides in the yard where she sunbathed in her youth, she believed that silicone was a health hazard.[56] When she learned that it encased the saline, she immediately had both implants removed. Although she was thin and had not had very large breasts, she had liked them, describing breasts as "important to men." When they were removed, her partner told her that she should have consulted him in the first place, before agreeing to the implants, as he would have told her not to have them. Jeanne thought she had now made the right decision, but she was still grieving over her flat chest at the time of the interview:

> I'm trying to convince myself that I'll live with it. I don't want to lean over. . . . You know it looks strange being perfectly flat. . . . I'm hoping that I'll eventually get used to it. I notice women's breasts, especially. I love when I see women who are flat-chested. . . . That's new. . . . You know like, "Oh boy, so maybe they won't notice me if there are others around. . . . The rest of my body I like. . . . But in terms of my chest, no, I don't feel comfortable.

Her women's group reminded Jeanne that she had not originally had the breast implants to please her partner. Rather, she had had them for herself, and this made sense to her. Still, now that they were removed, Jeanne was uncomfortable appearing nude in front of him. She believed that he was comfortable with her breast amputations, but she had been trying long and hard to have "a perfect body," and she "really worked at it." Her idea of a perfect body was a thin runner's body—Jeanne once ran a sixty-two-mile race—but like many thin women, she also wanted breasts.[57]

Most of the accounts of medical problems with reconstruction involved physical imperfections or minor health risks like a deflated implant.[58] In these cases, as we have seen, the problems were largely emotional. In a few cases, more serious issues arose. One of the most problematic accounts involved Sheila, a traditional responder, living in an older city neighborhood consisting mostly of row homes. Sheila was forty-two years old at diagnosis. When I met her, she was overweight and troubled by this. She had a clerical occupation and a husband working in a blue-collar trade for a utility company. Their home was small, neat, and attractive, and between them they made over seventy-five thousand dollars per year. Sheila had first had a lumpectomy, but when the surgeon could not get clean margins, he gave her a choice of radiation or a mastectomy and she chose the latter.

Sheila was one of the few women in my study to receive medical advice not to rush into reconstruction. Her female gynecologist recommended that Sheila not make any decisions about reconstruction until after having her breast removed. By her own account, Sheila did not listen. The surgeon sent her to a plastic surgeon and as Sheila described it, "He sold me a real bill of goods." Why was Sheila so anxious to have reconstruction? Like many women, particularly traditional responders, she colluded with doctors in her haste to recover her breast:[59]

More than anything else, it was not appearance. It was balance, because I was busty. . . . [He] sat in the office and talked with us, and he proceeded to show us a film. The film was fantastic. . . . You would never know that the woman had anything wrong with her. . . . I said to my husband, "Well, why wouldn't I do that? And besides I can have myself reduced, and then I'll be small. . . ." His information was what I wanted to hear. . . . My decision to go ahead with it is because I thought, "If I don't do this now, I'm not going to go back and do it."

While Sheila recognized her complicity in rushing to have a breast implant, she also noted that "there were a lot of things he did not tell us that we didn't know until after the fact." Sheila's silicone implant, she later learned, should have come with a pamphlet describing problems patients might have, but she never received one.

And Sheila began to have problems from the beginning, starting with instructions she had difficulty following:

> I had the implant put in, and I had the right side reduced, so I was sore. He had told me to try to massage it. Well, you're not stitched, you're wired, because it weighs so much that they don't want it to break through the skin. It was very painful.

In addition, she did not like the way it looked:

> I kind of looked like I had this zipper. It looked more like a bump than a breast. . . . I went back for my checkup, and I wasn't happy with it. . . . I didn't tell him at first. . . . He said, "Oh, everything looks good. . . ." I bought a prosthesis to put in my bra, so it looked like I had a breast. . . . I went to a corset shop. They don't make expressions on their face, because, obviously, they are trained not to, but you can still see it in somebody's eyes when they think, "Oooh, they really did a number on her."[60] When I went back, I said to him, "Oh, by the way, I had to buy a prosthesis." And he said, "What did you do that for? What do you think you came to me for? We can put a nipple on that and you'll feel differently." I said, "Yes, but we're not going to do that, because it doesn't fill out a bra." "I can fix that. . . . We're going to take that one out and put another one in." I said, "No, we're not." I was content with the prosthesis.

Things stayed this way until Sheila started to experience a lot of pain. In retrospect, once she had read some of the considerable press about silicone implants and their problems, Sheila decided that her body had been rejecting the implant.[61] A lot of her pain was caused by the large amount of scar tissue she developed. After struggling for a couple of years, Sheila went to a second plastic surgeon to have the implants removed, but she encountered lots of resistance:

> They won't just take it out. "No, that wouldn't be good. We need to replace it." "I don't want another implant. I don't want anything."

"Well, maybe we can do the tummy." I said, "No, we can't because we couldn't do it in the beginning." Then I went to see another plastic surgeon, and he was the most obnoxious man. . . . He made me feel like a piece of dirt, because I wanted it out. He said, "My mother has an implant." I said, "I just want to have this one removed." He said, "Well, I'll be the judge of that. . . . I think we'll do the tummy tuck."

Finally, in despair, Sheila went back to the gynecologist who had advised her to wait. She told the gynecologist that she was depressed because she could not find a doctor who would take out her implant: "It's just ripping and tearing. It doesn't do anything. It's there." The gynecologist sent Sheila to a female plastic surgeon who "listened to me. She didn't tell me what I needed, or what she thought I needed." Sheila's surgeon took the implant out. By this time there had been a lot of news coverage about the possible dangers of silicone implants. Although there is continuing controversy about the dangers of silicone implants, Sheila was convinced:

All this time, since this went in, I had been nothing but sick. . . . I slept all the time . . . sinus infections and bladder infections. . . . It was what they called encapsulated. . . . Once it was out of my body, I was a different person. . . . It came out at the time they were doing this—the lawyers were doing these commercials on these implants. . . . I went and talked to one, because it was too late to sue the doctor. Not that I wanted to sue the doctor; I wanted to kill the doctor. . . . There wasn't anything I could do with the plastic surgeon, but I could, in fact, become part of the class action suit.

After the ordeal was over, Sheila went back to the corset shop and got a full breast prosthesis. When I talked to her, she was fairly resigned to her outcome and was relieved to be feeling better. Still struggling some-what with depression, particularly over her weight gain, she continued to miss her breast. Noting that she was now in her fifties and "not look-ing for someone," she still got a little "envious, when you see the young girls." She had not anticipated this before her mastectomy. Instead, she had imagined that it would be "no big deal." Losing her breast, having cancer, and suffering an ordeal over surgical reconstruction, she said, "just changes your life completely." Like other traditional responders,

Sheila had been a woman who always trusted her doctors and who did as she was told, but now she had become quite suspicious of medical care. Her experience with the reconstruction and the doctors who expected her to cooperate with their plans had radicalized her and made her more critical of biomedicine.

Like other women, Sheila made it clear that her implants had been something she did for herself and not something her husband had demanded or even desired. When she lost her breast in the first place, "He kept saying to me, 'That's not you. That's nothing.'" Raised by a mother who stressed modesty, Sheila had always found nudity difficult. Now, although she was more self-conscious about her body than before, because "It looks so terrible," she had become much more comfortable exposing her body around her husband. She added, "It's a shame, because I wasn't this open when I was fine."

The way in which the breast defines what it means to be a woman is illustrated in Sheila's story. In retrospect, Sheila believed she would have done things differently. She would "still have had the mastectomy," but instead of reconstruction she would "have one large breast and one large prosthesis."[62] In this calculation, Sheila had come to understand that, given the fact of breast cancer, this combination would have produced the most realistic breasts possible. In the end, however, Sheila, like others in this study, willingly participated in breast reconstruction. Dorothy Smith describes women as viewing their bodies as objects to be fixed and improved.[63] When I interviewed her, Sheila was still working on her body and imagining the decisions she might have made and the outcomes she might have liked. And even now, she envied young women and their two "normal" breasts.

Almost every woman I interviewed had breasts that were permanently altered after treatment for breast cancer. This was the most visible reminder they had of the experience they had been through. It also reminded them of the possibility of a reoccurrence. In their article on cosmetic surgery, Diana Dull and Candace West distinguished between reconstructive plastic surgery and cosmetic surgery.[64] However, since reconstructed breasts are patterned after enhanced breasts, not actual breasts, the distinction is fuzzy. Part of the problem women experienced with breast reconstruction is that both they and their plastic surgeons envisioned breasts that looked like ones from central casting, rather than the breasts that had actually been removed.

While breast disfigurement was an ordeal experienced by every woman who had breast cancer, it was not the only bodily ordeal for women, at least in the short run. As is discussed in the next chapter, for many women, this was but one of several issues they faced after being diagnosed with breast cancer.

SEVEN Bodies after Cancer

After their treatment for breast cancer, the women I interviewed remained acutely aware of the changes to their breasts every time they looked in the mirror. Postlumpectomy breasts usually showed the damage clearly. For women who had a mastectomy, reconstruction could lessen its impact, but reconstructed breasts never looked or felt as they had before surgery. Most women mourned these permanent changes as constant reminders of what they had been through.

However, in addition to the direct effects of breast surgery, women experienced other bodily changes. These, too, were usually for the worse. Two of the most devastating were hair loss, which most women had anticipated, and weight gain, which they had not. Furthermore, the combined effects of a near-death experience, treatment, and these bodily changes had an impact on many women's emotional and sexual lives.

This was sometimes exacerbated when treatment put them into menopause. This chapter explores these issues and the interrelationships among them. Although there were some variations by response group, almost all the women in this study found these changes difficult to cope with.

Chapter 1 discusses the ways in which women's narratives about breast cancer follow predictable forms. This is most apparent in their stories about weight. Many women found weight gain to be the most unpleasant side effect of breast cancer. A number of them had struggled with excess weight even before diagnosis. Some women told what Douglas Degher and Gerald Hughes have called "fat stories." In these stories, women explained how breast cancer treatment had caused weight gain and why they were unable to lose weight. Other women told "eating stories," which excused excessive eating during breast cancer treatment.[1] These stories reflect the cultural obsession with weight, particularly women's weight, and this affected even those who claimed not to care. Kimberly, a biomedical expert introduced in chapter 6, was a beauty shop owner. She described herself as disinterested in her appearance, even though she was "in the beauty industry." In further discussion, however, she exhibited considerable ambivalence about her body, just as she had about her breasts. After saying "I'm comfortable enough with every shape I am, I think," she declared: "Oh God, who's satisfied with the way their body looks? No, I would like it to be beautiful, but it's not going to happen." This, she said, was because "I'm not a hard worker at making my body look good."

In *Unbearable Weight,* Susan Bordo documented the trend since the early 1980s in which women came to believe that they must do more than avoid excess weight; they must try to sculpt perfect bodies. A less than perfect body indicates that its owner has not dieted sufficiently hard or worked out with the necessary discipline, and others make negative judgments about this.[2] While these pressures affect both men and women, they are stronger, and negative evaluations are more disapproving, where women are concerned.[3] Judith Lorber has described the ways in which gendered social practices transform bodies—in the case of women, to fit an ideal of feminine beauty.[4] In a study of a commercial weight loss program, Kandi Stinson found that a strong work ethic was deemed essential to successful weight loss. Women who failed to lose weight were described as "lazy."[5] Kimberly had internalized the norm that the right look can be earned through hard work. Even though she described herself as unwilling to do this work, she had attended Weight Watchers for about a year before her diagnosis and had learned to "eat everything in moderation." In addition, she had walked at least three miles a day and lifted "little weights" four times a week.

In addition to its role as a signifier of discipline and hard work, weight has become a marker of health. Much of the rhetoric about weight and health comes from the medical profession, but it has become a generally accepted truth.[6] Nita McKinley has noted that a person's weight tells others whether or not that person is living a healthy lifestyle, that is, eating the right foods and engaging in an appropriate amount of exercise. McKinley further argued that women face additional scrutiny; they are under particular pressure to contain and control their weight.[7] Yet, as Deborah Lupton has observed, most women are more concerned about the appearance of an overweight and underexercised body than about the health aspects of excess weight.[8] Some studies have found that most women, including women of average weight, perceive themselves as too fat, whereas men often wish to gain weight.[9] Finally, there is research showing that overweight women manage their identities in ways that allow them to resist negative stereotypes; this was found among a few women in my study.[10]

Given Kimberly's struggle to attain the idealized thin female body, she became frustrated when she gained weight during treatment. Since she did not need chemotherapy, she started taking tamoxifen immediately after her surgery.[11] She became so upset when she "gained six pounds like gangbusters" in the first few weeks of taking this medicine that she stopped taking it. Slightly overweight at the time of the interview, she had been outraged with her male oncologist, who told her that the total weight gain on tamoxifen would be "not very much, like fifteen, thirty pounds." For Kimberly, even her six-pound weight gain was "worse than having breast cancer."

I judged about one-third of the women to be overweight at the time of my interview. Of these, many were quite obese, and most had been unhappy about their bodies for a long time.[12] Time and again, women told me that they had thought they would lose weight as a result of their treatment, and that this would be one of breast cancer's few benefits. Instead, half gained weight and less than a third lost. Gaining weight seemed like the ultimate breast cancer outrage. There was little difference, by response group, in weight before diagnosis or in the proportion who gained weight. However, biomedical experts were more likely to lose weight during treatment than any other group; in the other three groups less than one-quarter of the women lost weight, but among the biomedical experts over 40 percent did. As is discussed in chapter 3, biomedical experts had been particularly concerned about losing control, and, as a result, many had become vigilant about eating a low-fat, healthy diet after diagnosis and following an exercise program. This no doubt had an impact on their weight. Losing weight in the face of a high probability of gaining was a way of maintaining control. Pierre Bordieu has argued that there are class differences in attitudes toward the body, and that the upper middle class is particularly inclined to believe in the value of a slender body and to think that this can be achieved by self-control.[13] As we saw, biomedical experts were overwhelmingly affluent and well educated, and many held the views Bordieu described.

However, regardless of group, there was no difference in how women felt about weight gain. Women who gained weight were upset by it in every instance. Given the many similarities of experience among the women in the four groups, I decided to write about all their experiences of bodily changes in a single chapter, as with chapter 6 on the appearance of postsurgery breasts, rather than about each group separately. I wanted to avoid repetition and to explore the reasons these issues loomed so large for all women, regardless of class, race, or education. There were some differences in how each group coped with bodily changes, which I explore here.

Many traditional responders, for example, felt defeated by weight gain. They did not find it easy to control the body in the manner Bordieu described and had thought breast cancer might take care of the problem for them. However, they were just as upset as those in the other groups when they experienced weight gain. Gabrielle, introduced in chapter 2, put it this way:

I must have weighed maybe 180, and I went up to about—I remember them saying, "199," "200," "199." My thoughts—when you see someone with cancer—is people lose weight. And I'm thinking, "Okay, this is my chance. At least when I come out of this, I'm going to be thin." And I gained weight.

When a woman diagnosed with breast cancer sees a potential weight loss as a compensation for her illness, it marks the importance of weight in Western society and of the "spoiled identity"[14] associated with fatness. Indeed, men regard overweight women in especially negative terms,[15] and such women are discriminated against more than overweight men.[16] No wonder Kimberly was furious with the male physician who told her not to worry about weight gain. At a time in women's lives when their breasts were under assault, it should be no surprise that weight gain seemed an intolerable indignity.

Like Kimberly, Gabrielle's weight gain during breast cancer was one episode in a longer battle. She had long been an on-and-off participant in Weight Watchers, and, as she put it, she knew "about eating healthy and all that." After breast cancer, however, things became even more difficult. She was premenopausal when diagnosed at age forty-seven but reported that her "last menstrual period was the same weekend that my hair fell out." This meant that in addition to the weight gain from treatment, she also had to contend with the weight gain that is common among women after menopause.[17] After finishing chemotherapy, she lost the added pounds, because she "worked on it and walked . . . like a maniac." However, when she returned to the oncologist for a checkup, she had a low white blood cell count, "and the doctor told me I should just focus [on work], and in the summer, walk." As a result, Gabrielle stopped exercising for a while, and her weight jumped yet again. Like many traditional respondents, Gabrielle found that acting to benefit her own destiny was often harder in practice than in theory.

The next summer when Gabrielle was off from teaching, she started over: "I went on Weight Watchers and I must have lost forty pounds all last summer." However, she explained that she "got pneumonia last August" and once again, "Just about all of it has come back on now. So now I'm back on Weight Watchers again." Gabrielle understood that "It's not healthy to yo-yo and then gain and then take it off." She had gained an estimated twenty pounds from the time she started taking tamoxifen. When the doctor told her "You have to lose this," Gabrielle answered, "If you'd stop putting me on this medicine I would." Gabrielle's explanation of her weight gain mirrors the eating stories that Degher and Hughes heard in their study of how overweight people managed a "fat" identity.[18] Stories like Gabrielle's and Kimberly's medicalize the problem of weight, which lets women assuage their guilt over their presumed lack of self-control.

Gabrielle's frustration at the oncologist's mixed messages was understandable. In general, however, women were more likely to be told by doctors not to worry about weight gain than they were to be told to lose weight. Rosamund, met in the chapter on religious responders, had been somewhat overweight before diagnosis and gained fifteen pounds during chemotherapy:

> I was not pleased. And the doctor, he was good. He kept saying, "This is natural . . . when you're done with the treatments, then focus on the weight. . . ." One of the dieticians had also stressed that. She was saying with the mouth sores or whatever, "Gravy will help things slide down, so put gravy on stuff and don't worry about the calories."

Forty-five years old at diagnosis, Rosamund went into menopause as a result of chemotherapy, which did not help her avoid gaining weight. In addition, menopause made her feel "not good":

> I felt that I would've liked to have gone into it the way you normally would where it's a gradual thing. . . . The hot flashes and all were very embarrassing for me. And the vaginal dryness and all of that, that was very embarrassing for me. . . . I never had another period, once I had the chemo. . . . I wasn't even ready to start thinking about menopause yet, and then I'm in it.

Through a combination of diet and exercise, Rosamund was able to lose the weight she had gained after her treatment was over. Stinson has made the point that women's dieting experiences tell us about more than cultural expectations; they also tell us about the material nature of the body and the relationship of eating to the physical.[19] Narratives such as the ones told here underscore this point. The stories tell how illness had made control over bodies even more difficult than before. Women who long had had issues with weight had learned that eating could only be controlled through hard work. However, illness had taken this possibility away from many women.

Weight gain was not confined to women who had previously struggled with weight. Even some women who had been satisfied with their weight before diagnosis found themselves gaining weight through a combination of medication and menopause. Alicia, a thirty-nine-year-old real estate office manager and a traditional responder, had never really struggled with weight issues before cancer. During chemotherapy, she gained twenty pounds. She, too, received the message that she should not try to lose right now:

> I'm not too happy, but I figured if that is a side effect, and it is all part of me getting well, I'll deal with it later. . . . I'm still struggling. I'm taking it off very slowly, because I don't want to jeopardize my health. . . .
> I'd say I've taken off about five. My doctor said, "Don't worry about it, eat. . . . Please, whatever you do, don't diet. Don't start an exercise program. Don't start anything goofy, because the main thing is to keep your strength up."

Although Alicia was not happy about the weight gain, she was calmer about it than women whose weight had been an issue for much of their adult lives. Unlike them, she was confident that she would lose the additional weight after chemotherapy was over. She believed this even though "my chemo threw me into menopause," which "has been permanent so far." Alicia had been warned that this was a possibility and that, if she wanted to have more children, she should either "not continue with the treatment" or freeze her eggs. Since Alicia did not want more children, she was fine with her loss of fertility, but menopause was "not fun."

Many women experienced a loss of body definition in addition to weight gain; the combination of breast deformities and weight gain made them feel shapeless and, therefore, old. Lupton argued that the aging body is a source of anxiety in Western society because bodily signs of aging are seen as abhorrent.[20] We saw evidence of this in the last chapter, with women's reactions to their breasts becoming uneven or ill-shaped.

Dinah was a traditional responder, age fifty, postmenopausal, and "ten pounds overweight" at diagnosis. A large-breasted woman, she had worn "tailor-made clothes" to her job in the family-owned business and had liked getting dressed up every day. As Dinah put it, "You had the big breasts, so that, no matter what you had on your rib cage or your waist, you looked fabulous." Dinah saw her shape as a crucial marker of gender.

After a mastectomy and chemotherapy, Dinah gained twenty-seven pounds. She had reduction surgery on the healthy breast, because the plastic surgeon could not reconstruct her missing breast to be as large as it had been before surgery. So, now, she had a larger stomach and smaller breasts. Dinah had just come back from a trip and in the pictures they had taken, "I look like a fat old broad." Then she added, "But I'm a healthy fat old broad." Her assumptions that shapely breasts and body were signifiers of youth and that a youthful figure is desirable in women reflect the cultural messages discussed in chapter 1, in which breast cancer is portrayed as a young women's disease.

At the same time as she mourned the passing of her youthful feminine figure, Dinah was using a common coping strategy. She justified her weight by saying that she was healthy, and thereby, she moved herself away from negative assessments about weight and health.[21] She also hated her scars, but she found a way to come to terms with them as well. As she put it, "I went from always worrying about, 'How would someone identify me if I was in an automobile accident, because I have no identifying scars' to 'There's no mistaking me now.'" Dinah's body was replete with markers of the history of her illness.

In contrast to women who gained weight, some lost. Philomena, a biomedical expert, was forty-one years old when diagnosed and had felt her life was going well. Slim and attractive, she earned a comfortable income in pharmaceutical sales. During chemotherapy, she lost ten pounds. This gave her a feeling of being in control, but, in addition, there was another gain:

> I looked really good, I thought. Jeans looked really good. I knew it was a little too much, but it was that sort of borderline. With just only a couple of pounds more, I'd be model-perfect in my clothes.

Although Philomena put the weight back on slowly, and although she knew that this weight gain was a good thing, she experienced regret at never getting to be "model-perfect." Like almost everyone else in the study, she had internalized the values about perfect bodies. Much has been written about women who diet to excess, as is the case with anorexia.[22] Women with these illnesses are a more extreme version of the far larger group of women like Philomena, who do not really feel good about their appearance unless they are very thin.[23] Moreover, biomedical experts, like Philomena, were particularly susceptible to a desire to control their illness through weight loss.

Hedley, a biomedical expert discussed in chapter 3, was slender when I interviewed her and had a similar tale of the desire for thinness:

> I have always struggled with my body image, always felt too heavy. I was heavier. . . . I liked the fact that I lost weight, so I liked it when this breast got very small. I lost twenty-five, thirty pounds. I got terribly thin. . . . I have a full-length mirror upstairs, and I did not use it during that time. A couple of months after I finished chemo, I went on a trip and I was in a hotel, and I got out of the shower and there was a mirror right there. I remember being astounded at myself. I looked like I just got out of a concentration camp.

In spite of the painful honesty of this description, Hedley reported that she had not tried to gain any weight after treatment ended. Still, she had gained ten pounds back, and she ended her comments about weight by declaring, "I usually feel fat."

Perhaps the best way of illustrating the complicated relationship between breast cancer and weight is to look at women whose weight fluctuated during treatment. Madeline, a sixty-two-year-old biomedical expert, had been unhappy with her weight before diagnosis and was overweight when I met her. She had monitored her weight carefully during treatment and watched the changes:

> I had lost weight after I first found out, and I was happy to lose the ten pounds. Then during the chemo, the first week I couldn't eat well, so I lost weight. And then the second and third week, I was so happy to get my appetite back, I ate. So I never really ended up losing weight.

Madeline described her weight as a lifetime struggle: "I'm always trying to lose weight." Like many women in this study, she had a difficult relationship with food, and although she described eating a balanced diet, she added, "I have a sweet tooth that I'm trying to control." She saw her experience during chemotherapy as a particularly difficult episode in this battle. Like many others, she had thought cancer would produce the compensation of weight loss, a compensation she dearly wanted in this thinness-obsessed culture. Madeline talked the language of control and had been active in the decision-making throughout her illness, but her weight fluctuations felt like defeat.

Like Madeline, Trish, age thirty-six at diagnosis and an alternative expert met in chapter 6, had believed herself to be overweight by "about fifteen to twenty pounds." This was also my assessment of her weight, at our interview. Like other women in the study, she had been "trying to lose weight," but her weight fluctuated during treatment:

> At first I lost weight . . . on the AC.[24] Then I started gaining weight. It would go up and down. . . . For the five to seven days after the AC, I would lose weight, then I would compensate by, "Well, I'm gonna eat ice cream and make up for lost time. . . ." I gained weight on the Taxotere[25] . . . probably ten pounds lost on chemo, and then I gained it back plus probably another five pounds. . . . Nobody told me I should watch my weight. . . . I've probably lost about five pounds so far.

Like a number of women who gained weight, Trish held her doctor responsible for not warning her to watch her weight. Yet Trish had been fighting her weight for most of her life, so she might have been expected to anticipate the possibility of weight gain. Biomedical experts and alternative experts were more likely to blame doctors for weight gain than to blame themselves. This is understandable because these two groups were more critical of shortfalls in the medical care they received. In contrast, traditional responders and religious responders were more likely to blame themselves. This is undoubtedly related to the class differences noted among the groups. The more affluent and educated biomedical and alternative experts were more inclined to believe they were managing their illness admirably and therefore to blame the medical profession when things did not go according to plan.

Weight gain was not the only indignity to their bodies that women suffered when undergoing chemotherapy. For some, hair loss, not weight, was the most problematic side effect. As Rose Weitz has pointed out, American women are obsessed with their hair.[26] She noted that women who lose their hair as a result of breast cancer face a complicated set of psychological and social effects. Rita Freedman has described women's hair as "a source of hedonic power that can be used to attract attention."[27]

Women who did not have chemotherapy were spared the experience of hair loss. Sometimes chemotherapy caused hair to thin, and this was not always noticed. However, two of the most common chemotherapy drugs—Adriamycin and Taxotere—cause women to lose their hair entirely. And since Taxotere is typically taken after Adriamycin treatment finishes and hair has started to grow back, some women lose their hair twice. Approximately half the women in this study lost all their hair. This was difficult whenever it happened, but over half of those who lost their hair took it especially hard. This did not vary by response group. Hair was important to everyone not only because luxurious hair is a feminine signifier but also because of the association of hair loss with illness. As Ava, a religious responder who was fifty-six years old at diagnosis, put it:

> That was the most traumatic part of the whole thing. The day I looked in the mirror, and, I mean, it was coming out. I saved it, and I used to put it in a tissue. And the next day, when I'd get more, I'd throw that one away. . . . That day I could see the bald spots. I stood in front of the mirror, and I cried. My husband was here and he said, "What's the matter?" And I said, "You couldn't see the cancer, but you can see this."

Ella, a biomedical expert introduced in chapter 6, also stated that losing her hair "made me look sick—it made me look like I had cancer." Myra, a traditional responder met in chapter 2, described it even more graphically, saying, "You look at yourself, and I felt that I looked like a concentration camp victim."

For a minority of women, their hair had been one of the things they really loved about their appearance. Hedley described herself as having "very good hair . . . thick and wavy in adulthood." She added, "It has probably been one of two parts of my body that I did like, and it was a real part of my identity, so to lose it terrified me." Some women who had

loved their hair went to great lengths to ensure that its loss remained private. Dinah, the traditional responder discussed above, described herself
as "totally losing it" when she looked in the mirror and all she saw was
"a bald head." She was determined to keep her head covered at all times.
She wore her wig during the day and a turban at night:

> I would wear the turban to bed. . . . I had this fixation that [my husband]
> shouldn't see me without my hair. I woke up in the middle of the night,
> and the turban was off. I was like, "Oh, I've got to find my turban." This
> went on for about two or three weeks.

This added to Dinah's sense that she was aging rapidly. She had gone
from being ten pounds overweight with fabulous breasts and a full head
of hair—a woman who loved getting dressed up every day—to being a
"fat old broad" with shapeless smaller breasts, a bigger body, and no hair.
She no longer cared about her appearance as she once had.

For some women, adjusting to hair loss was painful but could be managed with the support of others. Aisha, a traditional responder, was only
thirty-four years old at diagnosis, the mother of two young sons and living in a small house in the outer suburbs. An African American who had
worn her hair long and straightened, she had gone to great effort to get it
the way she wanted, and she had been very proud of it. This is how she
described hair loss:

> In the beginning, it started coming out in handfuls, and every day my
> husband came home from work, and I would be crying because I would
> comb my hair and it would come out in brushes full. He said, "Aisha,
> why don't you just let me shave it off?" I fought him for a week, so
> finally I had this patch of hair on top. . . . I said, "You know, we should
> just cut it off. . . ." That was the best thing I did . . . and I kind of felt like
> it was okay for him to cut it off if I took charge, as opposed to the cancer
> taking charge.

Aisha had worried about her children's reaction to the hair loss, but
things turned out differently than she expected:

> My oldest came in the bathroom after my husband had shaved me. He
> says, "Hey, Mommy cut her hair—cool." And then my youngest one,

when he saw, he says, "Mommy, you look beautiful." And of course I cried. . . . It didn't matter to them. So when I was around the house I basically didn't wear anything.

Aisha had assumed that her children would react to hair loss as adults did, but her young sons were fans of Michael Jordan and really did think that bald heads were cool.

Adults realized only too well how our culture interprets hair loss. Honor, a traditional responder, found she had breast cancer at age fifty. Coming from a family with a history of this disease, she had responded calmly to treatment until she lost her hair. Before hair loss, a friend had advised her to buy a wig before she needed it:

> I had researched it . . . and even talked to a friend of ours who is a manu-facturer of wigs. His advice was to buy a synthetic wig, which I did, and I went with my sister to a place. . . . A very nice woman waited on me, who was obviously in tune to do this type of thing. And we tried to make fun of the whole thing. We tried different—you know, blondes, redheads and so on.

At this point, Honor thought she was proceeding in her usual calm man-ner. However, she continued:

> I'll never forget, when I walked out of there [the saleswoman] said to my sister, "You'd better take your sister for a drink, because she's in a state of shock." I had never really looked at it that way. But we did come home, and we were living in an apartment at the time, and I'll never forget when my sister pulled up. I was so hysterical that the poor door-man came to the door to open the car, and my sister said, "Forget it," and we just drove off.

Honor eventually came to terms with losing her hair. She bought three or four inexpensive wigs. Then she and her daughter-in-law bought hats and scarves, and when she was at the seashore she wore those. She was careful not to let anyone but family see her bald head, and, looking back, she still felt that "losing it was probably the most traumatic thing that happened."

Honor's experience in wig buying was fairly typical according to a beautician and professional wig fitter I interviewed, Maria Scarduzio. Half of Maria's business involved selling wigs to breast cancer patients. Her experience doing this led her to believe that many women were more upset about losing their hair than losing a breast. Women who experienced hair loss had a predictable set of fears: they worried about scaring their children, they wanted to continue working and felt the need to look their best during chemotherapy, and they worried about their appearance on special occasions such as weddings. Finally, they did not always know where to turn to get help. Some places, Maria reported, hung numerous wigs on the wall, and women got disoriented looking at them. Other places mixed breast cancer patients buying wigs in with women having their healthy hair done. All too frequently, buying a wig became one more burden for women when they felt especially fragile.

Maria took care to provide a private setting for wig consultations—women who were losing their hair did not want to sit next to beauty parlor clients. She also advised women to pick the wig closest to their natural hair color, even though many of them came in looking for something different. She sold every type of wig, from ready-made synthetic ones to custom-made natural hair wigs, for which women could spend up to two thousand dollars. Maria viewed breast cancer as a tremendous crisis for women and believed it was her responsibility to give them all the care and sympathy she could.[28] She saw herself as helping women maintain their femininity at a time when it was under assault. For most women, hair was an important part of being a woman, and they wanted to keep up the appearance of femininity, even through an illusion.

A few women coped with hair loss without too much trauma, sometimes even managing to find something positive in the experience. Jeanne, a biomedical expert who planned everything carefully, bought a natural hair wig, paid for by her insurance. Many insurance companies will pay for wigs, once again underscoring the idea that it is healthy for women to care so much about appearance. Jeanne's wig was dyed to match her hair color, so most people never realized she was bald. The wig salon advised her, "Get a sleep cap, because you'll find when you wake up in the morning, your loss will not be all over your pillowcase." Once she lost her hair, she wore the sleep cap every night because it kept her head warm. When she was with her family and close friends, she would ask them if she could take the wig off, because "I tried to educate them" about the effects of breast cancer.

In addition to her struggle with weight described above, Alicia lost all her hair. She described this as very strange, because you lose "even your nose hair." She delighted in the fact that her skin became very smooth, noting, "You enjoy the little things that you can get out of chemo." The most positive experience, however, was that her husband shaved his hair:

> So the next day is Sunday and all the guys [at church] are coming up to my husband, hugging my husband, crying . . . because what a sweet sentiment. . . . We had our picture taken. . . . The photographer did not know what to think at first . . . and we're talking and we're joking around. And we're telling him, "You know what this is? You know that I don't have AIDS. We're not skinheads. This is just part of our cancer treatment." And the next thing you know they're crying, and they said, "You can have the pictures for free."

Alicia grew quite comfortable with her bald head and told me that she only covered it when she went to work "because I did not want to offend or scare" anyone.

I noted that Philomena exulted in her weight loss in spite of losing her hair. Philomena's mother helped her style the synthetic wig she bought. Philomena did not like it even so, and instead she wore baseball hats whenever she could. But once her hair started to grow back, she faced another challenge:

> A whole bunch of us were going to a Halloween party. I said, "Gee, I just don't know what to be." And [my friend] said, "I know you hate that wig of yours, you would make an awesome GI Jane." And I said, "Done. That is when the wig is coming off. It's never going back on again. . . ." I went right to [the army surplus store and] got the tiniest little fatigues, and I thought, well, being Demi Moore, her breasts are definitely bigger than mine, so I put on a miracle bra and stuffed that a little more. I felt the world that night. . . . I was never wearing my wig again.

Sandra Bartky has described our culture as embodying a "tyranny of slenderness"—the idea that women should take up as little space as possible.[29] Philomena underscored this point; she could wear her hair very short without losing her femininity, because her body was that of an appropriately small woman.

When hair grew back, it often was different, typically curlier and grayer than before. Gabrielle had been blonde and straight-haired all her life. Hers grew back curly and dark:

> I went from being my father's daughter to my mother's. . . . It stayed curly for two years. . . . I loved the curly hair. There were ringlets. I just loved washing it and having it. . . . I thought God owed me this. Now I have waves and body. . . . I'll be walking by the mall, and I'll have this picture of myself, what I've looked like my whole life, and I expect to see a blond-haired person going by, and I'll still do a double-take if I catch myself in a mirror.

Gabrielle's beautiful hair was compensation for her struggles with weight. Like other women in the study, her worries about the performance of gender were so strong that she kept a private score sheet. She calibrated the loss of femininity from the weight gain and balanced it against the feminizing effect of ringlets.

Given their numerous physical changes, we might expect women's intimate relationships to change also, and, in many cases, they did. Almost half of those who were involved in an intimate relationship reported that they became closer as a result of breast cancer, while many of the rest commented that the relationship was already good before and stayed the same after. However, in the main, cancer did not have a positive effect on women's sexual relationships: over one-third reported losing interest in sex, and many women reported that their partners became hesitant about touching their breasts after surgery. Several writers have noted that the sexual effects of breast cancer are multiple and are connected to a number of the issues raised in this chapter and the previous one, including changes in the appearance of breasts, weight gain, the effects of treatment on well-being, and hair loss.[30] Women equate beauty with sexuality, and when they feel unattractive sexually, they often are disinterested in sex.

Changes in intimate relations varied by response group. Religious responders were more likely to report intimate relationships that increased in closeness than did those in any other group. Almost three-quarters of religious responders reported this. The other three groups were all fairly similar to each other in this regard, with about half reporting increased closeness. There was a greater range in the rates of loss of sexual interest by group. Almost two-thirds of the traditional responders reported losing interest in sex, compared to just over a third of the religious responders and less than a quarter of either the biomedical or the alternative experts.

How can we make sense of these differences? Traditional responders were women who felt a tremendous responsibility to care for family members, even while sick, and who found the diagnosis especially frightening. It is not surprising, therefore, that although almost half of them became emotionally closer to their partners, many were too exhausted by the whole experience to feel sexually responsive. Religious responders, in contrast, not only reported feeling closer to their partners, but also closer to God. They had experienced breast cancer as part of a religious journey with a better outcome at the end, and, not surprisingly, an outcome that was better for their families. Biomedical and alternative experts had steered their own ships through diagnosis and treatment. These women were evenly divided between those whose relationships improved and those whose relationships stayed the same, but most of them did not let a breast cancer diagnosis stand in the way of their right to sexual pleasure. Social class privilege allowed these women a level of care that left them sufficiently rested to enjoy sex.

Ella, an African American lawyer, was a traditional responder with a breast reconstruction that she found frighteningly ugly. This may have been part of the reason for the traumatic effect of breast cancer on her marriage. Her husband, she reported, did not know how to deal with her reaction to cancer:

> He pretends like it's not there and it doesn't bother him, but he won't touch it there, and he says he won't touch it there because I don't want him to touch it. . . . With these hot flashes, I just want to be left alone.

Ella's husband appeared unexpectedly in the middle of our interview. He had come home from his job saying he needed something. Ella explained:

He knew you were coming, and I knew he was gonna find an excuse to come here. . . . I mean, he really had to do a lot while I was sick and the baby was small, so he had a lot of burdens on him. . . . I think, now, he thinks I'm cured, and it's over, and it's done. . . . He knows that talking about it upsets me, so we don't talk about it. But if we do talk about it, his attitude is that there's nothing wrong with me and that it's all taken care of. I'm all better; nothing else is ever gonna happen.

So Ella and her husband both remained fearful of the future. She was still frightened about cancer and unhappy about her appearance. She did not feel attractive and could not imagine that he found her attractive. He also seemed to be frightened, wanting her reassurance, not her fears, so he coped by denying anything further could happen. Yet his wife was only thirty-four at diagnosis. Since breast cancer is more virulent in younger, premenopausal women, and Ella had had three positive lymph nodes, which increased her risk of metastasis, she had reason for continued vigilance and concern.

Aisha's narrative reflected that of a number of traditional responders. Even though Aisha's hair loss had been traumatic, she remained amorous throughout chemotherapy. However, she lost interest in sex once she started tamoxifen,[31] although in some ways, her marital relationship improved:

I honestly think if I didn't have my children and my husband, I would have lain down and just died, because I would have had nothing to fight for. . . . The chemo—it just takes everything from you. . . . In my eyes that was worse than actually losing the breast. I think [our relationship] has gotten a lot better. Throughout the cancer, he was there for me, and we've gotten a lot closer. . . . We still don't talk the way I'd like for us to talk. . . . I guess he had to help through the chemo, and he never really stopped helping since then. . . . It seems like I don't want [sex] quite as much as I did before . . . but I consciously try not to say no to him, because it's just not right. . . . We feel closer to each other. Or, I should say, I feel closer to him. With men, it's different, you know.

These two stories reflect many cultural beliefs about the differences between men and women. Both women reported that they wanted a different kind of talk than their husbands provided. This "feeling" kind of

talk, they believed, was difficult for men, and Ella, who was more traumatized by the whole experience than Aisha, found this particularly
hard. Aisha believed that she needed to be sexually responsive to her
husband even if she were not feeling amorous, because husbands need
physical passion rather than emotional talk. She believed that her sexual
relationship had in some ways improved, because she felt more loving
toward her husband. Aisha remained optimistic that things would continue to improve. When I interviewed her, a family birthday party was
soon to start. Aisha's husband was busily entertaining the boys and getting everything ready in the backyard as she and I talked.

Francesca Cancian has taken issue with the large number of studies
that see women as more interested and skilled in love than men.[32] She
finds these studies biased because they measure love by things like ver-
bal self-disclosure and emotional expression and do not include more
practical measures of love. Men, Cancian argues, show their love through
practical help, joint activities, and sex.[33] Aisha's relationship with her
husband reflected these differences, but Aisha interpreted this to mean
that she had become closer to her husband and that it most likely was not
reciprocated.

Shantal, the religious responder introduced in chapter 4, strengthened
her relationship with her spouse after diagnosis, even though they had
had a close relationship already. His care, including nursing care, brought
them together:

> He was there, my husband, twenty-four hours a day, every day. . . . [He]
> did whatever had to be done in the house for several weeks. No one else
> did anything, my husband did it. . . . When I first had the surgery, I had
> a drain there, and the next day . . . someone was supposed to pull the
> drain, and he offered to do it. . . . He didn't know whether it would
> hemorrhage or whether it wouldn't come out. . . . I didn't know that
> until later. . . . My husband was there for emotional support.

Shantal's positive outlook on her marriage was reflected in her assurance
that breast cancer had not changed her sexual relationship at all. Her husband provided both the practical support Cancian describes as normative
for men and the more womanly kind of emotional support. This is a man,
as mentioned in chapter 4, who cried when his wife was diagnosed.

Another religious responder, Glenna, felt that breast cancer had deepened her relationship with her husband. Like Shantal, she had had a fairly traditional marriage. With breast cancer, things changed at least temporarily:

> It offered us an opportunity to kind of reverse roles in terms of personal care, in terms of helping to support each other in that I'm the more emotional and physical supporter of around the house, whereas he provides for things outside the home like working and all. . . . [Breast cancer] put some stresses, but I think in hindsight it was healthy for our relationship, and we were able to talk through issues that we probably wouldn't have been able to talk about before.

In spite of this closeness, Glenna was like many respondents in that her interest in sex became "basically nonexistent" during chemotherapy, and afterward she developed vaginal dryness, which created a second set of problems. She added, "That corrected itself, but then I was tired from the radiation, so it's just been one kind of thing after another." She noted, however, that their improved communication was helpful in working through some of these sexual problems.

Eve, a biomedical expert first discussed in chapter 3, experienced no loss of interest in sex as a result of breast cancer. She described her husband as "wonderful" before breast cancer but said that, since her diagnosis, things had become even better. This was because time together seemed more precious than before:

> Sometimes, he'd be traveling around the world, get home late Friday night, and we would go to synagogue on Saturday afternoon. He would come into work, and, on Sunday he would be off around the world again. But that little Saturday morning always came to be time that we spent together, and that mattered.

Also, when Eve developed a painful thrush in her mouth as a result of chemotherapy, her "wonderful husband and the blender saved me from going into the hospital. He had to blend up everything . . . to get some nourishment."

Since the breast cancer, Eve said she was trying to take things "easy."

Because her husband had been "so nice all the time," her interest in sex increased during chemotherapy and had remained high since. Eve described herself as "dating my husband," adding that "We're having a good time" even though "He's a workaholic and so am I." Although her description of her husband's increased availability might not seem extensive, Eve and her husband had worked constantly throughout their marriage. After breast cancer, she noted, "We're putting in time for ourselves and not postponing things." Eve's story was one of managing her life and increasing her pleasures, now that she had faced her mortality. As a professional woman, Eve understood the career pressures on her husband and appreciated his willingness to set aside time for her. Neither she nor her husband had been used to the type of emotional self-disclosure described by Cancian. This is a woman who had to go to a psychotherapeutic support group to learn how to talk about her cancer and whose husband had not told his parents that his wife had been ill, for fear of distressing them. Only some couples were in the types of relationships where the husband showed his love by doing and the wife by being, and this most commonly occurred for the traditional responders.

Like Eve, Pearl, the biomedical expert whose resistance to breast reconstruction is discussed in chapter 6, described her husband as having been wonderful before breast cancer and continuing to be wonderful after diagnosis. Her sexual relationship had gone through some changes but had survived more or less intact. Like a number of respondents, her husband had been unsure about touching her remaining breast or her scar after surgery. She explained this by saying, "When you're recovering from surgery, you yourself aren't sure what you can tolerate, and they're certainly very cautious." Still, she added, "You get through it together, you know, you just take it slowly . . . and before you know it, nothing's changed." This nervousness about touching breasts was something biomedical experts often dealt with in a direct manner. For example, Annette, who had a "wonderful" and supportive husband, had said to him, "Do you realize you never touch my breasts anymore?" When her husband answered that this was because he thought it might hurt, she was able to put him straight. Even in this intimate aspect of their lives, biomedical experts described themselves as remaining in charge. They were more likely to view sexual pleasure as an entitlement like a man might rather than as contingent on their personal attractiveness. They were used to expressing themselves directly at work and in their personal lives.

Although alternative experts did not, in general, have as many close relationships as biomedical experts, this was not universally true. Laura had lived with the same woman for five years before being diagnosed:

> It was already an incredibly intense close relationship, and it [the bad news] just drew us even more closely together—the fear that perhaps I could die and we needed to spend time together. . . . It was hard for her, because she would have to go to work in the morning and I'd stand at the door going, "Goodbye," and looking pitiful.

At the time of the interview, Laura had just learned that her partner had a malignant tumor in her nasal passage, and the memories of her own cancer experience had come flooding back. When I interviewed her, her partner was present for the introductions, and the tenderness between the two women was palpable. Laura did not have close relationships with the rest of her family, so she relied on her partner for many things.

Many alternative experts did not have such a close long-term relationship, but even so they tended to report satisfactory sex lives. Jasmine was forty-seven years old at diagnosis and engaged in a passionate, sexual relationship with a younger man. One day, she told the oncologist that as soon as her appointment was over, "I am going to go home and have sex with my friend." The oncologist asked Jasmine, with some surprise, if she still was interested in sex, and Jasmine replied, "Sure I [am]. Is that supposed to change?" The oncologist answered, "Not necessarily, it may or it may not." Jasmine had the last word with, "Well, if something happens, I'm coming back to tell you, because we have sex quite often." Jasmine felt entitled to good sex whenever she wanted it, and in this way alternative experts were like biomedical experts. Jasmine's relationship ended shortly after this because, although it was sexually fulfilling, it lacked the emotional support Jasmine desired while undergoing treatment. Where traditional responders made excuses for the lack of emotional support from the men in their lives, alternative experts felt entitled to get the type of support they desired. They enjoyed seeing themselves as unique and different, and Jasmine told the story of the oncologist's reaction with relish.

Since many alternative experts were either divorced or never married, they did not always have the emotional support of a mate. However, this was something that most of them wanted. Hannah, introduced in chapter 5, had been divorced for years before her diagnosis but met someone early in her treatment:

> I think he was probably sent as an angel to me . . . and I went out to dinner with him, and he was very nice, and I said, "You know what? You're a nice man, but I'm not interested in dating you now. Call me in six months. I'm just starting to walk down this very difficult road in my life." And he said, "That's okay." I said, "You don't understand, I've just been diagnosed with breast cancer. . . . I don't really feel like dating, and I'm not going to be any fun. . . ." This man was a chemist, so he would do a lot of the research for me, and he hung in with me. He was really quite lovely throughout the whole thing.

Hannah described herself as having had a temporary lessening of sexual interest during treatment, but she added that she "didn't lose it totally" and that, after treatment, it came back completely.

In time, many of the issues around weight, hair, and sexual interest resolved themselves either by a return to the situation as it had been before or because the aging process, not breast cancer, came to be defined as the cause of changes. A number of women, for example, told me that while their sexual interest had waned during breast cancer, their husbands had since developed health issues—heart problems or diabetes, for example—that had made it hard to recover the sexual interest they had before breast cancer. In these cases, if a couple had become closer after breast cancer, this helped them survive other problems too. Edna, a traditional responder who had been a school cafeteria worker, reported that she had not had much interest in sex since the mastectomy. But her husband's interest had waned also. He was suffering from hepatitis C and could not have a liver transplant because he had heart trouble. Describing her relationship as closer than before breast cancer, she added,

"Between the two of us, right now, we're just happy with each other without our sex. Sometimes we just lie in bed and hold hands." Stories similar to Edna's were told by others, particularly older women.

Many, but not all, of the negative side effects of breast cancer waned over time, and women were free to return to their former lives. However, many women remained heavily involved in breast cancer issues even after some of the visible reminders had disappeared. We now turn our attention to some of the ways women became involved in the larger breast cancer movement. In America, this movement is multifaceted.

EIGHT

Breast Cancer Activism,
Education, and Support

In the *New York Times Sunday Magazine* for December 22, 1996, Lisa Belkin asked how breast cancer had become "this year's cause."[1] With the benefit of hindsight, the only problem with her question is that she should have asked how breast cancer became the cause of the 1990s. We might also ask why it remains so prominent. Pink ribbons still abound; if anything, they have become more ubiquitous.[2] And the plethora of support services and activities is such that, once a woman is diagnosed, she can make breast cancer education and activism a full-time avocation for the rest of her life.

Such a woman could attend or volunteer for a variety of support and educational services. She could get involved in activist organizations of every political persuasion, and she could attend numerous specialized programs about alternative treatments and diet, if she found conventional medicine lacking. Some of the women I interviewed did little of this during treatment, but others became involved in many activities. A number of women joined breast cancer organizations once their treatments ended.

Although the type and extent of activity women became involved in varied greatly by response group, I chose to write about breast cancer activism in a separate chapter, for several reasons. First, activism is the most visible face of breast cancer and a large part of the reason that the disease is so public. Most have heard of the Race for the Cure, for example, and women from every response group had participated in it. Second, not every woman I interviewed became active in the breast cancer movement after treatment, so this chapter deals with a subset of my respondents. Finally and most important, I wanted to examine the various activist organizations and their adherents because there has been so much written about them. It made sense therefore to devote a single chapter to the topic and to integrate my respondents' choices with the organizations' points of view.

Belkin noted that more money was raised for breast cancer than for any other disease, even though it was not the country's biggest killer— that distinction belonged to heart disease. It was not even the biggest killer among cancers—lung cancer was. Belkin explained the success in fund-raising with the argument that the dedication to breast cancer is about more than the disease itself. The many and varied programs organized around breast cancer remind us, once again, that this is not just another illness. It has enormous cultural and emotional significance, and it is saturated with gendered notions of femininity.[3] However, the assumptions underlying different programs vary, and their appeal varies depending on a woman's characteristic response to her breast cancer diagnosis. Women's involvement in breast cancer organizations varied according to response group.

In her article, Belkin listed the companies that had given money and other forms of support to breast cancer organizations: J. C. Penney, Pier 1 Imports, Tiffany, Ford Motor Company, New Balance, American Airlines, and Ralph Lauren, to name a few. Some of these companies put pink ribbons on their products, and Lauren designed the signature T-shirt for

"Fashion Targets Breast Cancer," which is used every October during Breast Cancer Awareness Month.[4] Because so many women find breast cancer terrifying, companies that identify themselves as supporting a cure create the image that they care about women. To quote *Adweek* magazine, breast cancer is a "dream cause" because "It's the feminist issues without the politics."[5]

Breast cancer activism involves more than raising money for research, even though this is a central activity for a number of organizations. Since Rose Kushner's time, the movement has become more complex. The more militant breast cancer groups have learned from AIDS activists that patients can influence medical research and protocols, if they inform themselves sufficiently well and are willing to insist on their rights.[6] Some even challenge the current emphasis on finding a cure. At the same time, many women are not comfortable with militancy and prefer to become involved with social service efforts providing help for women who do not know where to turn after diagnosis.

Much has been written about breast cancer activism in its various forms, and it is not my intention to reproduce that work.[7] What follows is a brief summary of the main organizations and their debates over the causes of breast cancer and over the appropriate ways to organize around the disease. This is provided to set the stage for a discussion of the different ways in which some of the women I interviewed became involved in activism and other volunteer activities. Gary Fine has conceived of social movements as "a bundle of narratives" that commits participants to shared goals and identities. As we will see, these narratives varied by organization.[8] Women became involved in those that most closely meshed with their personal narratives about their breast cancer experiences.

Organizations to educate women about breast cancer started in the early twentieth century and focused on early detection.[9] It was not until much later that fund-raising became central. The Susan G. Komen Foundation was one of the first to raise funds specifically for breast cancer research as opposed to cancer in general. Founded in 1984 by Nancy Brinker and named in memory of her sister, who died of breast cancer at age thirty-six, the Komen Foundation currently raises about 130 million dollars a year and gives out almost 100 million dollars in grants for research and community programs. Nancy Brinker is well connected to the Republican Party; her husband has been a generous contributor to national politics, especially to politicians from his home state of Texas. Brinker, who was diagnosed with breast cancer after her sister's death, was named ambassador to Hungary by President George W. Bush. Yet in spite of her Republican affiliations, her cause is such that politicians of all stripes have supported her organization. One of the attractions of breast cancer as an issue is that it cuts across all groups. Many prominent people have been touched personally by the disease, and supporting the cause has not drawn dissent or disapproval from the mainstream. Both the Quayles and the Gores have been honorary chairs of the Komen Foundation's Race for the Cure.

A number of more radical writers have argued that organizations like the Komen Foundation assume a traditional image of womanhood and position women with breast cancer as helpless victims who need to learn self-advocacy. Organizations like Komen and the American Cancer Society, these critics charge, hold women responsible for their cancers if they do not use self-help techniques that can prevent breast cancer or at the very least ensure early diagnosis.[10] While the Komen Foundation does take this position, its overall stance is more complex. It is true that the organization has emphasized the importance of femininity and the pain caused by the loss of a breast, but it is less clear that women have been viewed as helpless. Furthermore, from the start, Komen has been run largely by women, top to bottom, and these women have been highly effective at raising money and awareness. The organization does, however, retain an individualistic perspective, arguing that the disease must be fixed one woman at a time, which is not a surprising viewpoint in such an individualistic society as America.

The goal of the Komen Foundation is to find a cure for breast cancer. In line with its gendered view of the world, its Web site and materials are replete with pink images, particularly pink ribbons. The organization promotes the long-standing argument that the solution to breast cancer is to raise money for research, so that the pace of research can accelerate and a cure can be achieved more quickly. Using the slogan "The Race Is On for a Cure," in 2005 the Komen Foundation's Race for the Cure raised money and awareness in over 110 cities. At each event, crowds turned out to participate in a road race or a walk, for those who could not run. All participants wore "Race for the Cure" T-shirts—those of breast cancer survivors are always bright pink to create visibility around the issue of survival. In each city, the race was organized by local activists, many of whom were either survivors or friends or relatives of women who had had breast cancer.[11] The three messages on display were that breast cancer is an urgent issue, that it can be cured with enough determination, and that women who have breast cancer should be open about their heroic battles. The local groups raise money in many different ways, but the Race for the Cure is always the biggest and most public draw.

The oldest and most visible cancer organization is the American Cancer Society. Its mandate extends to all cancers, but, from its beginning in 1913 when it was called the American Society for the Control of Cancer, it has placed particular emphasis on breast cancer as the most feared of women's cancers.[12] In 2006, the most striking image on its Web site's home page was a pink ribbon and the pink words "Making Strides Against Breast Cancer."[13] The American Cancer Society combines government lobbying with advice about the diagnosis and treatment of numerous cancers. In its section on breast cancer, the Web site provides information about breast reconstruction, in which the pros and cons of each surgical procedure are weighed in a balanced, biomedical manner. Since the organization began, its mantra has been early diagnosis. One approach to this is through its Tell a Friend program, which has placed the burden of cancer detection on individuals and their social networks. Like the Komen Foundation, the American Cancer Society is committed to finding a cure for breast cancer.

One of the longest running programs is Reach to Recovery, founded in 1954 by Terese Lasser, and taken over by the American Cancer Society in 1969.[14] In this program, volunteers—breast cancer survivors "who have fully adjusted to their breast cancer treatment"—visit patients matched with them for age and experience.[15] They pay special attention to mastectomy patients, providing information and support after surgery as well as a temporary prosthesis for women to use while waiting for their wounds to heal and a more permanent solution to be decided upon.

This emphasis on the individual's responsibility for preventing and surviving breast cancer does not appeal to all women. A number of organizations have raised awareness and funds by using the argument that the prevention and cure of breast cancer necessitates a more aggressive thrust. The National Breast Cancer Coalition (NBCC) featured the title of its public service campaign, "Not Just Ribbons, Revolution," prominently on the home page of its Web site and used this line in print advertising to push the point home.[16] Instead of ribbons, these advertisements showed a bulldozer, toolbox, and hard hat to make the point "that symbols must be aligned with effective advocacy to win the fight against breast cancer."[17] Instead of focusing on the individual woman's responsibility, NBCC argues that collective political action is necessary if a cure is to be found. Furthermore, the organization argues that individual fundraising, no matter how successful, can never provide the financial support necessary for the massive amount of research needed.

NBCC president Fran Visco is a Philadelphia lawyer and breast cancer survivor. Visco used her experience in the women's movement to organize NBCC's militant approach to breast cancer funding. In the early 1990s, NBCC joined others in pushing the claim that the federal government had underfunded women's health issues. With the help of Iowa senator Tom Harkin, the organization achieved an annual increase in breast cancer funding of nearly 300 million dollars.[18] NBCC has trained thousands of its members to lobby for breast cancer funding at the state and national levels and to understand enough about the biomedical issues to participate in funding decisions.[19] Their most successful lobbying effort to date has been to include breast cancer research funding in the Department of Defense budget and to obtain agreement that trained NBCC volunteers would participate in its grant decisions.[20]

The coalition has criticized the National Cancer Institute (NCI) for neglecting research on breast cancer. The NCI and its supporters have responded that focusing on individual cancers would take away from essential basic research. NBCC has answered this with the rebuke that its goal is to open up "NCI's cliquish inner circle and bring in new faces."[21] So while more militant in its tactics and more critical of the medical profession than the American Cancer Society or the Komen Foundation,

NBCC still has focused most of its efforts on biomedical research as the route to eradicating breast cancer.

A more radical organization based in California, Breast Cancer Action (BCA), has also taken aim at pink ribbons. While BCA has criticized what it calls the "breast cancer establishment," its main target has been corporate capitalism. Key to its critique is the argument that there exists a link between environmental toxins and breast cancer. Furthermore, BCA claims that this link has been ignored by the breast cancer establishment: the NCI, the American Cancer Society, the pharmaceutical companies, and the comprehensive cancer centers that the NCI funds.[22] San Francisco activist Judy Brady, who was diagnosed with breast cancer in 1980, was one of the first to push this connection. Brady explained her own breast cancer as the result of exposure to ionizing radiation, which is produced in a variety of locations in her native California.[23]

BCA is not the only environmental group; the oldest is the grassroots organization called "1 in 9" located on Long Island where breast cancer rates are high.[24] This organization has successfully pushed the federal government to investigate environmental links to breast cancer.[25] BCA, however, has taken on the cancer establishment in a more confrontational way. Calling themselves the "bad girls of breast cancer," BCA's Web site declaimed, "Think Before You Pink" and added, "Breast cancer is about women's lives, not a marketing opportunity."[26]

BCA has removed the responsibility for breast cancer from individual women to an even greater degree than NBCC by taking the position that efforts should be directed to preventing breast cancer, instead of focusing on a cure. Noting that nonindustrialized countries have lower breast cancer rates than industrialized countries,[27] its explanation for this has been environmental. Although there is controversy about the extent to which increased rates of diagnosis in the West result from an epidemic rather than from earlier diagnosis and increased longevity, BCA has argued that the rates show a connection between environmental toxins and breast cancer. In BCA's view, the risk of breast cancer has increased and continues to increase. BCA's solution has been to fight for more money to be spent researching breast cancer causes as opposed to breast cancer cures. In BCA's opinion, the reason most research money has been allocated toward finding a cure is because cures benefit the drug companies and the medical profession, whereas prevention indicts the former and lessens business for all. Thus the leadership of BCA has blamed the cancer establishment for focusing on biomedicine at the expense of social change.

The American Cancer Society along with the NCI have both long been targeted as apologists for a medical-industrial complex. This complex is deemed responsible for the environmental hazards that, activists argue, have led to an epidemic of breast cancer, among other medical problems. The loudest, longest, and most persistent critic of "the politics of cancer" has been Samuel Epstein, a physician and emeritus professor at the University of Illinois at Chicago. Since 1978, he has produced numerous books and articles stating that cancer is increasing, that the ability to treat cancer is virtually unchanged, and that this is due in large part to the policies and priorities of the cancer establishment, in particular the NCI and the American Cancer Society.[28] Only occasionally has either the NCI or the American Cancer Society deemed it necessary to respond to his charges, but environmental breast cancer activists cite his work frequently.[29]

This debate over the type of activism that would be most effective in dealing with breast cancer was further fueled in November 2001, when longtime activist and writer Barbara Ehrenreich wrote about her experiences with breast cancer and breast cancer organizations in *Harper's Magazine*.[30] Ehrenreich lashed out at what she saw as mainstream activism's negation of the women's health movement, a movement that could claim credit for forcing doctors to replace the debilitating radical mastectomy with less invasive surgery.[31] She castigated the infantilizing mess of pink teddy bears and ribbons and the breast cancer establishment's promotion of a resolutely upbeat attitude that banished all fear, even when fear was appropriate.

Ehrenreich joined forces with BCA to push her arguments that most breast cancer activism was misplaced and that more effort should be focused on the causes of breast cancer, particularly environmental causes. She cited Epstein in support of this view.[32] Given Ehrenreich's visibility as a best-selling author, the media picked up the story, particularly after BCA launched advertisements in the *New York Times* starting in 2002.[33]

These advertisements harshly criticized mainstream breast cancer activism. Corporate sponsors started raising questions about this negative publicity, which caused the Komen Foundation to respond sharply. In its response, Komen did not answer critics directly but instead lauded corporate sponsorship for bringing in millions of dollars for breast cancer and declared its goal to be the eradication of "breast cancer as a life-threatening disease."[34] BCA has continued to push its argument against pink ribbons every October during Breast Cancer Awareness Month, and the media have continued to pay attention to these arguments, particularly to their connection to Ehrenreich.[35]

In addition to its pro-environmental arguments, BCA has taken a militant position on social inequities in breast cancer diagnosis and treatment.[36] Finally, the organization has criticized standard diagnosis and treatment modalities. Where the Komen Foundation and the American Cancer Society have urged women to have regular mammograms, because they view early diagnosis as the sine qua non of survival, BCA has questioned the efficacy of mammograms in reducing mortality.[37] And BCA has echoed Susan Love's description of cancer treatment as little better than "slash, burn and poison."

This range of activist groups provides many opportunities for women diagnosed with breast cancer to become involved. In addition, women may volunteer to work for support organizations. In my study, whether and where women chose to become involved varied by response group. In each group, some women tried to put cancer behind them once it was over, even if they had used the services of activists and volunteer organizations during treatment. Others felt the need to stay involved. While many women stayed somewhat involved by attending educational programs from time to time or participating in the Race for the Cure each year, I defined activists as women who helped organize events or programs either for activist groups or for support organizations. So a woman who attended an organizing meeting for the Race for the Cure would be considered an activist, but a woman who simply attended the race and/ or the survivors' luncheon the weekend before the race would not.

The women least likely to become involved in activism were, not surprisingly, the traditional responders; only seven of these thirty-two women became activists. This compared with twelve of the thirty-two biomedical experts, and three of the ten religious responders. Alternative experts were the group most likely to become involved; eleven of these seventeen became activists after diagnosis. It is not surprising that women who had an outsider's viewpoint would be most likely to work toward social change. Also, many alternative experts had a history of activism.

When they did become involved, groups differed in the types of social action they chose. Traditional responders usually selected organizations that did not conflict with women's long-standing roles of caring and support. Honor, the traditional responder met in chapter 7, became involved in the organizations she had found most helpful while she was having treatment. This started when a Reach to Recovery volunteer visited her after her mastectomy. Honor had been offered the option of a lumpectomy plus radiation, but since her mother had died of breast cancer, she elected to have a prophylactic double mastectomy with subsequent reconstruction. In addition to helping her go through this process, the Reach to Recovery volunteer "encouraged me to use—besides the wig— the hair bands and bandannas and hats and to make it fun."

A number of hospitals also hold programs to help women maintain their appearance while going through breast cancer—something more radical activists disparage. Honor attended one of these and found it helpful. The typical program is like the one I attended at a university comprehensive cancer center.[38] In a pleasant room in a hotel near the university hospital, an elaborate cold lunch was available before the seminar, and the speaker, who specialized in hair and skin, showed wigs and other head coverings. She also showed products that prevented hair loss, demonstrated how to draw eyebrows when real ones disappeared, and recommended a variety of skin products. She handed out free samples and answered women's numerous questions. Barbara Ehrenreich, in a speech to BCA, found it odd that no one complained "about the strange idea that you can fight a potentially fatal disease with eyeliner and blush,"[39] but it was clear from the questions that no one attending this session was under this illusion. Rather, they asked about sore, dry hands, or chest skin that had become so thin that wearing a prosthesis was painful, or a wig that looked terrible because its wearer had received no instructions about how to care for it. These women certainly cared about their appearance as do most women, but their questions showed an engagement with the consequences of treatment that went beyond mere vanity.

Honor was so impressed with Reach to Recovery that she decided to become a volunteer once she recovered:

> The first thing is that you must be a year after your surgery, and you must go through an interview process to make sure you're emotionally ready. . . . Once I did get through the training, then I had a mentor who took me on what they call a "buddy visit" to make sure I was comfortable and to see how the program worked. . . . I might do six a year or something like that. . . . That is the goal of the program, to try to match you up with somebody similar, because otherwise you can't relate.

Honor was very comfortable with the idea that providing each woman with individual help tailored to her needs included the need for compatible personalities, but she wanted to do more than visit new patients a few times a year. Like many traditional responders, she wished her work to focus on human relationships. She had little desire for technical information, because she did not want "to dwell on it."

Honor's solution was to get involved with the Komen Foundation's local affiliate, which she learned about from having attended the Race for the Cure with her daughter in the first year after diagnosis. The next year she took a number of women relatives to the race. Like many traditional responders, Honor "liked the idea of doing a walk and being surrounded by other women who have breast cancer." She expanded on this point by saying, "Once someone has had breast cancer, and they meet someone who has breast cancer, there's just a natural bond." Her attitude that the experience was a collective one affecting many women is an antidote to the emphasis on personal responsibility that organizations like Komen often seem to emphasize.

When I interviewed Honor, she and her daughter were co-chairs of the annual Race for the Cure. Honor explained her involvement this way:

> The first time I did the Race, I just loved everything it stood for. . . . My friend, who subsequently died, was involved and was a speaker for them. A year or two after doing the Race for the Cure, I started getting

involved with the group. . . . I subsequently moved up and did the survivors' luncheon, which was at the Ritz Carlton, and this year I'm the co-chair. . . . I'm on the phone constantly. This time of year, starting now, I go in one day a week to the office. . . . I think I raised about twenty-five thousand dollars this year . . . just reading about things in the paper and making calls. So it's very gratifying as far as that goes. . . . I was asked to go to Texas, where we have meetings twice a year . . . for the whole Foundation and for all the Races. . . . So I got indoctrinated into that, and I've made some wonderful friends from it as well.

I attended a Race for the Cure meeting co-chaired by Honor and her daughter. There was a huge turnout with lots of eating and social activity continuing throughout the formal presentations. The meeting started with volunteers making requests for help with the many different fundraising activities, not only for the Race. Lots of people signed up for each request, many times interrupting side conversations to do so. The level of energy in the room was high, and the joie de vivre and humor in getting people to volunteer were abundant. There was also a strong sense of group solidarity that I found quite contagious.

Although the group was largely white and upper middle class—a fact frequently commented on by those who write about breast cancer activism in general—those who did not fit this demographic profile were clearly welcome and comfortable in their surroundings.[40] This was confirmed when I interviewed Amber, an African American woman and a traditional responder, like Honor. She had become involved in volunteering for the Race, after Honor visited her for Reach to Recovery. She told me she loved volunteering, and that she and Honor had become good friends.

The executive director of the local Komen affiliate, Elaine Grobman, told me in an interview that her organization raises money not only for the national organization but for the local branch. Each branch makes its own decisions annually about which local groups and activities to support. For example, about twenty hospitals in the local area had agreed to give mammograms to low-income women in return for a twenty-five-dollar processing fee from the Komen Foundation. Grobman also spent a lot of time getting women without health insurance into treatment. She estimated that they obtained funding for about six uninsured patients a week, each one taking several hours of her time.[41]

It is hard to categorize the political impact of the Race for the Cure. The Komen Foundation has a conservative ideology of not criticizing bio-medicine or corporate America, a source of much of its support, and it takes an individualistic approach, helping one woman at a time rather than trying to fix the system. Yet a number of more radical organizations use their largesse to fund programs for poor women and others not well served medically. Among the local activities supported by the Race for the Cure the year Honor was co-chair were an educational support group for black women, another for Latina women, and a program to sensitize physicians to meet the medical needs of lesbians. And the reasons local women become involved have to do with more than pink teddy bears and ribbons. In a study of the varieties of breast cancer activism in the San Francisco Bay area, Maren Klawiter charged that the Race for the Cure validates survivors at the expense of the dead. Their message, she argued, was, "The proactive survive, and only the unaware and the irresponsible die."[42] This may be true at the level of national policy, but as Faye Ginsburg discovered in her study of abortion activism, local activists' agendas may differ from those of the leaders of national organizations.[43] Honor never forgot that her mother had died of breast cancer and that her close friend had also, and she did not assume that either death could have been avoided if the victim had worked harder to survive. In fact, Honor commented, "I think I handled [breast cancer] like my mother handled it. I felt like she was kind of looking over my shoulder and really giving me guidance."

Honor gained emotional support from contact with other survivors. At the same time, she worried about her daughter's chances of getting breast cancer and, in fact, had postponed genetic testing because her daughter, her sister, and her niece had all asked her not to have it done. So death was present in Honor's mind all the time. Yet in becoming a volunteer, she focused on living, and like many women I interviewed, she described herself as more interesting and more likable than she had been before cancer. Ehrenreich takes issue with women who find the breast cancer experience ennobling. She declared that breast cancer had not made her "prettier or stronger, more feminine or spiritual—only more deeply angry." Still, it is not unreasonable to look for a larger meaning after going through a death-defying experience. Nor does it mean that a woman is ignoring the real possibility that breast cancer might return and take her life.

Honor's response is an example of what Verta Taylor and Marieke Van Willigen term "women's self-help." Its core, they say, is "getting and giving support." The activities Honor became involved in served to "confirm shared experiences and open windows in new identities."[44] Traditional responders such as Honor gained satisfaction from working alongside other survivors. They received support as they gave it. They did not regard themselves as experts. Honor was a high school graduate. And she felt privileged to be involved with the Race for the Cure, not entitled.

Many biomedical experts also became involved in the Race for the Cure, in part because of its emphasis on biomedicine, but also because it was the most accessible breast cancer organization. After becoming involved in this way, many biomedical experts moved on to organizations more focused on developing and disseminating scientific knowledge. Joann, introduced in chapter 3, was such a person. Joann, like Honor, had lost her mother to breast cancer, and she tried a number of coping mechanisms before focusing on an organization at the forefront of breast cancer education. For example, she went to several support groups "only to walk away from each of them." She also went to hear alternative medical guru Bernie Siegel. She had listened to his tape, *Love, Medicine and Miracles,* but attending the presentation proved disappointing:

> At a break he was taking questions, and I ran and got to the front of the line. . . . I said, "Dr. Siegel, I just finished four cycles of AC, what do I do now? I feel totally vulnerable. . . ." He told me to go get a good therapist. It was totally against what he writes. . . . I was appalled. I wasn't crying. I wasn't showing any angst. I was very clinical. I literally walked away with my jaw hanging.

Like most biomedical experts, Joann focused intensely on her illness throughout her treatment. When treatment was over, she felt the need to stay involved with breast cancer, at least in part because staying informed could help her control her own health. Breast cancer had been a part of her life for so long. Three months after treatment ended, she decided to make it her career. She started out by persuading the hospital that had treated her that they needed psychosocial support programs and that she was the right person to develop them. She also joined the board of Reach to Recovery, and she started attending the Race for the Cure. Eventually, she obtained her current position working with a breast cancer educational organization. This job has provided her with the opportunity to develop the kinds of programs she is most interested in— those that support biomedicine and biomedical research. She described her hiring process when I interviewed her in the organization's meeting room:

> I spent two hours interviewing. . . . They called me the day after. . . . "You know we would be honored to have you on staff. . . ." NSABP [National Surgical Adjuvant Breast and Bowel Project] actually just offered me to serve on their advocacy committee, which they are creating brand new. . . . I'm a huge advocate for what they do. I'm actually presenting at their conference. . . . NSABP . . . is a national cooperative oncology group, and the bulk of their clinical trials are breast cancer. . . . They are the organization that launched the Breast Cancer Prevention Trial and now the STAR trial.[45]

As part of her work, Joann had also been involved with the local affiliate of the National Breast Cancer Coalition.

The organization Joann worked for runs conferences regularly. These often consist of one or two keynote speakers plus breakout sessions where a variety of topics are discussed. The keynote address usually covers the latest research findings or sometimes diet or other topics of particular interest to women, such as sexual functioning.[46] Whatever the topic, the keynote speaker is typically an M.D. and is affiliated with traditional biomedicine. For example, Dr. Mitchell Gaynor, who spoke at one of the conferences, was a board-certified oncologist affiliated with Cornell University's Center for Complementary and Integrative Medicine at the time of his speech.[47] In a definitive manner that brooked no argument, he spoke about how women could improve their immune systems by eating foods containing antioxidants and "detoxifying enzymes." Although he cautioned that everything he said was not yet proven, he undermined this caution by the certainty with which he spoke and his frequent disparagement of other doctors who disagreed with him.

This pattern of using the aura of biomedical science to present alternative treatments is becoming increasingly common and makes the information palatable to some who believe in biomedicine. A number of hospitals now have departments of integrative medicine—even though many physicians in those same hospitals are uncomfortable about the lack of scientific evidence involved—and almost all hospitals now use such alternative treatments as acupuncture and relaxation therapy.[48] I attended a typical program about breast cancer given at a hospital center for alternative medicine. The presentations were on how alternative medicine works, mindfulness meditation, support groups and coping skills, movement therapy, and acupuncture.[49]

Hospitals also run more traditional programs. Philadelphia's university-based comprehensive cancer center runs them frequently; in the space of a couple of months it ran a conference on breast cancer, a conference on breast cancer and diet, and a conference on women's cancers in general. The one on breast cancer started with a prominent physician/medical historian describing the historical controversies over breast cancer.[50] This was followed by lectures on changes in surgical treatment as well as in chemotherapy. The final lecture was by an epidemiologist, and the speaker took the position that it is unclear whether a breast cancer epidemic really exists. This conference was unusual in its academic tone. The other programs run by this hospital were more typical, with discussions focused on diet and nutrition, the importance of clinical trials, evidence about tamoxifen, and help in coping with the stress of cancer.[51] At these conferences, the emphasis was on what individual women can and should do for themselves. It is no surprise, therefore, that many women in the audience asked the kinds of questions that biomedical experts might ask, because biomedical experts believe in taking responsibility for their own recovery.

Joann believed in mainstream biomedicine, and she was somewhat skeptical about alternative treatments. Throughout her experience, she remained a true believer in medical science, as her enthusiasm about the NSABP indicates. She held on to this belief in spite of the fact that the longtime head of the NSABP, Bernard Fisher, had been forced to resign several years before I interviewed Joann, after one of his centers admitted to falsifying data in an important clinical trial, but she did not mention this.[52] In contrast to Honor, Joann had undergone genetic testing because she believed she had a breast cancer gene, given the amount of breast cancer in her family, and she wanted to know everything.

Joann was so busy providing information to women with breast cancer that she rarely thought about her own mortality, even though she realized that she might die of cancer. She acknowledged this by saying, "Maybe I should have let other people see more of the sadness." Her mother had lived twenty-six years after a breast cancer diagnosis, only to succumb to a different kind of cancer. Joann believed that her own breast cancer had enabled her to focus on the important things in life and to take each day as it came. She did not exhibit the anger of more radical activists; she was like Honor in that her involvement demonstrated an agency that translated into personal action.

While some biomedical experts focused on education, others became involved in political activism through the National Breast Cancer Coalition (NBCC) or its local affiliate. Fran Visco, the president, is the quintessential biomedical expert.[53] In her frequent speeches, she rouses her audience to action with her personal history.[54] Visco recounts her career as a lawyer and as a veteran of the women's movement. She first became involved in the breast cancer movement as a volunteer with a local organization in her community. While she believed such activity was important, her heart was not in it. Having become outraged at what she saw as indifference on the part of both politicians and the medical establishment to this serious issue of women's health, she found a perfect home with NBCC. NBCC engages in political action, in particular in pushing the government to provide more funding. It does this on the grounds that individual donors, such as those solicited by the Komen Foundation, cannot provide the resources needed. Visco views NBCC as having changed the world of breast cancer. Support and advocacy had operated on a one-to-one basis prior to NBCC.

In their study of the postpartum support and breast cancer movements, Taylor and Van Willigen noted that personal narratives can be used to transform individual experiences into collective action.[55] This is why Visco's account of her path into breast cancer politics has been so effective in developing a systemwide structure of advocacy. NBCC takes a middle ground between Breast Cancer Action and the Komen Foundation; its leadership is sympathetic to support groups and to educational organizations but not to gestures like wearing pink ribbons. As Visco joked during the Republican primary in 2000, "There was a dispute between McCain and Bush over who had the biggest pink ribbon." Adding that "That's typical of the kind of arguments men have," she used this story as an example of how not to engage in political action. "Bush," she said, "wore a pink ribbon. He stood on the stage and has done nothing" about breast cancer.

Visco's themes were repeated in an interview I had with Judy Wallace, then education director of NBCC.[56] She, too, had been an archetypal biomedical expert. A research psychologist before her breast cancer diagnosis, she had learned so much during her treatment that she decided to link with an organization that would use her skills. NBCC was perfect. Wallace described NBCC as an organization dedicated to teaching women enough science so that they can design research studies and, when funding is given out, sit "at the table making decisions." Her description of the women who take NBCC's training corresponded closely to my descriptions of biomedical experts: "Those who want to be part of the decision-making with their doctors, and who want to be able to call with questions—they make good activists."

While NBCC prides itself on its independence, it receives funding from pharmaceutical companies and corporations of the type that BCA disparages. At NBCC's 2000 conference in Washington, for example, Fran Visco gave an award to Avon, a company that licenses its own pink ribbon. Avon has supported NBCC since 1996. This makes for a touchy issue. It takes a lot of money to maintain a staff of twenty, and while much of this comes from individuals, the organization needs additional financial support. Even though some of this comes from companies with agendas of their own, Judy Wallace insisted that NBCC stays independent of its sponsors and focused on its own goals.

Although Joann had only been marginally involved with NBCC, several of the biomedical experts I interviewed had become active in this organization. I met one such woman, Iris, at their national conference and she agreed to an interview. Iris, who was a teacher and forty-one years old when first diagnosed, described herself as someone who "didn't go into all those wellness type of things, because they seemed to me to be the Bernie Siegel type of thing, and I was interested in everything on the cancer itself." She first became involved in breast cancer activism through Reach to Recovery; she reported that, after she took their training, "Every time I would go out, I felt so good about it." In fact, "Whenever the phone called and they said can you make a visit, I dropped everything." She was so interested in learning everything she could about her disease that when *MAMM,* a new magazine devoted to women's cancer appeared, she became a charter subscriber and learned that she could get even more training:

> I remember reading about Project LEAD and it just sounded interesting. . . . They were aiming to make people more knowledgeable, really understand the science behind breast cancer. They wanted to get you involved in being more than just an active support person. . . . I wanted to get into the senior high school. . . . My message was early diagnosis. . . . I tried as much as I could, and I haven't been able to do that much. . . . I am a support, where there are mothers of the children in my school who are diagnosed.

Iris loved the Project LEAD training:

> I think we had fourteen scientists teaching . . . people who were in the area of cancer research who came to speak. We talked about genetics . . . case studies, how they're designed, what are the problems. . . . We would be meeting as a whole group and then break into small groups, each group led by one of these scientists, so the feeling was amazing. Everybody stayed together most of the time, so you had meals with the scientists. . . . When I came back . . . they said, "There's a commitment." They wanted you to work as an activist. I knew that I wasn't really doing activism. I was doing more support.

When I talked to Iris, she had made some attempts to become an activist doing what she had been trained for, but she was still struggling to find her way. Her husband, who had an office in New York, had sub-leased space to a breast cancer support organization, had given them months of free rent, and had donated furniture. This is not quite what NBCC has in mind for activists. Iris exemplified the point that local activists may have different goals than those of the national organization. Many biomedical experts love the LEAD training because they learn so much, but they are more interested in education than political activism. They support the goals of NBCC but tend to be uncomfortable in the difficult world of lobbying. They want to help women manage their own treatments, and they believe the route to this is knowledge. They had used their education to inform their own treatment, and now they wanted to enhance it to help others.

Religious responders had different motivations for activism than biomedical experts. Those who became involved did so because they heard a calling from God. Not surprisingly, they were more interested in social service activism than in politics. They were similar in some ways to traditional responders, but the religious component in their service made for a major difference. Ulrike Boehmer, in a study of women's breast cancer activism, has argued that while white women activists tend to be those who have had cancer, African American activists are professionals, without a history of cancer, employed to provide services.[57] This was not the case in the current study. All three of the religious responders who became activists were African American, and there were African American activists in the other groups as well.

Shantal, like Honor and Joann, had a mother who died of breast cancer. As noted in chapter 4, Shantal formed a support group for African American women with breast cancer after her own treatment ended. She spent a great deal of time fund-raising for this group, and she received money from both the Komen Foundation and the American Cancer Society. She believed that founding the support group was part of God's plan for her, and she described how she got started:

> My friends and coworkers and church workers—if they had heard someone was diagnosed with breast cancer—asked me if I would talk with them. . . . They said, "We observed you going through and you did so well. . . ." And I did, and I saved their phone numbers, and I sent

a card to them. Later my pastor asked . . . if I would have a program about breast cancer at the church, and I said to myself, "He's asking me to do that? I don't know what to do." So I call these people: the Cancer Society, [a breast cancer support organization], and [a comprehensive cancer center], and asked them if they would come. . . . I invited these ladies, who I had maintained on the list. . . . We had a great outcome. . . . [A second breast cancer organization] sent out the mobile van outside the church and we did forty-two mammograms.

At the end of the year, Shantal assumed she was finished with the program, only to be told by those who had attended, "Oh no, you can't be." She added:

All this was just so amazing to me, and empowering to me, knowing that at that point I had learned the death rate for African American women, and I was driven. . . . I didn't realize at the time, but the breast cancer world . . . had been trying to enter the African American community. . . . They wanted this to continue. . . . I said to my husband, "I can't continue to work. . . . I have enough years to retire, and I have some income," and he said, "Well go ahead, and do it then. . . ." I told my coworkers what I wanted to do, and one of the gifts they gave me was a brand-new briefcase. . . . I went in to the Cancer Society with this briefcase and a breast cancer Avon pin with the breast cancer ribbon on it, and I had my high heels and hose, and I was ready. And I guess they said, "This lady is serious."[58]

Shantal's story shows that even pink ribbons can be more than just a feel-good symbol. A woman with great persuasive ability, Shantal has received support from almost all the breast cancer funding organizations in the city, as well as other groups. She has asked each for specific things: a room for the program from her church, office space from one cancer organization, free mammograms from another, ongoing financial support from a third, and support for a weekend retreat from a fourth. Every group in the city knows her work. Other organizations, including the one Joann works for, pay special attention to minority women because of their lack of services and high mortality rates. However, these groups do not have the rapport with the community that Shantal has. She not only gets constant individual requests for help, which she never turns away, but as she noted above, she has become a conduit for other groups to enter the black community.

When asked to explain her success, Shantal described her program as a combination of educational speakers and, more important, self-help, because "You pretty much help each other." Also, "Since you have a spiritual center, you help in that way." This spiritual element was very important to the African American women Shantal served. Indeed, although the city's other major support group for African American women was held in a hospital, it also had a strong spiritual component. Each meeting started with women standing in a circle, while the leader prayed and thanked God for his blessing. At a meeting I attended, the main speaker was the wife of a minister, who informed the audience that she had been supposed to die three times, but the Lord had always pulled her through. One time a doctor had actually told her she was going to die. This typifies religious responders' view of God as all-knowing and doctors as fallible.[59] Religious responders and traditional responders who became activists wanted to provided care and support. For traditional responders, that meant human fellowship, but the audiences for religious responders wanted a divine intervention as well. African American women do not trust human intervention to be sufficiently caring without the backing of God. This is a continuation of the themes about race and class discussed in chapter 4.

As is discussed in chapter 5, while alternative experts shared with religious responders a desire to look outside biomedicine for breast cancer recovery, they looked in very different places. For example, Hannah had tried numerous alternative treatments. She was particularly interested in understanding the environmental connections to breast cancer. Among the programs she had attended were those at the Center for Advancement in Cancer Education (CACE). Its executive director, Susan Silberstein, has spoken at numerous venues in Philadelphia and elsewhere. In a typical presentation, she claimed, "No one needs to die of breast cancer, if she chooses not to."[60] The solution she recommended was diet, in particular avoiding a high-fat diet. High levels of fat, she said, would cause the dangerous type of estrogen to increase. This was compounded by "xenobiotics," which she defined as foreign chemicals such as pesticides and antibiotics, and which, she said, mimicked estrogen in the breast. "They love fat, live in it, and don't metabolize out of it." Silberstein supported these definitive claims by citing unnamed studies. She rarely acknowledged that some of her statements were hypotheses rather than demonstrated truths. Hannah followed Silberstein's recommendations carefully while undergoing treatment, as did a number of other alternative experts.

The most remarkable thing about alternative experts is the extent to which, after treatment finished, they became involved in breast cancer activism; it was much greater than for any other group. Two-thirds of these women were actively engaged in some kind of activism at the time of the interview, and several others said that they intended to become involved in the future. And when they did become involved, alternative experts were inclined to join more radical organizations than were activists from the other groups. Their skepticism about biomedicine and their frequent critical stance toward society helped to explain this.

Hannah had been concerned about environmental causes of breast cancer during her treatment, but she first became involved as an activist by volunteering for the local affiliate of NBCC. While there, she met another survivor, Charlotte, who shared her interest in the link between hormone replacement therapy and breast cancer. While both of them supported NBCC's advocacy, they did not think enough was being done in terms of prevention, so they formed a local organization to promote awareness of the health dangers of environmental degradation. Other survivors, as well as relatives of women who had died of breast cancer, soon joined the group. Their arguments were similar to those of Breast Cancer Action (BCA), and they focused on a collective response rather than individual solutions to the disease. They differed from BCA in that they did not confine themselves to breast cancer, although this was a major focus. One of their goals was to train physicians to take environmental histories of their patients. They believed that asking questions about environmental exposure, work history, residential history, and other activities would help physicians understand the causes of patients' illnesses.[61] Unlike NBCC, this environmental organization would not take money from any group or business it considered responsible for polluting the environment.

When Hannah's organization realized it wanted "to be broader than just breast cancer," the group linked up with a women's advocacy organization, the Women's Environment and Development Organization (WEDO), founded by former congresswoman Bella Abzug before she died of breast cancer in 1998. It, too, focused itself more broadly than breast cancer. Even so, Hannah told me, "Breast cancer is clearly in the forefront, because most of the research related to environmental links has really been in breast cancer." Becoming involved in this organization had changed Hannah's view of herself and her goals:

> Since I started to do the environmental work, I don't refer to myself as a breast cancer survivor, I don't call attention to myself in that way, and, for years, I really did. . . . The research is astounding, when you look at where the pockets of breast cancer are, when you look at where it is in the world. . . . I felt stronger and stronger that, maybe by looking at environmental risks, it would open up a door that not enough people were opening.

In discussing her transformation, Hannah noted that she had originally experienced her cancer in a more personal way, but now that treatment was over, she was able to look beyond herself to the larger social causes. Like other alternative experts, she had long been critical of American society and she now turned her critical gaze onto breast cancer.

While there are lots of suggestive findings of a connection between breast cancer and the environment, as Gina Kolata noted in the *New York Times*, "The links are elusive."[62] Although there has been much recent research about whether exposure to pesticides, for example, could cause cancer, showing such a connection is very difficult. This is further confused because many epidemiologists have argued that increases in recorded cases of cancer of the breast do not result from an epidemic but are an artifact of improved screening.[63] For example, epidemiologist Richard Peto noted that, "When healthy people are screened, the tests find not only cancers that would be deadly if untreated, but also a certain percentage of tumors that would never cause problems if left alone."[64] This poses a difficulty for those who wish to argue for environmental causes of breast cancer, since to do so presupposes an increase. That is, as environmental degradation has increased, it has led to an increase in breast cancer. Not surprisingly, therefore, Kolata found that the arguments against the existence of an epidemic did not convince those living in areas like Long Island, where rates of breast cancer are higher than average. Nor did they convince activists like Barbara Brenner, the executive director of Breast Cancer Action, who having had breast cancer twice has stated, "We think there is something going on, and we'd like to find out what it is." Writer Sandra Steingraber has taken a middle ground, estimating that between 24 and 40 percent of the recent upsurge is attributable to early detection, with the rest representing a real increase, particularly among African American women and the elderly.[65] Robert Bullard has documented how African Americans are exposed to a disproportionate amount of environmental toxins.[66]

Although the Komen Foundation's local affiliate in Philadelphia was largely staffed by traditional responders working as volunteers, women in all of the other groups benefited from their fund-raising. For example, they had funded support for lesbians with breast cancer through the Philadelphia Community Health Alternatives (PCHA). This organization was founded in the late 1970s to address the health needs of the city's gay and lesbian population. While many of its activities involve support for persons living with AIDS, in 1997 PCHA added a women's program after first initiating a lesbian health needs assessment survey. The director told me that one of the things its respondents were most concerned about was breast cancer, because many lesbians had heard that it was something they had a higher than average risk of developing.[67] This belief evolved out of concerns that some of the purported risk factors for breast cancer—childlessness, higher than average weight, alcohol consumption, and a lack of medical care—might be higher among lesbians.[68] This possible risk was publicized in a study by Susan Haynes. Haynes made a conceptual leap, based on assumptions about the incidence of these risk factors among lesbians, which led her to state that lesbians have a one-in-three lifetime risk of developing breast cancer. Even though there are almost no data on the actual health risks of lesbians, a number of writers have taken Haynes's assertions to be true, and several organizations have supported special task forces or conferences on breast cancer risk.[69]

As Susan Yadlon noted, in the absence of data, lesbians were conflated with demographic factors that are not themselves synonymous with breast cancer.[70] The possibility that lesbians had higher rates of breast cancer translated into assumptions that there was a lesbian cancer epidemic.[71]

In an early study of breast cancer activism, Theresa Montini argued that women involved in breast cancer advocacy found themselves engaging in a difficult balancing act between the expectation that they would present a feminine and, therefore, emotional response, and the realization that emotional appeals were often discredited.[72] In the current study, while some women in all groups challenged some aspects of gender—for example, the assumption that they should hide the effects of breast cancer[73]—they responded to this dilemma differently depending on the response group they belonged to.

Most traditional responders did not become activists, because they preferred to put cancer behind them. Those who did become involved used the womanly virtues of care and nurturance and the long history of women's volunteerism to raise funds for breast cancer and to provide emotional support to one another while they did so. This was in keeping with the desires for the social support these women had obtained from similar organizations during treatment. This is a point made by Barron Lerner in a letter to the editor of *Harper's Magazine* after the appearance of Barbara Ehrenreich's article criticizing mainstream breast cancer treatment and activism. While agreeing with Ehrenreich's argument, Lerner noted that current priorities reflect "the cultural and political choices" of American society in general. After all, "Just as healthy women may be more interested in fashion or exercise than in cleaning up industrial waste, the same is often true for breast cancer survivors."[74] Certainly, the traditional responders felt this way. They had not felt entitled during treatment, and most of them wanted to put cancer behind them once it was over. Many had heavy family responsibilities that they needed to return to and little assistance. The few who became involved were most comfortable in organizations that emphasized the personal touch and that raised money for a biomedical miracle.

Biomedical experts were typically professional women who had benefited from second-wave feminism and the affirmative action programs that movement helped spawn. Most had professional careers, and if they became involved in the breast cancer movement, they used the skills they had learned in school and at work to demand a larger share of the research pie and to obtain the latest in expert education for themselves and others. In doing this, they turned their backs on emotion and frequently decried its use.[75] When they became activists, they stayed focused on research and education. They saw increased research funding as the long-term solution to breast cancer, and better education as an immediate way to help individual women make their own vital medical choices. When they became involved in breast cancer activism, as many of them did, their professional backgrounds and the expertise they had gained in managing their own treatments made them confident that they could put these skills to good use. They had long idealized science, and it was to science and its possibilities that they now turned.

Religious responders were closer to traditional responders than biomedical experts. They located themselves firmly in providing support networks and in taking care of others like themselves. Having survived their own treatment, they worked hard to help others survive theirs. They did this because they believed that in bringing them through breast cancer, God intended them to serve the community by taking his support to others. Some religious responders did not stray outside their own religious communities. Those who became involved in providing help to others were African American women who wanted to help their communities. They did so by combining faith and prayer that God would bring other women through treatment safely, just as he had for them, and by giving other women the emotional support to maintain their faith.

Finally, most of the women who became involved in the environmental breast cancer movement were alternative experts. Theirs was the most militant response of the four groups and the one most dependent on collective action—"a collective expression of rage," according to Klawiter.[76] Many of the women in this group had held negative opinions about corporate America long before they were diagnosed, and breast cancer simply galvanized their existing worldviews. The women in this group were the most inclined to become activists. They were comfortable organizing, and their educational backgrounds enabled them to develop a more sophisticated analysis of what needed to be done. Yet, although they eschewed individual responses to their diagnoses, the anger and emotion shown by the women in this group and by the organizations to which they were attracted, led to the risk, noted by Montini, that their response would be dismissed as a typical woman's response.

A few women, particularly those whose cancers had metastasized, could not be fitted into any of the four response groups. In the final chapter, these women's stories are examined, as a prelude to a summary of the findings of this book and a discussion of the larger implications.

Conclusion

Of my ninety-six respondents, three had metastatic breast cancer at the time of the interview.[1] These women were not able to put their illness experiences behind them; the illness stretched before them endlessly. All three had response patterns that differed from those of other women in this study, because each had moved from one response category to others as the disease progressed.

One of the three was Jo-Ellen, whose story is discussed at the beginning of chapter 1. Jo-Ellen had started out as the perfect example of a biomedical expert. A nurse with a master's degree in a related medical field, she had been a true believer in the power of medicine as well as in her own ability to make decisions about her health. She did all the things that typified biomedical experts: learning about her treatments, going for second opinions, attending educational programs, eating a healthy diet, and giving money to the National Breast Cancer Coalition (NBCC).

When she had reconstruction, she chose saline implants in order to avoid the major surgery that a tramflap would have necessitated. She was unsure about why she had developed cancer. Her adoptive mother had also had breast cancer, but Jo-Ellen did not conclude from this coincidence that the cause was environmental contamination, as an alternative expert might. Rather, she imagined that her biological mother might have had breast cancer and unknowingly passed the gene on to her.

Before diagnosis, Jo-Ellen had been trying to get pregnant—she stopped trying during treatment—and after treatment ended, she began again. However, this proved difficult:

> I was on the tamoxifen and the chemotherapy. I had lost my period for a couple of months, but then it came again. . . . When I was evaluated by the reproductive gynecologist, he was happy that I was getting my period. . . . I wasn't in menopause. When we did the first round of fertility drugs—when I didn't produce more eggs—he had the suspicion that I had some obvious ovarian failure.

Jo-Ellen had been so anxious to become pregnant that she had come off tamoxifen after only a few months, rather than taking it for the five years for which it was prescribed. She did this before starting fertility treatment.

Then another problem intervened with Jo-Ellen's pregnancy plans—she began to experience hip pain. Because she knew that breast cancer frequently metastasizes to the bones first, she visited an orthopedic oncologist, who diagnosed bursitis. However, when she saw her regular oncologist and told him that the pain was no better, he sent her for a bone scan, which confirmed her fears. At this point, her faith in biomedicine was somewhat shaken, but still she clung to the hope that she could recover with treatment. She started taking Taxol,[2] a fairly new chemotherapy drug at the time, and she had radiation to the bone metastasis. This treatment caused other problems:

> When I started with the radiation and the Taxol, I haven't had a period since last March. . . . I'm not completely in menopause, but it's basically like, it's almost there. . . . When [fertility injections] did not work, that was the low point. . . . My husband and I had always talked about our plans to have children.

When Taxol failed to stop the metastasis, Jo-Ellen continued trying new procedures. She had the now-discredited stem cell transplant, and she convinced her surgeon, against his advice, to perform a prophylactic mastectomy on her second breast.

Jo-Ellen was thirty-four years old and five years from her first diagnosis when I interviewed her. She recounted her aggressive attempts to treat her cancer. She was also well informed about her prognosis. Since she was being treated at the hospital where she worked, "If I have a study done, I'll go and get the report." Yet biomedicine seemed to have failed her, both in recovering from cancer and in getting pregnant. Jo-Ellen was finally losing faith in its ability to save her life, and she was reluctantly moving toward alternative practices, trying things she would have had no patience with earlier.

Jo-Ellen started taking a number of supplements bought from a health food store, like folic acid, vitamin C, and gentian,[3] although she had some ambivalence about which ones she should take and how they would interact. She had also been having massages and going to meditation classes—she justified the latter by explaining that she had learned about meditation in nursing school. She was even contemplating a consultation with a physician who ran a program in alternative medicine at a top medical school. She was hesitant about doing this, because her oncologist apparently disapproved and her biomedical habits died hard. In addition, she had given up on getting pregnant, and she and her husband had contacted a lawyer about adoption.

Jo-Ellen was not the only person who followed this pattern. Petra was thirty years old at diagnosis, with an MBA and a job she loved. Like Jo-Ellen, Petra was diagnosed shortly after getting married. At this point in her life, the future had looked rosy, but since Petra's mother had died of breast cancer when Petra was seven years old, she had decided to have a baseline mammogram before getting pregnant. Her thinking was that, if anything changed or looked suspicious in a subsequent mammogram, the baseline would be available for comparison. However, this first mammogram showed calcifications—usually an indication of ductal carcinoma in situ (DCIS), which is a precancerous condition that doctors often treat as breast cancer but which generally is not serious. In Petra's case, they decided to remove the calcifications surgically, rather than keep an eye on them, because of her family history.

After that, things deteriorated quickly. The biopsy of Petra's calcifications led to a mastectomy, and when the doctor examined her lymph nodes, one was positive. So she had chemotherapy and radiation to maximize her chances of recovery from what was no longer a precancer. A biomedical expert, like Jo-Ellen, Petra had gone for a second opinion after the first biopsy. Anxious, as she put it, to "be at the place that is known and has a reputation," she chose the university comprehensive cancer center for her treatments rather than the local hospital she had gone to first.

Although her doctors had recommended tamoxifen, Petra realized that taking it would probably put her into menopause, and since she still planned on getting pregnant, she decided against it. When things seemed to be fine after the chemotherapy ended, Petra and her doctors agreed that she was safe having her breast reconstructed. Like Jo-Ellen, she chose an implant rather than the tramflap; her decision was also predicated upon the expectation of a future pregnancy and the need for stomach muscles during delivery.

Shortly after her chemotherapy ended, Petra's periods returned, and she resumed the life that she had anticipated living at the time of her marriage. She went to a friend's wedding and had a wonderful time dancing, but, afterward, she thought she had pulled a muscle in her leg. When it did not get better quickly, she told the doctor who was treating her father's terminal cancer. This doctor suggested getting a bone scan just to be sure. When the pain proved to be caused by a metastasis, Petra still kept her faith in biomedicine and immediately went on tamoxifen and Aredia,[4] as well as planning another bout of chemotherapy. When I interviewed her, she was somewhat self-critical, because she believed that she could have been more aggressive in pursuing the latest medical treatments:

> There are things you wish you knew beforehand. . . . People I have met and talked to after, say, "I did a trial" or "I did something where they were testing stronger CA [Cytoxin and Adriamycin]. . . ."[5] When I think back, my focus was that I wanted to be pregnant. Maybe I wouldn't have wanted to be faced with the choice of doing something harsher.

Like most biomedical experts, Petra had attended lots of educational programs, including those at the university hospital where she was treated and at Living Beyond Breast Cancer (LBBC). She had lots of help from friends, who made meals and took her for doctors' visits. She described herself as the kind of person who talked about the clinical aspects of her illness and treatment rather than the emotional aspects. This led to some trouble with her husband, because he assumed she was coping better than she was:

> The first diagnosis, we had a rocky time in our relationship. He didn't understand that, if I would physically handle myself, emotionally I still needed him. . . . I called him one night. He was at work at eleven o'clock at night. Crying, I called my girlfriend and she said, "Call him, and tell him to come home. . . ." Finally, I said to him, "We could go to counseling and work on a lot of issues related to you working so much, but I will never forgive you for this. . . ." I was ready to leave him. . . . After that issue, it has been fine. Now he is even going to a support group.

Here, we see Petra's biomedical response to problems at the beginning of her treatment, including therapy for relationship issues. No doubt, her husband had not anticipated that "for better or worse" meant an almost immediate immersion into the world of chronic cancer, but his wife quickly educated him.

By the time I interviewed Petra, however, she, like Jo-Ellen, was losing faith in biomedical expertise, and she was incorporating more and more alternative practices into her life. She had changed from her former instrumental, goal-oriented self and had become focused on obtaining interested emotional help. She no longer went to meetings of LBBC's Young Survivors' Network, because she did not view herself as a survivor anymore—she could no longer have children, and at age thirty-two, she was hoping to live until her forties. Petra was now trying other programs. She was attending support group meetings at the Wellness Community, a national organization providing all kinds of help and support to cancer patients, but especially emotional support to individuals and their families living with serious and life-threatening cancers. Its support groups are attended mostly by seriously ill people with different kinds of cancers. Petra had also joined an online breast cancer group, telling me, "I have been doing that every day. I am addicted to it. Women reach out to each other—that's a major resource to me now."

Petra was trying several alternative techniques, mostly to cope with the stress of her illness. Like Jo-Ellen, she tried massage as a way of relaxing and had taken meditation training at the Wellness Community. In the future, she planned to have acupuncture and to learn yoga. Her whole focus had shifted from recovery to making it through each day as it came and dealing with the sadness and pain that clouded her life. So, for example, where she had previously been a healthy eater and had loved regular exercise, she now ate anything she fancied as long as it took minimal effort, and she could not exercise because the metastasis had weakened her hip.

Perhaps the most extreme example of a person who had changed response categories was the third woman in my study with metastatic cancer. June was forty-six years old when I interviewed her, and she had been struggling with breast cancer and subsequent metastases for six years. A mother of two young sons with an alcoholic husband when diagnosed, she was originally a traditional responder and followed the doctor's orders. June had her first mammogram after an annual gynecological visit, when the nurse-practitioner found a lump. This led to a cancer diagnosis. Because she had no health insurance, June went to a hospital clinic using Medicare, and they performed a lumpectomy with radiation. She then had chemotherapy. The doctor, she explained, said, "This is what we are going to do. This is what I recommend for you." June added, "I knew nothing. He's well trained, so I listened to him."

Although June had a college degree and might have been expected to be more assertive, she described herself as passive about treatment. As is discussed in the chapter on traditional responders, some women in this group had personal responsibilities that caused them to rely on doctors for treatment decisions. June had to cope with a husband who "just went full tilt with the alcoholism" after diagnosis, and she also had sole responsibility for her children. The children had a difficult time when June became ill, and their problems increased when their father told them they were going to be orphans. June excused his behavior, in part, with "I think if I had not had the cancer, he would have not been drinking as heavily as he did." However, "His drinking led to hepatitis. . . . He now has cirrhosis of the liver." Not surprisingly, June felt too overburdened to make treatment decisions. In particular, she needed to pay close attention to her grieving children.

Although June remained cancer-free for a while after the original bout and was soon back working and supporting her family, she was careful to go for checkups because they had found "two to three" positive lymph nodes during the first surgery. After two years, June started to have back pain, which became so severe that, fearing it was metastasis, she returned to the oncologist, who confirmed the worst. He arranged for more radiation to her back, but the disease progressed.

June's husband increased his drinking as her cancer worsened, and eventually, she separated from him. When I interviewed her, she was critical about his treatment of his family. The years of struggle with her illness had fueled her anger because, instead of supporting her, he had become an increased burden.

June became a biomedical expert in spite of herself. Living with a chronic disease, she learned more about treatment than she ever intended to. The year before I interviewed her, she had undergone a stem cell transplant. At that time, this treatment was being lauded as a last chance for desperately sick breast cancer patients. It was an expensive operation for an unemployed, uninsured woman to obtain, but by then, June had become more assertive. She talked to her oncologist and persuaded him to help her:

> My oncologist really had to fight hard for me, because I have medical assistance and, you know, they don't want to approve anything. I went through the whole stem cell process, and . . . I was the lowest count that they had ever had at [the hospital], as far as what stem cells they collected.[6] I was one of the lowest in the nation. So they were thinking of not finishing it, but I went through the whole thing. . . . I was the sickest I have ever been in my whole life. It was atrocious.

After coming home and being too weak to even to climb the stairs for about a month, June slowly started feeling better. But unfortunately, "It didn't knock all the cancer cells out," so, she added, "I have been in active cancer treatment basically all along."

By the time I interviewed her, June could give me detailed descriptions of the many cancer drugs she had taken or was taking. She knew about all the side effects, and she knew a lot about experimental drugs still in development. Cancer, June said, had changed her:

> I developed a lot more self-sufficiency, and that helped me draw the line and, you know, make a decision about separating from my husband and stay with it and not go back and forth. People tell me that I've changed an awful lot. I'm not as quiet. I'm not shy. I'm not withdrawn like I used to be. I am more outgoing. . . . I won't take anybody's stuff. . . . I'm more able now to fight for something that has to be fought for. I never, never knew that I had all this strength. . . . I thought that I didn't.

One of the things that June had learned to do was to fight on behalf of her children:

> It's been very hard; it really has. My little one knew that something was really going on. He had taken a really long time to talk, and as soon as I got sick again, he stopped talking. . . . He's seven and a half now, and since then he's been in speech therapy. . . . He's gotten a lot better, but everything stays inside. . . . The older one is fourteen and a half now. He handled it well the first time. . . . He's having an enormous number of problems right now. . . . It's a good portion of his life that his mom has been sick and his dad has been sick. [He] has lots of issues like, "What's going to happen to me, if something happens to you and Dad?"

Where other women with this kind of family stress handed over treatment decisions to their doctors, June's prognosis had become too frightening for her to continue to take this course. So she needed to find the personal resources to handle everything with the help of her mother and siblings. June was someone whose illness had truly transformed her. She did not have any choice when her situation became so dire. Her husband had exacerbated the family's problems both through his insensitivity and by his slowly killing himself, so June had to take charge of her children's crises while she battled her own disease. Even though she viewed herself as passive and even timid in the face of authority, she rose to the occasion.

She reassured her older son that, no matter what their father told them, he and his brother would be well looked after:

I've told him, and I put it in the will. . . . If something happens to me, and [their father] is not well, both children will go to my sister and her husband. . . . I'm in the process of trying to find the right placement for my older son in school. I have to fight for my son—we just found out he has some learning disabilities. I took them to a children's support group at [a comprehensive cancer center]. . . . [The older one] really got a lot out of that. He really felt good, because he had been dealing with it for a long time. . . . I think he really helped the other kids, and that helped him a lot.

June also paid additional attention to her younger son, and he was doing much better in school as a result. The year I interviewed her, she was volunteering as a room mother along with another parent. She planned this activity carefully; she was still very tired much of the time. For example, since she could never be sure when she was going to get sick, she told the other room mother, "You know I can handle Christmas, because I am doing really well right now. Let me do the Christmas party, because I don't know what's going to happen."

June's descriptions of her children and their problems took on the kind of psychotherapeutic tone that was common among biomedical experts—a language she had learned in coping with her own grief and that of her children. She had also become strategic about obtaining things for her children that she did not have the personal resources to provide. Her concern about making sure they enjoyed Christmas caused her to contact the Breathing Room Foundation, an organization that provides services for the families of people with cancer. She had been able to get various kinds of help for her children there, including the Christmas presents that she could not afford.

June had moved from being a traditional responder overburdened with her private life, to a biomedical expert taking part in medical decisions. But she did not stop there. When I interviewed her, she was quite skeptical about the ability of medicine, alone, to cure her. Like Jo-Ellen and Petra, she was now interested in alternative medicine but had already tried more radical treatments than they had used. Telling me that "I like the whole idea of alternative medicine and traditional medicine trying to work things out," June described the programs in which she had participated. These included support groups, nutrition seminars, and a course on the mind/body connection. She had also tried several radical diets:

> With my second diagnosis, I went to a homeopathic doctor, and he put me on a very strict diet. Lots of it was basically vegetarian with an egg a week, and the rest was tofu, and tempeh, and stuff like that. I was also juicing carrot juice every day and drinking that. . . . I was very, very tired. . . . I was trying to follow the vegetarian diet and trying to cook a regular meal, and it wasn't going. . . . [Now] I have medicinal tea. I take homeopathic medicine. I take lots of supplements. [The homeopathic doctor] does magnetic responses, and he holds the medicine up to you and does a muscle test to see the right dosage, or whether this item will help or not, and that is how he decides what I should have.

June's dietary experiments were not, however, her most unusual foray into alternative medicine:

> I go to get doctored and do a spiritual healing with American Indians. I'm being treated by . . . two different medicine men. They have helped me tremendously. The first time was when I was rediagnosed last November with metastatic cancer. My uncle came over and said, "I have been involved with this for a couple of years, and we just worked with a woman who had cancer, and she seems to be doing great. Would you be interested in trying this out?" I said, "Yeah, sure." So by Thanksgiving . . . we brought the medicine man from South Dakota. . . . [He] came for four or five hours a day for four days in a row to do healing with me. The first day, I was in excruciating pain, even with the morphine. I could not move. . . . By the fourth day, I was lying on the floor kicking my legs up and stretching my arms over my head. . . . And I have not taken morphine since. . . . I haven't been in the hospital since.

June used this success with alternative medicine to hold on to some optimism about the future. As I was leaving, she told me that her energy had increased and that she felt that she was getting better.

We can learn a lot about how women respond to breast cancer by looking at these three cases. It is not just chance that they all ended up moving toward alternative expertise. All three women had good reasons to believe that biomedicine was not going to cure them. No matter how much they learn about their disease or how thoughtful they are in making medical decisions, most women whose breast cancers metastasize simply cannot be saved by biomedicine. Such women's cancers are considered to be at Stage IV—there is no stage V—and the five-year survival rate at this stage is 16 percent.[7] Jo-Ellen, Petra, and June all had slim chances of surviving much longer, and so they had become willing to try extreme treatments or to do whatever it took to cope with the tragedy of their lives. In this, biomedicine was of little help.

Furthermore, although June had started out as a traditional responder, the work of managing successive cancer episodes had forced her to gain expertise, and the problems of her personal life had changed the way she handled crisis. June still had some ambivalence about her appropriate role in decision-making. She knew that "a lot of people feel they should have as equal a hand in it" as the doctors, but she did not really agree with this sentiment, because her oncologist "had graduated in the top 5 percent of his class at MIT." No matter how much she read, she would not know as much as him because, "That is what the oncologist is educated for." June remained willing to listen to her doctor and to follow his advice, but she justified this with biomedical reasoning, such as his elite medical background. And she went in another direction completely with her South Dakota medicine men and the magnet therapy from her homeopathic healer.

These three stories show the structural basis of women's responses. No matter what their personal backgrounds or ideologies, if they were sick enough, women learned the biomedical options available for treating their disease, and if this did not work they eventually turned elsewhere for help. Their life circumstances forced them into behaviors that they might not have anticipated.

Two other women fit into more than one response category, but, unlike the three women above, they did this simultaneously, not serially. Both panicked at diagnosis. They acted like biomedical experts: they went for several opinions and read and learned a great deal about cancer. At the same time, they tried many alternative practices. Finally, they believed God was guiding them from start to finish. When asked for their theories as to why they got cancer, both gave religious responses—that it happened for a reason and that it was in God's hands. Perhaps they found their illnesses so frightening that they turned to every kind of support they could find. And while it is probably a coincidence, both were nurses. They had lots of biomedical training, they made their living in this industry, and they also knew all the terrible things that could happen with a cancer diagnosis. It is possible that a larger, random sample would produce other women like them.

We have taken a long journey through the narratives of women diagnosed with breast cancer. We have seen that education, income, race, and marital and sexual identities influence these narratives. What else, if anything, can we learn from the stories women told about living with a serious illness? As Deborah Lupton has observed, there is a growing interest in analyzing firsthand accounts of disease and illness.[8] From this perspective, the views of doctors become only one source of data about sickness. By understanding patients' narratives such as those described in this book, sociologists have come to realize how frequently military metaphors shape illness narratives.[9] This is particularly true in the case of breast cancer, as Susan Sontag discovered when she was diagnosed in the 1970s.[10] Women in the current study talked about fighting their cancers, and they saw cancer as an outside agent that had somehow attacked their bodies. Some thought this had happened because they had let their defenses down, while others thought defense had been impossible against such an aggressive enemy. Either way, they saw themselves as brave in the face of invasion.[11]

Women believed that a fighting attitude was an important aid to recovery. It became the prime weapon in each battle they won against cancer. In a study of the military metaphors used in illness narratives, Deborah Oates Erwin found that, in spite of a continuing stigma about cancer and cancer treatment, most patients showed great optimism. They believed that they would achieve victory over cancer, and they had great faith in their doctors and in their treatment.[12] Lupton argued that patients, especially women, believe they can change the course of their disease through hope, particularly the hope for a medical cure. Given the nature of my sample, I cannot generalize to the population, but it should be no surprise that the majority of those I interviewed (67 out of 96) were believers in biomedicine. Deborah Gordon, in an analysis of long-standing assumptions in Western medicine, noted that medicine offers a strong message that humans can overcome nature. Believing this makes women feel that they have some agency and are not merely victims.[13]

Biomedicine, as many have noted, turns treatment into a trial that each woman—even those who have the support of loving others—experiences alone. Only the sufferer faces death and deals with the pain and problems of treatment. Given this individual nature of illness, it is not surprising that physicians' status has been so high. Doctors treat patients one at a time, treating effects rather than causes. Patients come to rely on doctors to understand what they're going through, since doctors have seen every illness and used every treatment before. The high status of doctors is especially evident in the United States, a society where individual explanations for disease are more accepted than elsewhere. In a study of French cancer patients, Patrice Pinell found that most saw the cause of cancer as outside their individual behaviors. Many saw it as a product of social disorder or as a result of environmental decay.[14] This perspective contrasts with the views of many of the women in my study, who frequently thought their own activities or attitudes had caused their cancer. Even when they had an explanation outside themselves, it was still an individual mishap they described, rather than a societal problem. A number of writers have noted that Americans are more likely to emphasize their personal responsibility for illness, especially for hidden illnesses like cancer.[15] Americans are expected to act preventively, or risk being seen as irresponsible. In chapter 1, for example, the frequency with which women's magazines ran stories on how to prevent breast cancer is noted.

These differential attitudes toward cancer reflect more general differences in culture between Americans and Europeans. American have long had a strong mistrust of government and a belief that individuals have the responsibility to make their own way in the world. This has led to a general mistrust of government spending on anything except defense and, as well, a mistrust of social programs. The French, however, and Europeans in general, have long believed that the government has the responsibility to ensure a reasonable quality of life for all citizens. It is interesting to see these cultural differences reflected in attitudes toward the causes of illness, with Americans showing their individualistic bias . and the French taking a more collective approach.

While American cultural attitudes about illness hold sway over all in the United States, they do so differentially. Women diagnosed with breast cancer respond in ways that fit the circumstances of their lives. Traditional responders had been caregivers for most of their adult lives. They had lower than average levels of education among the women interviewed, and they often had demanding personal responsibilities. No wonder they wanted doctors to make decisions for them. These were women who felt that their lack of vigilance had caused the cancer to happen. Had they done more to avoid illness, they might have prevented it. Yet they also had a psychological need to leave decision-making to doctors.

According to Lupton, social class differences help to preserve medical authority, and most of the traditional responders were less educated and informed than doctors.[16] Even in the modern world, where patients have access to a wide array of information, the treatment of illness still relies on the ability to interpret the evidence, and traditional patients believed that this was the job of the doctor. This adherence to medical authority is most common among those with a class position lower than that of doctors.[17] This is not an unreasonable position because no doubt doctors do frequently behave in a patronizing manner to less-educated patients, so traditional responders were making things less stressful for themselves by giving doctors their expected due. This was exacerbated by the other demands on them, demands that sometimes increased when they became ill.

Deference was not the only reason traditional responders relied on doctors in this way. Lupton noted that while the patient's involvement in her illness can be empowering, it can also constrain her and increase her anxiety. Lupton used Michel Foucault's perspective in her statement that patients frequently acquiesce in offering their bodies to the doctor's surveillance and control.[18] Doing this enabled traditional responders to undergo cancer treatment in a way that lessened their anxiety. It also allowed them to attend to other aspects of their lives. As a group, they had been terrified when first diagnosed, so minimizing stress was important to them. While focusing on their families and relying on their doctors, these women found comfort in media stories about others who recovered from breast cancer. When they recovered from their treatment, most of the women in this group turned their backs on cancer. They maintained their new identity of "cancer survivor," but they did not typically take on the role of activist, and when they did, it was more for companionship and to provide comfort than with the expectation that they could drastically change the world of cancer.

Biomedical experts were in a different position in the social structure than traditional responders. They were better educated, usually had professional careers, and believed in women's right to lead independent lives. Most were married to supportive partners, and with two high incomes in the family, these women could afford the health care and other support they desired. Influenced by the moral imperatives of the women's health movement, they felt obliged to partner doctors rather than to unquestioningly accept medical recommendations. In Gordon's discussion of the assumptions of modern medicine, she noted that, in American society, the individual is seen as culturally distinct—not so much a product of society as in conflict with it. Biomedical experts saw health as a project that they needed to manage. They could not turn this over to their doctors but instead resisted what they saw as overbearing medical authority. To Gordon, this stance is most common among those who live privileged lives, like the biomedical experts in my study.[19] For these women, doctors were their social equals.

Biomedical experts had the background and resources to learn about the latest treatment protocols and to get second opinions, and they wanted to feel they had done everything possible to ensure survival. While they were being treated for breast cancer, they did not hesitate to take center stage among family and friends, and they expected others in their lives to provide any support they needed. They did not believe in women's traditional role of nurturing and service to others. They followed the tenets of liberal feminism by pursuing the best care possible at the expense of others, if necessary, with an individualistic explanation of their disease and its treatment. That is, they believed that women are entitled to the same rights as men. When they became involved in breast cancer activism, and a number of them did, they pushed for a larger share of research resources because they believed that women's health had been neglected by the federal government. Theirs was an activism that demanded inclusion into the existing system rather than fundamental change.

Ironically, their strong sense of entitlement often led biomedical experts to focus on breast cancer to a degree that left little time for other, more pleasurable things while undergoing treatment. Sometimes, this focus continued afterward, as these women strove to stay educated about every new discovery. They attended conferences, visited new physicians even after treatment ended, made sure they exercised, and were careful about what they ate. In a study of alternative medicine, Rosalind Coward described how extensive the commitment has become to dietary change in response to illness.[20] While biomedical experts did not believe in alternative medicine, the imperative to take control of their illness found one of its greatest outlets in diet. They accepted the cultural mantra that dietary change is an essential accompaniment to medical treatment. Controlling what they ate allowed biomedical experts a chance to actively resist their illness several times a day, even if diet was not part of their prescribed cancer protocol. But diet alone was not sufficient prevention for many women in the group. Some of them had such a need to control their cancer that, after everything was over, they wanted additional treatment just to be sure. These were the women who talked surgeons into performing prophylactic mastectomies on the second breast.

Both traditional responders and biomedical experts—like the majority of Americans—accorded authority to biomedicine. Medicine has remained one of the most prestigious and successful professions in America, even in a time of rising costs and pressure on doctors from insurance companies.[21] It was not surprising, therefore, that the majority of women I interviewed were in these two groups. Even though I did not have a probability sample, I would expect the majority of Americans to have faith in biomedicine.

Some women, however, had reasons to be suspicious of the power of doctors and their allies to save them from breast cancer. Religious respond-ers, for example, did what the doctor told them but believed that faith, not medicine, was the most important avenue to survival. In this sense, they harkened back to an earlier era when religion, not science, held authority over people's lives. Claudine Herzlich and Janine Pierret have described an earlier belief in illness as a punishment from God.[22] While no one in the current sample explained their illness quite so starkly, reli-gious responders did believe either that God had given them breast can-cer for a reason or that he had not stepped in to prevent it. And they were often quite fatalistic about the progress of the disease, although they did believe that their prayers and the prayers of others would help. Where respondents who believed in biomedicine had personal explanations for why breast cancer had happened to them and described their fight against breast cancer in military terms, religious responders did not use such language. Instead they believed their cancer had a divine purpose rather than resulting from a biological mishap of some sort.[23] They also believed that their recovery would take divine intervention, not just medical skill.

In seeking an explanation for why some women had this prescientific understanding of illness, we should note that most of the women in the religious responders' group were African American. No doubt many had experienced discrimination in American society and endured a lack of respect from doctors and so had less reason than most to put all their faith in biomedicine. While only half of the African American women I interviewed were religious responders, those who were had less than a college degree, and many had struggled with poverty and other difficul-ties. Bella, for example, fit this profile well. The African American women who were not in this group distributed themselves among the other three response categories and tended to be better educated than the reli-gious responders.

We need to be careful in assuming that we know the direction of causality. Some religious responders were neither African American nor disadvantaged in any way. The two white women in the group were affluent stay-at-home wives of successful men. Religious belief may have caused such women to take less personal responsibility for their actions.

However, it is equally possible that married women who depended on busy husbands felt unable to take charge of their destinies and looked outside themselves for assurances about survival.

Black women did not always fall into the expected response category. I have written at length about Shantal, a woman in a longtime happy marriage with a loving extended family. To an outsider, she does not appear to fit the profile of disadvantage. The first time I met her, she had reluctantly agreed that I might attend her support group. At that meeting, she spoke bitterly about white female academics who wish to include information about women of color in their work. She viewed women like me as exploiting groups such as hers, for their own gain. Shantal and I have since become friends, but the memory and essential accuracy of her words have stayed with me. For many women trying to survive racism in America, a loving and egalitarian God is a great comfort.

Because they saw themselves as God's agents, when religious responders became activists, they focused on helping others and the help they provided included spiritual help. Their activism confirmed their belief that God loved them. He had allowed them to face a terrible illness so that they could further his goals in service to others. Such women continued to follow this path long after their treatment ended.

Like religious responders, alternative experts had reasons to distrust the medical profession. In their case, this resulted either from bad personal experiences or from a more generalized distrust of corporate America and its institutions. In addition, if their illnesses did not respond well to conventional medicine, women tended to end up trying alternative techniques in a desperate effort to obtain help. As James Olson explained, "when standard treatments fail, patients seek alternatives."[24] Furthermore, some lesbians distrusted doctors because they had had difficulties with them in the past. Yet other women came to breast cancer with an existing critical analysis of the way the health system works. These women were well educated and had professional careers in the main. They differed from biomedical experts in that they wanted to change the system rather than to achieve greater inclusion.

Lupton has stated that women who try alternative medicine feel disaffected by the strictures of scientific medicine, and this was certainly the case for alternative experts. According to Barbara Willard, where biomedicine views the body as an object to be repaired by an expert, alternative medicine puts agency in women's hands.[25] Many of the alternative experts I interviewed felt this way. When illness is medicalized, women cannot think of it without recourse to a doctor, even if, as in the case of biomedical experts, the patient wishes to partner the doctor.[26] It is hard to escape this viewpoint in our culture, and in the current study everyone subscribed to it to some degree. However, under biomedicine, being sick means submitting to medical rules, and alternative experts had a more oppositional stance. They compromised the rules in different ways, obeying only those they chose or using supplementary measures to counteract what they saw as the lethal aspects of their medical treatments. These women were more radical in their feminism than biomedical experts. They saw science as male and the alternative approach as more natural and therefore female. They also had fewer family resources than biomedical experts. They were less likely to be currently married, in part because a number of them were lesbians and also because their relationships were more transient.

Coward described those who are attracted to alternative health procedures as believing in a nature that is pure and clean.[27] This is a different perspective on nature than the scientific, rational one, which allows no room for sentiment. Alternative experts have a view of nature as self-regulating and healthy if left alone. In this view, science has disturbed nature's purity and brought illness in its wake. Chemotherapy, invented by man, is toxic, and "natural" ingredients have the ability to counteract these toxic effects. Alternative experts believed in what Coward called natural therapies. They saw such methods as nontechnological, non–drug based, and noninvasive.

Yet this alternative approach, just like that of biomedical experts, suggests that the individual has the ability and even the responsibility to control her own health. And alternative experts did think this to a large degree. At the same time, they saw social causes of cancer in ways that the other groups did not. Herzlich and Pierret described two conceptions of cancer: that it is an illness of the individual and that it is a disorder of our way of life and of society. They added that these two views are not necessarily mutually exclusive but can exist side by side. When alternative experts took personal responsibility for cancer, they did so by seeing it as an illness of individuals in their relations with a sick society. So they believed that if they fixed this relationship, they might fix their cancer. But at the same time, they thought that cancer would continue to increase as long as society was so damaging to its members. That is, they saw a complex configuration of threats.[28]

The alternative experts I interviewed had educational backgrounds similar to biomedical experts. And like biomedical experts, they often became involved in managing their illness to the extent that they excluded other things. Alternative experts also had professional careers, but their worldview differed. It was more like the view Pinnel ascribed to the French than the American worldview. Their worldview was also similar to that of many academics who have written about breast cancer. Sociologists, for example, have had a long-standing critical analysis of American biomedicine.

The academic literature on breast cancer, as cited throughout this book, has focused more on political activism than on any other aspect of breast cancer. Most of these authors are sympathetic to the environmental breast cancer movement—the activism of alternative experts—while critical of mainstream organizations' support of current breast cancer protocols. When alternative experts became involved—and they were the group most likely to do so—they did not join a fight against cancer. Instead, they participated in a fight against a greedy, materialistic social system that disregards the health of its members. Because of the way I drew my sample—carefully ensuring that I interviewed activists of all kinds as well as lesbians—this group is undoubtedly a larger proportion of my study than of the population in general. Surveying breast cancer activism in America shows, as Barbara Ehrenreich observed, that most women who become activists do not get involved in radical politics.[29] They are more comfortable with helping biomedicine extend its reach and gain the resources researchers say they need to "win the war" on breast cancer.

It was striking to see that all women struggled with breast and body issues after surgery and treatment, regardless of response group. As Lupton noted, with cancer, it is treatment and not illness that mutilates. She described the modern body as marked by silent illnesses. Women are not just responsible for their health but for finding illnesses hidden within.[30] Such illnesses lead to bodily changes, which women are encouraged to conceal. But concealment is not as easy as it seems. After surgery, every woman worried about how her breasts looked, and many worked hard to reconstruct the bodies they had before cancer or to continue working on bodies that they had already seen as imperfect. This effort was only partially successful for most women, and after breast cancer, their damaged bodies continued to remind them of what they had been through and what could reoccur at any time. For women in all groups— even alternative experts—gendered sexuality challenged their self-identity when their bodies changed as a result of illness. Many women felt less sexually attractive after treatment, and consequently they were less interested in sex.

Women who underwent mastectomies found themselves lined up for reconstruction—often without really deciding. Almost all the premenopausal women with mastectomies had their breasts reconstructed. While there were differences by group in the rates of mastectomy and of reconstruction (some of which were explained by age differences) as well as in the ways those who had a reconstruction arrived at a decision as to which procedures to use, all women felt the same pressures to enhance the appearance of their breasts.

It is tempting to view the response groups described here as simply a product of social structure and culture. Women typically responded in predictable and explainable ways. Some had more opportunities than others to go for second opinions and to become well informed about their treatment. Some women had more reason than others to be skeptical of biomedicine. All had access to cultural arguments in the media and in the stories they had heard from families and friends about the meaning and treatment of cancer. They could use these stories to create their own versions of the experiences they had been through. However, to describe women only in this way is to present them as foolish and passive, and one of my most important findings is that women showed considerable agency in dealing with breast cancer. For example, they did not always fall into the groups that their demographic profile might have predicted. Kimberly, introduced in chapter 6, was a beautician with a twelfth-grade education. Thus she might have been expected to be a traditional responder, but instead, she was a biomedical expert. Furthermore, it is not easy to explain why some well-educated and independent women became biomedical responders but others became alternative responders. As a group, alternative experts had made life choices that put them on the margins, but to acknowledge this simply begs the question. We can only conclude that education enabled women to make choices about their worldview and that they responded to breast cancer in line with views they already held about American society and the place of biomedicine in it.

In one of the first and most provocative pieces of writing on the medicalization of women's bodies, Barbara Ehrenreich and Diedre English gave an account of the history of the problematic ways in which these bodies have been portrayed—in particular, as threatening to social stability and social morality.[31] Where this was once a religious problem—women's bodies were replete with sin—it is now a medical problem.[32] This transformation from sin to sickness has been both empowering and oppressive to women. Some feminists have argued that medicalization has privileged doctors' knowledge of women's bodies over women's own authentic understandings. This may be true, but its effects are offset when women are able to verify these "authentic understandings" with medical diagnoses. Yet, when women's problems are legitimated through the medical process, the old sin of womanhood, promulgated in the story of Eve and her agency in the expulsion from Eden, changes into gender pathology. And when women have access to health care, sickness and wellness become consumer items.[33]

Peter Conrad has described medicalization as a process affecting both men and women.[34] Yet, as several feminist sociologists have noted, medicalization is highly gendered and has led, in some instances, to the overtreatment of women.[35] An example of this appeared in a short article in a *New York Times* weekly medical column called "Vital Signs." Writer Eric Nagourney described research showing that when older women tell doctors that they have mammograms at least once every two years—80 percent of them say this—one-quarter are lying. Nagourney then added parenthetically that "As a practical matter . . . there is no firm evidence that mammography has any value for women 69 and older. But doctors still recommend that they have the screening, unless they have an illness that is likely to shorten their life."[36] Thus, mammography joins the long list of practices that women should engage in to stay healthy in our bio-medicalized culture.

Some of the women in my study found medicalization more comforting than did others. Where alternative experts preferred the more nurturing treatments they received elsewhere, biomedical experts often pushed for treatments that even their doctors were hesitant to provide. We have seen that several women insisted on prophylactic mastectomies on their second breasts, in some cases arguing down demurring doctors. These women approached breast cancer not as a collective problem but as something they needed to manage for themselves, and they were relieved to be able to insist on all that medicine had to offer. The founders of the women's health movement believed they were working to end the collective oppression of women, but like many social movements, this one has been transformed largely into a commodity that individual women may purchase for themselves.[37]

Even the most ardent critic of medicalization would acknowledge that breast cancer is not merely a social construction, yet it too has been subject to the tendency of biomedicine to expand its borders. Ductal carcinoma in situ (DCIS) and lobular carcinoma in situ (LCIS) were formerly considered precancers that surgeons should just watch, with the understanding that typically they would not turn into full-blown cancer necessitating treatment. Now, most surgeons operate on these precancers.[38] Those women I interviewed who had either DCIS or LCIS certainly considered themselves to have had breast cancer. In a couple of cases, it was in a very early stage and doctors had suggested watching it. Instead, the women consulted other surgeons until they could find one who was willing to operate. On the other hand, as in Petra's case described at the beginning of this chapter, DCIS can occasionally be very serious, especially for a woman with breast cancer in her immediate family.

As Deborah Gordon has convincingly argued, scientific medicine is not always very scientific. Some physicians resist medically proven techniques—the classic example is lumpectomy with radiation, which took over a decade to be generally accepted by American doctors. Scientific studies are frequently criticized for poor design and practice, and there is disagreement about the best way to design clinical trials, especially in situations where it is not possible to perform a double-blind trial. An example of the debate about clinical trials occurred in the response to a study published in the American Medical Association journal, which appeared to demonstrate that women whose cancers are estrogen-receptor positive do not benefit from chemotherapy. Since 70 percent of cases are of this type, if the study is true, its implications for breast cancer treatment are revolutionary. The study, conducted by a group of leading breast cancer researchers led by biostatistician Donald Berry, analyzed existing data from three large clinical trials that had tested the efficacy of chemotherapy regimens. Berry and his researchers found that all of the benefit of any of these regimens applied only to women whose breast cancer was impervious to estrogen.[39]

When published, opinions varied as to the scientific veracity of this research. In a story in the *New York Times* about how doctors were responding, physicians had differences of opinion over what to tell patients. A critic of the research was John Glick, director of the Abramson Cancer Center at the University of Pennsylvania. Noting that the research involved "an after-the-fact analysis of selected clinical trials," Dr. Glick argued, "We're in an era where evidence-based medicine should govern practice." Glick is not a neutral observer. His oncology practice must contain many breast cancer patients who are estrogen-receptor positive. Glick's strict standard for evidence-based medicine does not appear to have been followed by his counterpart, oncologist Larry Norton of the Evelyn H. Lauder Breast Cancer Center at Memorial Sloan-Kettering Cancer Center. In commenting on a study proclaiming the safety of chemotherapy for pregnant women—something that has long been held to damage the fetus—Norton agreed that "Chemotherapy can be used safely as long as you avoid certain agents." Since the study was based on the outcome of only fifty-seven pregnancies, it would be hard to describe the result as conclusive, given the potential seriousness of an inaccurate finding. While different experts were cited in the different stories, both men run comprehensive cancer centers funded by the National Cancer Institute.[40]

When even doctors cannot agree about the best treatment, women diagnosed with breast cancer must find comfort wherever they can. Although the various groups did so in different ways, in the end, all the women I interviewed had actively participated in making decisions about how to handle their illnesses, even if those decisions were to leave it to the doctor. In telling me about how they coped with breast cancer, they used the language they had heard in the media or elsewhere. They created illness narratives from cultural messages, and they used these narratives to come to terms with what was happening to them. Over half a century ago, Talcott Parsons described how patients had to learn the sick role.[41] His classic research has been modified by Herzlich and Pierret, who have described the invention of the modern chronic-sick role. Individuals who are chronically sick may look fine but may have an illness that is a silent killer unless treated.[42] Once diagnosed, patients who take on the chronic-sick role are permanently transformed into vigilantes about their disease. This was true for the women in my study. In learning this frightening role, they tried to adapt with dignity and grace. The real story of breast cancer is about how brave women become when they have no choice but to face directly the possibility of their dying from this disease.

Notes

INTRODUCTION

1. In a series of interviews with nine breast cancer patients, Jennifer R. Fosket makes the point that women may come to rely on biomedicine as the best hope for a cure, while simultaneously recognizing that this knowledge is unstable and up for debate. See "Problematizing Biomedicine: Women's Constructions of Breast Cancer Knowledge," in *Ideologies of Breast Cancer: Feminist Perspectives*, ed. Laura K. Potts (New York: St. Martin's Press, 2000), 15–36.

2. This theory received support with the finding that since many women abandoned such treatment after a national study concluded it slightly increased breast cancer risk, rates for estrogen-receptor-positive cancer dropped by 15 percent. Gina Kolata, "Reversing Trend, Big Drop Is Seen in Breast Cancer," *New York Times*, December 15, 2006.

3. In order to interview survivors in leadership positions in breast cancer organizations, I interviewed some women diagnosed earlier than 1994. In a few special cases, for example women who had had a reoccurrence or who experienced ongoing problems with breast reconstruction, these also had been diagnosed before 1994.

4. M. Lethbridge-Cejku and J. Vickerie, "Summary Health Statistics for U.S. Adults: National Health Interview Survey, 2003," *Vital and Health Statistics* 10 (10 January 2006): table 5; www.cdc.gov/nchs/data/series/sr_10/sr10_225.pdf (last accessed 6/28/07).

5. Anne S. Kasper, "Burdens and Barriers: Poor Women Face Cancer," in *Breast Cancer: Society Shapes an Epidemic,* ed. Anne S. Kasper and Susan J. Ferguson (New York: St. Martin's Press, 2000), 184–212; Michael S. Simon and Richard K. Severson, "Racial Differences in Survival of Female Breast Cancer in the Detroit Metropolitan Area," *Cancer* 72 (1996): 208–314.

6. Mary K. Anglin, "Working from the Inside Out: Implications of Breast Cancer Activism for Biomedical Policies and Practices," *Social Science and Medicine* 44 (1997): 1403–15; Maureen Hogan Casamayou, *The Politics of Breast Cancer* (Washington, DC: Georgetown University Press, 2001); Patricia A. Kaufert, "Women, Resistance, and the Breast Cancer Movement," in *Pragmatic Women and Body Politics,* ed. Margaret Lock and Patricia A. Kaufert (Cambridge: Cambridge University Press, 1998), pp. 287–309; Verta Taylor and Marieke Van Willigen, "Women's Self-Help and the Reconstruction of Gender: The Postpartum Support and Breast Cancer Movements," *Mobilization: An International Journal* 1 (1996): 123–42.

7. Laura K. Potts, "Publishing the Personal: Autobiographical Narratives of Breast Cancer and Self," in *Ideologies of Breast Cancer: Feminist Perspectives,* ed. Laura K. Potts (New York: St. Martin's Press, 2000), 98–127.

8. Audre Lorde, *The Cancer Journals* (San Francisco: Aunt Lute Books, 1980), 16.

CHAPTER 1. TELLING STORIES

1. The term "survivor" to describe a woman still living is not strictly accurate, as many breast cancer activists note. It is not possible to know that someone has survived breast cancer until they die of something else. Arthur W. Frank, in *The Wounded Storyteller: Body, Illness and Ethics* (Chicago: University of Chicago Press, 1995), 8, uses the term "remission society" to describe people who are well but cannot be considered cured, and he includes in this group everyone who has had cancer. From time to time, I will use the term "survivor" as a useful shorthand to describe women who no longer had active cancers.

2. Tamoxifen is a medication in pill form that interferes with the activity of estrogen. Estrogen promotes the growth of breast cancer cells. Tamoxifen works against the effects of estrogen on these cells. It is used as adjuvant, or additional, therapy following primary treatment for early-stage breast cancer. In women at high risk of developing breast cancer, tamoxifen reduces the chance of developing the disease.

3. Ellen Leopold, *A Darker Ribbon: Breast Cancer, Women, and Their Doctors in the Twentieth Century* (Boston: Beacon Press, 1999).

4. American Cancer Society, *Breast Cancer Facts and Figures 2005–2006* (Atlanta: American Cancer Society, Inc.); www.cancer.org/downloads/STT/CAFF2005BrF.pdf (last accessed 6/28/07).

5. Susan Sontag, *Illness as Metaphor* (New York: Farrar, Straus and Giroux, 1977).

6. Steven Epstein, *Impure Science: AIDS, Activism, and the Politics of Knowledge* (Berkeley: University of California Press, 1996).

7. Robert A. Padgug, "Gay Villain, Gay Hero: Homosexuality and the Social Construction of AIDS," in *Passion and Power: Sexuality in History,* ed. Kathy Peiss and Christina Simmons (Philadelphia: Temple University Press, 1989), 293–313.

8. See, for example, Victoria Brownworth, *Coming Out of Cancer: Writings from the Lesbian Cancer Epidemic* (Seattle: Seal Press, 2000); Sue Buchanan, *I'm Alive and the Doctor's Dead: Surviving Cancer with Your Sense of Humor and Your Sexuality Intact* (Grand Rapids, MI: Zondervan Publishing House, 1994); Zillah Eisenstein, *Manmade Breast Cancers* (Ithaca: Cornell University Press, 2001); Katherine Russell Rich, *The Red Devil: To Hell with Cancer — and Back* (New York: Crown, 1999).

9. In this text, "end of treatment" does not include hormone treatment. Patients may still continue taking tamoxifen or another hormone for five years after other treatment has ended.

10. Barron H. Lerner, "Inventing a Curable Disease: Historical Perspectives on Breast Cancer," in *Breast Cancer: Society Shapes an Epidemic,* ed. Anne S. Kasper and Susan J. Ferguson (New York: St. Martin's Press, 2000), 25–49.

11. Leopold, *A Darker Ribbon.*

12. Leopold, *A Darker Ribbon.*

13. Leopold, *A Darker Ribbon.* For a more general history of women's relationship with surgeons, see Ann Dally, *Women under the Knife: A History of Surgery* (New York: Routledge, 1991).

14. Although individual women were silent about their diagnoses until the 1970s, the Women's Field Army, founded by the American Cancer Society in 1935, consisted of over two million women who went door to door warning women about cancer of the breast and uterus and urging early diagnosis. See Marcy-Jane Knopf-Newman, *Beyond Slash, Burn, and Poison: Transforming Breast Cancer Stories into Action* (New Brunswick, NJ: Rutgers University Press, 2004).

15. Rose Kushner, *Breast Cancer: A Personal History and Investigative Report* (New York: Harcourt Brace Jovanovich, 1975); Betty Rollin, *First You Cry* (New York: Harper Collins, 1976).

16. Nancy Brinker, *The Susan G. Komen Story,* January 30, 2006; www.cms.komen.org/komen/AboutUs/SusanG KomensStory/index.htm (last accessed 6/28/07).

17. Theresa Montini and Sheryl Ruzek, "Overturning Orthodoxy: The Emergency of Breast Cancer Treatment Policy," *Research in the Sociology of Health Care* 8 (1989): 3–32; Karen Stabiner, *To Dance with the Devil: The New War on Breast Cancer* (New York: Delta, 1997).

18. Barron H. Lerner, *The Breast Cancer Wars: Hope, Fear, and the Pursuit of a Cure in Twentieth-Century America* (New York: Oxford University Press, 2001).

19. Lerner, *Breast Cancer Wars*, 172–73.

20. The Boston Women's Health Collective, *Our Bodies, Ourselves: A Book by and for Women* (New York: Simon and Schuster, 1971). This first edition notes "though standard procedure for many surgeons, a radical mastectomy is not always the best treatment" (265). This edition goes on to briefly describe both lumpectomies and simple mastectomies. By 1984, the new edition of *Our Bodies, Ourselves* contained a longer section describing the controversies around the radical mastectomy and around lumpectomies versus mastectomies. At this time, they noted that the modified radical mastectomy was the most common method. The 1998 edition contains an even longer section on breast cancer, giving some of the same history and describing women's various options. More recent editions have continued to add information.

21. Lerner, *Breast Cancer Wars*.

22. Stabiner, *To Dance with the Devil*.

23. Stabiner, *To Dance with the Devil*.

24. National Cancer Institute, "Cancer Research Funding, 1993," National Cancer Institute, 30 January 2006; last available at www.cis.nci.nih.gov/fact/ 1_1.htm (last accessed 10/12/05). The current NIH Web site is www.cancer.gov.

25. Victoria Mock, "Body Image in Women Treated for Breast Cancer," *Nursing Research* 42 (1993): 153–57.

26. Marilyn Yalom, *A History of the Breast* (New York: Knopf, 1997).

27. American Society of Plastic Surgeons, "2003 Quick Facts: Cosmetic and Reconstructive Plastic Surgery"; www.plasticsurgery.org/media/statistics/ loader.cfm?url=/commonspot/security/getfile.cfm&PageID=13619 (last accessed 6/20/07).

28. Amy Bloom, "When Breasts Were Fun," *Self*, August 1998; Susan Seligson, "Your Breasts: How to Keep Them Healthy and Beautiful," *Redbook*, September 1997.

29. The magazines were *Glamour, Good Housekeeping, Ladies' Home Journal, McCalls, Redbook,* and *Self*. Each was examined from January 1994 to December 1998. I also examined two magazines geared toward African American women— *Essence* and *Ebony*—but they contained few breast cancer stories.

30. Cherise Saywell, with Leslie Henderson and Liza Beattie, "Sexualized Illness: The Newsworthy Body in Media Representations of Breast Cancer," in *Ide-*

ologies of Breast Cancer: Feminist Perspectives, ed. Laura K. Potts (New York: St. Martin's Press, 2000), 37–62.

31. Jennifer R. Fosket, Angela Karran, and Christine LaFia, "Breast Cancer in Popular Women's Magazines from 1913–1996," in *Breast Cancer: Society Shapes an Epidemic*, ed. Anne S. Kasper and Susan J. Ferguson (New York: St. Martin's Press, 2000), 303–23.

32. Saywell et al., "Sexualized Illness," 38.

33. "Breast Cancer Handbook," *Self*, October 1999.

34. Saks supported the Fashion Targets Breast Cancer campaign in this way for four years starting in 1999. Saks's sponsorship has since been replaced by that of other stores.

35. *New York Times*, September 19, 1999.

36. Lisa Belkin, "Charity Begins at . . . the Marketing Meeting, the Gala Event, the Product Tie-in," *New York Times Sunday Magazine*, December 22, 1996.

37. Sandra Butler and Barbara Rosenblum, *Cancer in Two Voices* (San Francisco: Spinster Book Co., 1991).

38. Christina Middlebrook, "Before I Die," *Ladies' Home Journal*, April 1996; Joanne Kaufman, "Will I Inherit My Mother's Disease?" *Redbook*, February 1997; Dixie King as told to Diana McLellan, "Do I Have the Breast Cancer Gene?" *Ladies' Home Journal*, April 1998.

39. Julia Glass, "A Baby after Breast Cancer," *Glamour*, July 1997; Ellen and Joel Bren as told to Margaret Jaworski, "A Man, a Woman, and Breast Cancer: One Couple's Story," *Redbook*, December 1997; Deborah Kent, "My Life or My Baby's," *Redbook*, May 1997.

40. Arthur W. Frank, *The Wounded Storyteller: Body, Illness and Ethics* (Chicago: University of Chicago Press, 1995), 5.

41. Peter Conrad and Joseph W. Schneider, *Deviance and Medicalization: From Badness to Sickness* (Philadelphia: Temple University Press, 1992), 1–16.

42. Bruno Latour, *Science in Action* (Cambridge, MA: Harvard University Press, 1997).

43. Charles L. Bosk, "Social Controls and Physicians: The Oscillation of Cynicism and Idealism in Sociological Theory," in *Social Controls and the Medical Profession*, ed. J. P. Swazey and S. R. Sheer (Boston: Oelgeschlager, Gunn, 1985), 31–48.

44. Anne Karpf, *Doctoring the Media: The Reporting of Health and Medicine* (London: Routledge, 1988).

45. James T. Patterson, *The Dread Disease: Cancer and Modern American Culture* (Boston: Harvard University Press, 1987).

46. *Charting the Course: Priorities for Breast Cancer Research* (Washington, DC: Report of the National Cancer Institute's Breast Cancer Progress Review Group, 1998), 113.

47. Sontag, *Illness as Metaphor.*

48. Lerner, *Breast Cancer Wars,* 294; Robert A. Aronowitz, "Do Not Delay: Breast Cancer and Time, 1900–1970," *The Milbank Quarterly* 79 (2001): 335–86.

49. Last tried January 30, 2006.

50. Emma F. Segal, "The Nine Top Ways to Prevent Breast Cancer," *Redbook,* September 1998; Susan M. Love, "Your Best Defense against Breast Cancer," *Good Housekeeping,* May 1995; John Michnovicz and Diane S. Klein, "The Anti–Breast Cancer Diet," *Ladies' Home Journal,* July 1994.

51. Christiane Northrup, M.D., *The Wisdom of Menopause* (New York: Bantam, 2001).

52. Marshall H. Becker, "The Tyranny of Health Promotion," *Public Health Review* 14 (1986): 15–25.

53. Susan Yadlon, "Skinny Women and Good Mothers: The Rhetoric of Risk, Control, and Culpability in the Production of Knowledge about Breast Cancer," *Feminist Studies* 23 (1997): 645–69.

54. Susan Sherwin, "Cancer and Women: Some Feminist Ethics Concerns," in *Gender and Health: An International Perspective,* ed. Carolyn F. Sargent and Caroline B. Brettell (Upper Saddle River, NJ: Prentice Hall, 1996), 167–86.

55. Michael S. Goldstein, *The Health Movement: Promoting Fitness in America* (New York: Twayne, 1992).

56. Bernie Siegel, *Love, Medicine, and Miracles* (New York: Harper Perennial, 1986), 94, 99.

57. Catherine Clifford, "Boost Your Immunity," *Redbook,* February 1995; Martha Barnett, "Think Yourself Well," *Good Housekeeping,* November 1997; Elaine Greene, "A Woman of Valor," *Good Housekeeping,* January 1998. Elizabeth Austin's "The Dark Side of Wellness" in *Self,* November 1997, was the only article to note the lack of empirical evidence about the relationship between attitude and breast cancer.

58. Judith Lorber, *Gender and the Social Construction of Illness* (Thousand Oaks, CA: Sage Publications, 1997).

59. American Medical Association, *Physician Characteristics and Distribution in the U.S.* (Chicago: American Medical Association, 2003).

60. Sarah E. Brotherton, Frank A. Simon, and Sandra C. Tomany, "U.S. Graduate Medical Education, 1999–2000," *Journal of the American Medical Association* 284 (2000): 1121–26, 1159–61.

61. Peter Conrad, "Medicalization and Social Control," *Annual Review of Sociology* (1992): 209–32.

62. Emily Martin, *The Woman in the Body: A Cultural Analysis of Reproduction* (Boston: Beacon Press, 1992); Deborah Lupton, *Medicine as Culture: Illness, Disease and the Body in Western Societies* (Thousand Oaks, CA: Sage Publications, 1994).

63. Simon J. Williams and Michael Calnan, "The 'Limits' of Medicalization:

Modern Medicine and the Lay Populace in 'Late' Modernity," *Social Science and Medicine* 42 (1996): 1609–20.

64. Nora Jacobson, *Cleavage: Technology, Controversy, and the Ironies of the Man-Made Breast* (New Brunswick, NJ: Rutgers University Press, 2000); Nora Jacobson, "The Socially Constructed Breast: Breast Implants and the Medical Construction of Need," *American Journal of Public Health* 88 (1998): 1254–61.

65. Elianne Riska, "Gendering the Medicalization Thesis," *Advances in Gender Research* 1 (2003): 57–87.

66. Richard Podell and William Proctor, "Ten Mistakes Your Doctor Could Be Making," *Glamour,* February 1995; Ford Fessendon, "The Mastectomy Question," *Ladies' Home Journal,* July 1995; Constance Costas, "'You're Too Young to Have Breast Cancer' and Nine Other Things Doctors Should Never Tell You," *Ladies' Home Journal,* October 1998; Laura Muha, "Is Your Breast Exam Good Enough?" *Good Housekeeping,* October 1996; Karen Stabiner, "What Price Pregnancy?" *Good Housekeeping,* July 1998; Nancy Snyderman, "Breast Cancer False Alarms," *Good Housekeeping,* September 1998.

67. Karpf, *Doctoring the Media.*

68. Mary Alice Kellog, "Both Worlds," *Self,* November 1996; Juliet Wittmat, "In Search of Life," *Ladies' Home Journal,* March 1994.

69. The hospital is Doylestown Hospital in Doylestown, Pennsylvania.

70. Yadlon, "Skinny Women and Good Mothers."

71. Robert N. Proctor, *Cancer Wars: How Politics Shapes What We Know and Don't Know about Cancer* (New York: Basic Books, 1995).

72. Christy Simpson, "Controversies in Breast Cancer Prevention: The Discourse of Risk," in *Ideologies of Breast Cancer: Feminist Perspectives,* ed. Laura K. Potts (New York: St. Martin's Press, 2000), 131–52.

73. Natalie Angier, *Natural Obsessions: Striving to Unlock the Secrets of the Cancer Cell* (New York: Warner, 1988); Sharon Batt, *Patient No More: The Politics of Breast Cancer* (Charlottetown, Prince Edward Island: Gynergy Books, 1994).

74. John Sedgwick, "The Estrogen Report," *Self,* March 1994. Similar findings are reported by Phil Brown et al., "Print Media Coverage of Environmental Causation of Breast Cancer," *Sociology of Health and Illness* 23 (2001): 747–75.

75. One of the first to make this argument was Audre Lorde in *The Cancer Journals* (San Francisco: Aunt Lute Books, 1980). Others include Roberta Altman, *Waking Up, Fighting Back: The Politics of Breast Cancer* (Boston: Little Brown, 1996); Batt, *Patient No More;* Sandra Steingraber, "The Environmental Link to Breast Cancer," in *Breast Cancer: Society Shapes an Epidemic,* ed. Anne S. Kasper and Susan J. Ferguson (New York: St. Martin's Press, 2000), 271–99; and Eisenstein, *Manmade Breast Cancers.*

76. See Breast Cancer Action, "Policy on Breast Cancer and the Environment," at www.bcaction.org (last accessed 1/30/06). There is a debate about whether the

increase in breast cancer rates is due to real increases in the incidence, to the early diagnosis of small precancerous tumors that may never have developed into full-fledged breast cancer, or to the aging of the population and the improvement in death rates from other causes. That is, if women do not die of, for example, heart disease, they stay alive long enough to eventually contract breast cancer.

77. Phil Brown, "Popular Epidemiology and Toxic Waste Contamination: Lay and Professional Ways of Knowing," *Journal of Health and Social Behavior* 33 (1992): 267–81; Epstein, *Impure Science;* Sherwin, "Cancer and Women."

78. For a discussion of treatment options for breast cancer, see Susan M. Love, *Dr. Susan Love's Breast Book* (Cambridge, MA: Perseus, 2000).

79. Sherwin, "Cancer and Women."

80. Aronowitz, "Do Not Delay."

81. Patricia A. Kaufert, "Women, Resistance, and the Breast Cancer Movement," in *Pragmatic Women and Body Politics,* ed. Margaret Lock and Patricia A. Kaufert (Cambridge: Cambridge University Press, 1998), 292.

82. Mildred Blaxter, "The Causes of Disease: Women Talking," *Social Science and Medicine* 17 (1983): 59–69.

83. Irving Kenneth Zola, "Medicine as an Institution of Social Control," *Sociological Review* 20 (1972): 487–504.

84. Adele E. Clarke et al., "Biomedicalization: Technoscientific Transformations of Health, Illness, and U.S. Biomedicine," *American Sociological Review* 68 (2003): 161–94.

85. Martha Balshem, *Cancer in the Community: Class and Medical Authority* (Washington, DC: Smithsonian, 1993).

86. Michael Bury, "Chronic Illness as Biographical Disruption," *Sociology of Health and Illness* 4 (1982): 168–82.

87. Deborah Lupton, "Consumerism, Reflexivity, and the Medical Encounter," *Social Science and Medicine* 45 (1997): 373–81.

88. Tovia G. Freedman, "Prescriptions for Health Providers: From Cancer Patients," *Cancer Nursing* 26 (2003): 323–30.

89. Simpson, "Controversies in Breast Cancer Prevention."

90. Martin, *The Woman in the Body.*

91. Bury, "Chronic Illness as Biographical Disruption."

92. Arthur Kleinman, *The Illness Narratives: Suffering, Healing, and the Human Condition* (New York: Basic Books, 1988).

93. Gareth Williams, "The Genesis of Chronic Illness: Narrative Re-Construction," *Sociology of Health and Illness* 6 (1984): 175–200.

94. Kleinman, *Illness Narratives.*

95. "TMJ" is the commonly used acronym for disorders of the temporomandibular joint and associated muscles of the jaw.

96. Linda C. Garro, "Narrative Representations of Chronic Illness Experience:

Cultural Models of Illness, Mind, and Body in Stories Concerning the Temporo-mandibular Joint (TMJ)," *Social Science and Medicine* 38 (1994): 775–88.

97. Jackie Stacey, *Teratologies* (New York: Routledge, 1997).

98. Lucy Yardley, "Introducing Material-Discursive Approaches to Health and Illness," in *Material Discourses of Health and Illness,* ed. Lucy Yardley (New York: Routledge, 1997), 1–24.

99. Erving Goffman, *The Presentation of Self in Everyday Life* (New York: Anchor Press, 1959).

100. Catherine Kohler Riessman, "Strategic Uses of Narrative in the Presentation of Self and Illness: A Research Note," *Social Science and Medicine* 30 (1990): 1195–1200.

CHAPTER 2. FOLLOWING THE DOCTORS' ORDERS

1. Doctors check the lymph nodes of women with breast cancer to determine whether it has metastasized. "The axillary (armpit) lymph nodes are the main passageway that breast cancer cells must use to reach the rest of the body. Their involvement at any time strongly affects the prognosis." From www.nlm.nih.gov/medlineplus/ency/article/000913.htm (last accessed 1/30/06).

2. Marcy E. Rosenbaum and Gun M. Roos, "Women's Experiences of Breast Cancer," in *Breast Cancer: Society Shapes an Epidemic,* ed. Anne S. Kasper and Susan J. Ferguson (New York: St. Martin's Press, 2000), 153–82.

3. Mildred Blaxter, in a study of working-class women in Scotland, found that they rarely explained the causes of illness by using self-blaming theories. This contrasts with the traditional responders described here, most of whom were working class or lower middle class. See Mildred Blaxter, "The Causes of Disease: Women Talking," *Social Science and Medicine* 17 (1983): 59–69.

4. Anne M. Kavanagh and Dorothy H. Broom, "Embodied Risk: My Body, Myself?" *Social Science and Medicine* 46 (1998): 437–44.

5. Linda L. Layne, "Unhappy Endings: A Feminist Reappraisal of the Women's Health Movement from the Vantage of Pregnancy Loss," *Social Science and Medicine* 56 (2003): 1881–91.

6. Paul Martin, *The Healing Mind: The Vital Links between Brain and Behavior, Immunity and Disease* (New York: St. Martin's Press, 1997).

7. Susan Sontag, *Illness as Metaphor* (New York: Farrar, Straus and Giroux, 1977), 50; Bernie Siegel, *Love, Medicine, and Miracles* (New York: Harper Perennial, 1986). For a discussion of the relationship between the mind and disease, see Martin, *The Healing Mind.*

8. In *The Reproduction of Mothering: Psychoanalysis and the Sociology of Gender* (Berkeley: University of California Press, 1978), Nancy Chodorow argues that

women learn to be passive and dependent in relation to men but not to children. We might expect therefore that women would not feel they could take charge of their recovery, particularly since most cancer physicians and surgeons are men.

9. Deborah Lupton, "Consumerism, Reflexivity, and the Medical Encounter," *Social Science and Medicine* 45 (1997): 373–81.

10. Ann Dally, *Women under the Knife: A History of Surgery* (New York: Routledge, 1991). For a discussion of the gendered nature of the doctor-patient relationship, see Judith Lorber, *Gender and the Social Construction of Illness* (Thousand Oaks, CA: Sage Publications, 1997).

11. Sue Fisher, *In the Patient's Best Interest: Women and the Politics of Medical Decisions* (New Brunswick, NJ: Rutgers University Press, 1986).

12. Robert A. Aronowitz, "Do Not Delay: Breast Cancer and Time, 1900–1970," *The Milbank Quarterly* 79 (2001): 335–86.

13. Barron H. Lerner, *The Breast Cancer Wars: Hope, Fear, and the Pursuit of a Cure in Twentieth-Century America* (New York: Oxford University Press, 2001).

14. After surgery, a tube is inserted in the breast so that excess fluid can drain.

15. In *The Myths of Motherhood: How Culture Reinvents the Good Mother* (New York: Penguin, 1994), Shari L. Thurer documents centuries of pressures on women to take on caregiving, especially for children. In the final chapter, she notes that even though women now have opportunities for careers outside the home, motherhood is still seen as their primary responsibility. See also Martha McMahon, *Engendering Motherhood: Identity and Self-Transformation in Women's Lives* (New York: Guilford Press, 1995). Psychotherapist Ellen McGrath, in *When Feeling Bad Is Good,* argues that women have learned a traditional core set of values about serving others and putting themselves last (New York: Henry Holt, 1992).

16. The reason smoking complicates breast reconstruction is due to an increased risk of skin necrosis among smokers. As a result, surgical wounds are slower to heal. Arvind N. Padubidri et al., "Complications of Postmastectomy Breast Reconstruction in Smokers, Exsmokers, and Nonsmokers," *Plastic and Reconstructive Surgery* 107 (2001): 350–51.

17. Susan M. Love, *Dr. Susan Love's Breast Book* (Cambridge, MA: Perseus, 2000), 462.

18. Michael Hardy, "Doctor in the House: The Internet as a Source of Lay Health Knowledge and the Challenge to Expertise," *Sociology of Health and Illness* 21 (1999): 820–36.

19. Anthony Giddens, *Modernity and Self-Identity* (Cambridge, UK: Polity Press, 1991).

20. Helen Lambert and Hilary Rose, "Disembodied Knowledge? Making Sense of Medical Science," in *Misunderstanding Science: The Public Reconstruction*

of *Science and Technology*, ed. Alan Irwin and Brian Wynne (Cambridge: Cambridge University Press, 1996), 65–83.

21. Marisa Weiss's book is full of technical information. Marisa Weiss, M.D., and Ellen Weiss, *Living beyond Breast Cancer: A Survivor's Guide for When Treatment Ends and the Rest of Your Life Begins* (New York: Random House, 1997).

22. David Spiegel, Joan R. Bloom, and Ellen Gottheil, "Effects of Psychosocial Treatment on Survival of Patients with Metastatic Breast Cancer," *Lancet* 2 (1989): 888–91; Joachim Weis, "Support Groups for Cancer Patients," *Support Cancer Care* 11 (2003): 763–68.

23. Robin Saltonstall, "Healthy Bodies, Social Bodies: Men's and Women's Concepts and Practices of Health in Everyday Life," *Social Science and Medicine* 36 (1993): 7–14. In contrast to women, men mentioned exercise first.

24. Love, *Dr. Susan Love's Breast Book*, 521.

25. Robert Crawford, "A Cultural Account of 'Health': Control, Release, and the Social Body," in *Issues in the Political Economy of Health Care*, ed. John B. McKinley (New York: Tavistock, 1984), 60–103.

26. In the stem cell transplant procedure, since discredited, severely ill women received massive doses of chemotherapy after having their stem cells removed first. These were replaced after treatment so women did not lose the capacity to produce red blood cells as a result of chemotherapy. See Katherine Russell Rich, *The Red Devil: To Hell with Cancer — and Back* (New York: Crown, 1999).

27. Laura K. Potts, "Publishing the Personal: Autobiographical Narratives of Breast Cancer and Self," in *Ideologies of Breast Cancer: Feminist Perspectives*, ed. Laura K. Potts (New York: St. Martin's Press, 2000), 98–127.

28. Ellen Leopold, *A Darker Ribbon: Breast Cancer, Women, and Their Doctors in the Twentieth Century* (Boston: Beacon Press, 1999).

29. Sheila Ruth, "Women's Personal Lives," in *Readings for Sociology*, ed. Garth Massey (New York: W. W. Norton, 2003), 139–49.

CHAPTER 3. PATIENTS AND DOCTORS AS PARTNERS

1. A small percentage of women, especially women of Jewish heritage, inherit mutations of the *BRCA1* or the *BRCA2* gene. For women who have either of these genes, the lifetime risk of breast cancer is estimated to be 67 percent. Mary-Claire King, Joan Marks, and Jessica Mandell, "Breast and Ovarian Cancer Risks Due to Inherited Mutations in *BRCA1* and *BRCA2*," *Science* 302 (2003): 643–46.

2. Jennifer R. Fosket, "Problematizing Biomedicine: Women's Constructions of Breast Cancer Knowledge," in *Ideologies of Breast Cancer: Feminist Perspectives*, ed. Laura K. Potts (New York: St. Martin's Press, 2000), 15–36.

3. Dorothy Smith, *The Conceptual Practices of Power: A Feminist Sociology of Knowledge* (Boston: Northeastern University Press, 1990).

4. Deborah Lupton, "Consumerism, Reflexivity, and the Medical Encounter," *Social Science and Medicine* 45 (1997): 373–81.

5. Anne M. Kavanagh and Dorothy H. Broom, "Embodied Risk: My Body, Myself?" *Social Science and Medicine* 46 (1998): 437–44.

6. Michael S. Goldstein, *The Health Movement: Promoting Fitness in America* (New York: Twayne, 1992).

7. Robert Crawford, "A Cultural Account of 'Health': Control, Release, and the Social Body," in *Issues in the Political Economy of Health Care,* ed. John B. McKinley (New York: Tavistock, 1984), 60–103.

8. The one-step procedure was the standard in the United States in the 1970s. Women would go under anesthesia not knowing if they would wake to find they had had a biopsy showing the lump to be benign or a radical mastectomy because the biopsy proved malignant. Kushner continued to rail against this procedure in subsequent years, but to Kushner's dismay, when Nancy Reagan found a lump in 1987, she underwent the one-step procedure. Barron H. Lerner, *The Breast Cancer Wars: Hope, Fear, and the Pursuit of a Cure in Twentieth-Century America* (New York: Oxford University Press, 2001).

9. When Rose Kushner published her book, *Breast Cancer: A Personal History and Investigative Report* (New York: Harcourt Brace Jovanovich, 1975), she angered many doctors who disagreed with her arguments and felt unfairly criticized.

10. There is considerable evidence for an association between percentage of body fat and breast cancer risk among postmenopausal women. See Petra H. Lahmann et al., "A Prospective Study of Adiposity and the Postmenstrual Breast Cancer Risk: The Malmo Diet and Cancer Study," *International Journal of Cancer* 103 (2003): 246–52.

11. Donald B. Ardell, *High Level Wellness: An Alternative to Doctors, Drugs, and Disease* (Emmaus, PA: Rodale Press, 1977); John H. Knowles, "The Responsibility of the Individual," in *Doing Better and Feeling Worse: Health in the United States,* ed. John H. Knowles (New York: W. W. Norton, 1977), 57–80.

12. Susan Bordo, *Unbearable Weight: Feminism, Western Culture, and the Body* (Berkeley: University of California Press, 1993), 209.

13. Susan M. Love, *Dr. Susan Love's Breast Book* (Cambridge, MA: Perseus, 2000), 250.

14. In an excisional biopsy, the surgeon removes the whole lump instead of removing only a few cells.

15. Clean margins are achieved when the edges of the removed tissue contain no cancer cells, thus increasing the surgeon's confidence that no cancer cells have been left behind. Sometimes surgeons will take a wide excision to try to ensure clean margins.

16. The National Cancer Institute designates as "comprehensive cancer centers" approximately sixty hospitals in the United States with major cancer research programs. The NCI describes these hospitals as the "centerpiece of the nation's effort to reduce morbidity and mortality from cancer." More detail is provided at www.cancer.gov/cancercenters/description.html (last accessed 1/30/06).

17. Bone marrow transplant was a radical procedure used at the time of Eve's surgery, but it has since been discredited as a treatment for breast cancer. The body is bombarded with massive doses of chemotherapy; the procedure was only used in the most severe cases because of the trauma to the patient and her general health. Eve knew how dangerous it was and did not want to have such a treatment unless there was no other option.

18. At the time of Eve's surgery, the bone marrow transplant was the subject of a large, multisite clinical trial in which this hospital was participating.

19. For a more detailed definition of evidence-based medicine, see www .ebmny.org/thecentr2.html (last accessed 5/22/06).

20. Steven Epstein, *Impure Science: AIDS, Activism, and the Politics of Knowledge* (Berkeley: University of California Press, 1996).

21. Memorial Sloan-Kettering Cancer Center is a comprehensive cancer center in Manhattan and is possibly the most famous in the country.

22. Because of the risk of bilateral breast cancer in patients whose cancer is sufficiently developed to necessitate a mastectomy, mirror image biopsies are sometimes performed on the unaffected breast. For more information, see H. J. Wanebo et al., "Bilateral Breast Cancer: Risk Reduction by Contralateral Biopsy," *Annals of Surgery* 201 (1985): 667–77.

23. Atypical hyperplasia is a precancerous condition that does not necessarily lead to breast cancer. For details, see Love, *Dr. Susan Love's Breast Book*, 260–63.

24. Fosket, "Problematizing Biomedicine."

25. A study of women who used the Internet to learn about breast cancer found that women who did so experienced psychological benefits. Joshua Fogel et al., "Internet Use and Social Support in Women with Breast Cancer," *Health Psychology* 21 (2002): 398–404.

26. Emily Martin, *The Women in the Body: A Cultural Analysis of Reproduction* (Boston: Beacon Press, 1992).

27. Elianne Riska, "Gendering the Medicalization Thesis," *Advances in Gender Research* 1 (2003): 57–87; Catherine Kohler Riessman, "Women and Medicalization: A New Perspective," in *Inventing Women: Science, Technology, and Medicine,* ed. Gill Kirkup and Laurie Smith Keller (Cambridge, UK: Polity Press, 1992), 123–44; Michael Hardy, "Doctor in the House: The Internet as a Source of Lay Health Knowledge and the Challenge to Expertise," *Sociology of Health and Illness* 21 (1999): 820–36.

28. Hardy, "Doctor in the House," 827.

29. Helen Lambert and Hilary Rose, "Disembodied Knowledge? Making Sense of Medical Science," in *Misunderstanding Science: The Public Reconstruction of Science and Technology,* ed. Alan Irwin and Brian Wynne (Cambridge: Cambridge University Press, 1996), 65–83.

30. Another book that a lot of women relied on was Marisa Weiss, M.D., and Ellen Weiss, *Living beyond Breast Cancer: A Survivor's Guide for When Treatment Ends and the Rest of Your Life Begins* (New York: Random House, 1997).

31. Adriamycin and Cytoxin are commonly prescribed drugs that have debilitating side effects, especially nausea, tiredness, and, in the case of Adriamycin, a tendency to burn the veins where it is administered, leading to the need in many cases for oncologists to surgically insert a catheter.

32. The Web site used to check costs of discounted drugs in Canada was www.rxnorth.com (last accessed 6/18/06).

33. Reach to Recovery is a program of the American Cancer Society.

34. When lymph nodes are removed under the arm, it affects the lymph system's ability to drain swelling from the arm, hand, or breast—all these areas drain into the lymph nodes under the arm. So anything that can cause swelling— shots, bites, injuries, infections, or even heavy physical exertion where the arm muscles swell to take on the extra work—can cause lymphedema, which is a painful swelling of the arm or breast. Some doctors advise women to avoid using the affected arm as much as possible, but a more recent trend is to send women for physical therapy and to have them exercise the arm and slowly build its strength. In newer surgical techniques the sentinel node—the first node to be infected by breast cancer—is located and removed; as a result, fewer lymph nodes are removed, lessening the problem of lymphedema. However, the surgery has been somewhat slow to catch on because it is more difficult for surgeons to learn and some do not believe in its effectiveness. For more information see Weiss and Weiss, *Living beyond Breast Cancer.*

35. Therapeutic support groups have been associated with increased longevity after cancer. These support groups are run by clinically trained leaders and follow the principles of group therapy.

36. For more information on Living Beyond Breast Cancer, the National Breast Cancer Coalition, and the American Cancer Society, see www.lbbc.org, www .natlbcc.org, and www.cancer.org, respectively.

37. Reach to Recovery trains women volunteers who have had mastectomies to visit new mastectomy cases in the hospital and offer to help patients recover from the trauma of losing a breast.

38. The program Look Good . . . Feel Better is run by the American Cancer Society. In this program women are taught how to wear wigs and scarves, what

kinds of moisturizers to use, and how to apply makeup to disguise the loss of eyebrows and so on during chemotherapy.

39. The Wellness Community is a national organization running many different support services for cancer patients of all kinds.

40. Larry Norton is one of the most well-known oncologists in America. He holds the Norna S. Sarofim Chair in Clinical Oncology at Sloan-Kettering; he pioneered the value of using sequential combinations of drugs, as well as the drug Taxol for the treatment of breast cancer.

41. Bob Arnot, *The Breast Cancer Prevention Diet* (Boston: Little, Brown, 1998). This book has been criticized by many in the medical profession for what they see as its overly optimistic claim that by eating right one can prevent either breast cancer or a reoccurrence.

42. Some experts recommend tofu as a breast cancer preventive because Japanese women have high levels of soy consumption and a low incidence of breast cancer. However, others are uncertain about the effects of soy's estrogen-like properties on already diagnosed women.

43. Susan Yadlon, "Skinny Women and Good Mothers: The Rhetoric of Risk, Control, and Culpability in the Production of Knowledge about Breast Cancer," *Feminist Studies* 23 (1997): 645–69.

44. Bruno Latour, *Science in Action* (Cambridge, MA: Harvard University Press, 1997).

45. For more information on possible links between breast cancer and lack of exercise, see www.cancer.gov/cancertopics/wyntk/breast/page4 (last accessed 1/30/06).

46. Susan M. Love, *Dr. Susan Love's Menopause and Hormone Book* (New York: Three Rivers Press, 1998), 103.

47. Ibid.

48. Bordo, *Unbearable Weight*.

49. Gantt charts are used in project management. They are graphical representations of the duration of tasks over time.

50. Barron H. Lerner, *The Breast Cancer Wars: Hope, Fear, and the Pursuit of a Cure in Twentieth-Century America* (New York: Oxford University Press, 2001).

CHAPTER 4. FAITH IN THE ULTIMATE AUTHORITY

1. Robert Joseph Taylor, "Structural Determinants of Religious Participation among Black Americans," *Review of Religious Research* 30 (1988): 114–25; Arthur H. Miller and Martin P. Wattenberg, "Politics from the Pulpit: Religiosity and the 1980 Elections," *Public Opinion Quarterly* 48 (1984): 301–17.

2. Cornel West, *Race Matters* (Boston: Beacon Press, 1993).

3. Stephen B. Thomas et al., "The Characteristics of Northern Black Churches with Community Health Outreach Programs," *American Journal of Public Health* 84 (1994): 575–79.

4. Cathy J. Cohen, "Contested Membership: Black Gay Identities and the Politics of AIDS," in *Queer Theory: Sociology,* ed. Steven Seidman (Cambridge, MA: Blackwell, 1996), 362–94.

5. Hollie I. West, "Down from the Clouds: Black Churches Battle Earthly Problems," *Emerge* 1 (1990): 48–56.

6. C. Eric Lincoln and Lawrence H. Mamiya, *The Black Church in the African-American Experience* (Durham, NC: Duke University Press, 1990).

7. This literature is summarized in *Unequal Treatment: Confronting Racial and Ethnic Disparities in Health Care,* ed. Brian D. Smedley, Adrienne Y. Smith, and Alan R. Nelson (Washington, DC: National Academies Press, 2003).

8. Thomas, "Characteristics of Northern Black Churches with Community Health Outreach Programs."

9. Theresa Hoover, "Black Women and the Churches: Triple Jeopardy," in *Black Theology: A Documentary History, Volume One: 1966–1979,* ed. James H. Cone and Gayraud S. Wilmore (New York: Orbis Books, 1993), 293–303.

10. Mary Abrums, "'Jesus Will Fix It after Awhile': Meanings and Health," *Social Science and Medicine* 50 (2000): 89–105.

11. Lisa C. Richardson, "Treatment of Breast Cancer in Medically Underserved Women: A Review," *Breast Journal* 10 (2004): 2–5.

12. P. Diehr et al., "Treatment Modality and Quality Differences for Black and White Breast Cancer Patients Treated in Community Hospitals," *Medical Care* 27 (1989): 942–59.

13. W. D. Hobson, *Racial Discrimination in Healthcare Project — A Special Report* (Seattle: Seattle and King County Department of Public Health, 2001).

14. The Henry J. Kaiser Family Foundation, *Health Insurance Coverage in America — 1999 Data Update* (Washington, DC: The Kaiser Commission on Medicaid and the Uninsured, 2000).

15. Jean V. Hardisty and Ellen Leopold, "Cancer and Poverty: Double Jeopardy for Women," in *Myths about the Powerless: Contesting Social Inequalities,* ed. M. Brinton Likes et al. (Philadelphia: Temple University Press, 1996), 219–36.

16. Anne S. Kasper, "Burdens and Barriers: Poor Women Face Cancer," in *Breast Cancer: Society Shapes an Epidemic,* ed. Anne S. Kasper and Susan J. Ferguson (New York: St. Martin's Press, 2000), 184–212; Michael S. Simon and Richard K. Severson, "Racial Differences in Survival of Female Breast Cancer in the Detroit Metropolitan Area," *Cancer* 72 (1996): 208–314.

17. Holly F. Matthews, Donald R. Lannin, and James P. Mitchell, "Coming to

Terms with Advanced Breast Cancer: Black Women's Narratives from Eastern North Carolina," *Social Science and Medicine* 38 (1994): 789–800.

18. Anne M. Kavanagh and Dorothy H. Broom, "Embodied Risk: My Body, Myself?" *Social Science and Medicine* 46 (1998): 437–44.

19. Bryan S. Turner, *The Body and Society* (Oxford: Basil Blackwell, 1984); Bryan S. Turner, *Medical Power and Social Knowledge* (London: Sage, 1987).

20. Malcolm Bull, "Secularization and Medicalization," *British Journal of Sociology* 2 (1990): 245–62.

21. Tovia G. Freedman, "Prescriptions for Health Providers: From Cancer Patients," *Cancer Nursing* 26 (2003): 323–30.

22. Abrums, "Jesus Will Fix It after Awhile."

23. American Cancer Society, *Breast Cancer Facts and Figures 2005–2006* (Atlanta: American Cancer Society, Inc.); www.cancer.org/downloads/STT/CAFF2005BrF.pdf (last accessed 6/28/07); Dolores Davis-Penn, "Rural Black Women's Knowledge, Attitudes, and Practices towards Breast Cancer: A Silent Epidemic," in *African American Women's Health and Social Issues,* ed. Catherine Fisher Collins (Westport, CT: Auburn House, 1996), 149–63.

24. For more information about the organization Living Beyond Breast Cancer, see www.lbbc.org (last accessed 1/30/06).

25. Deepak Chopra, M.D., is a well-known authority on mind-body medicine. For more information, see www.chopra.com (last accessed 1/30/06).

26. Christy Simpson, "Controversies in Breast Cancer Prevention: The Discourse of Risk," in *Ideologies of Breast Cancer: Feminist Perspectives,* ed. Laura K. Potts (New York: St. Martin's Press, 2000), 131–52.

CHAPTER 5. OPPOSING THE MAINSTREAM

1. James S. Olson, *Bathsheba's Breast: Women, Cancer and History* (Baltimore: Johns Hopkins University Press, 2002).

2. Heather Hartley, "'Big Pharma' in Our Bedrooms: An Analysis of the Medicalization of Women's Sexual Problems," *Gender Perspectives on Health and Medicine* 7 (2003): 89–129.

3. For a series of essays from this perspective, see Judith Brady, ed., *One in Three: Women with Cancer Confront an Epidemic* (Pittsburgh: Cleis Press, 1991).

4. Zillah Eisenstein, *Manmade Breast Cancers* (Ithaca: Cornell University Press, 2001), 1.

5. Laura K. Potts, "Publishing the Personal: Autobiographical Narratives of Breast Cancer and Self," in *Ideologies of Breast Cancer: Feminist Perspectives,* ed. Laura K. Potts (New York: St. Martin's Press, 2000), 103.

6. Sharon Batt, *Patient No More: The Politics of Breast Cancer* (Charlottetown,

Prince Edward Island: Gynergy Books, 1994); Audre Lorde, *The Cancer Journals* (San Francisco: Aunt Lute Books, 1980); Jo Spence, *Cultural Sniping: The Art of Transgression* (London: Routledge, 1995).

7. Michael S. Goldstein, *The Health Movement: Promoting Fitness in America* (New York: Twayne, 1992).

8. Peter Conrad and Joseph W. Schneider, *Deviance and Medicalization: From Badness to Sickness* (Philadelphia: Temple University Press, 1992).

9. Deborah Lupton, *Medicine as Culture: Illness, Disease and the Body in Western Societies* (Thousand Oaks, CA: Sage Publications, 1994); John A. Astin, "Why Patients Use Alternative Medicine," *Journal of the American Medical Association* 279 (1998): 1548–53; Richard L. Nahin, "Toward Integrated Medicine," *Journal of the American Medical Women's Association* 54 (1999): 171–73; Anne Scott, "Homeopathy as a Feminist Form of Medicine," *Sociology of Health and Illness* 20 (1998): 191–214; Analee E. Beisecker and Thomas D. Beisecker, "Using Metaphors to Characterize Doctor-Patient Relationships: Paternalism vs. Consumerism," *Health Communication* 5 (1993): 41–58; Donna L. Richter et al., "Developing a Video Intervention to Model Effective Patient-Physician Communication and Health-Related Decision-Making Skills for a Multiethnic Audience," *Journal of the American Medical Women's Association* 56 (2001): 174–76.

10. Christy Simpson, "Controversies in Breast Cancer Prevention: The Discourse of Risk," in *Ideologies of Breast Cancer: Feminist Perspectives*, ed. Laura K. Potts (New York: St. Martin's Press, 2000), 131–52.

11. Brady, *One in Three*.

12. Batt, *Patient No More*; Eisenstein, *Manmade Breast Cancers*.

13. Susan Sherwin, "Cancer and Women: Some Feminist Ethics Concerns," in *Gender and Health: An International Perspective*, ed. Carolyn F. Sargent and Caroline B. Brettell (Upper Saddle River, NJ: Prentice Hall, 1996), 167–86.

14. John B. McKinlay and Lisa D. Marceau, "The End of the Golden Age of Doctoring," *International Journal of Health Services* 32 (2002): 379–416.

15. Research on environmental causes of breast cancer is ongoing and inconclusive. See, for example, the NCI Web site on epidemiology and genetics research: http://epi.grants.cancer.gov/LIBCSP/Overview.html (last accessed 1/30/06).

16. Ralph W. Moss, *Questioning Chemotherapy* (New York: Equinox, 2000); Samuel S. Epstein, *The Politics of Cancer Revisited* (Freemont Center, NY: East Ridge Press, 1998); Roberta Altman, *Waking Up, Fighting Back: The Politics of Breast Cancer* (Boston: Little, Brown, 1996); Richard Walters, *Options: The Alternative Cancer Therapy Book* (New York: Avery, 1993).

17. The Dana Farber Cancer Institute, affiliated with Harvard Medical School, cites a 25 percent chance of metastasis after ten years. See www.hms.harvard.edu/news/pressreleases/df/0702post_surg_chemo.html (last accessed 1/30/06).

18. Elianne Riska, "Gendering the Medicalization Thesis," *Advances in Gender Research* 1 (2003): 69.

19. Walters, *Options*.

20. Deepak Chopra, *Quantum Healing: Exploring the Frontiers of Mind/Body Medicine* (New York: Bantam, 1989). For more information on this and other books, see www.chopra.com (last accessed 1/30/06).

21. Bernie Siegel, *Love, Medicine, and Miracles* (New York: Harper Perennial, 1986), xii.

22. Jennifer Fishman, "Assessing Breast Cancer: Risk, Science, and Environmental Activism in an 'At Risk' Community," in *Ideologies of Breast Cancer: Feminist Perspectives*, ed. Laura K. Potts (New York: St. Martin's Press, 2000), 181–204; Steven Epstein, *Impure Science: AIDS, Activism, and the Politics of Knowledge* (Berkeley: University of California Press, 1996); Phil Brown, "Popular Epidemiology and Toxic Waste Contamination: Lay and Professional Ways of Knowing," *Journal of Health and Social Behavior* 33 (1992): 267–81.

23. For a description of alternative therapies for cancer, see Walters, *Options*.

24. Katherine S. Mangan, "Take Two Herbal Remedies and Call Me in the Morning," *Chronicle of Higher Education*, 18 November 2005.

25. See the Center for Advancement in Cancer Education's Web site: www .beatcancer.org/purpose.html (last accessed 1/30/06).

26. An example of the kind of diet described here can be found in Cristina Pirello, *Cook Your Way to the Life You Want* (New York: HPBooks, 1999).

27. Visualization, also known as guided imagery, is a technique in which individuals create mental images of healing. For more information, see Marion M. Lee et al., "Alternative Therapies Used by Women with Breast Cancer in Four Ethnic Populations," *Journal of the National Cancer Institute* 92 (2000): 42–47.

28. See www.healthjourneys.com (last accessed 1/30/06).

29. See www.joanborysenko.com (last accessed 1/30/06).

30. Jane Roberts was a founder of the New Age movement. She claimed to "channel" a young man named Seth, who existed outside space and time and provided words of wisdom through Roberts's voice. For more information on Jane Roberts and Seth, see www.sethcenter.com (last accessed 1/30/06).

31. Steven Levine, *A Gradual Awakening* (New York: Anchor, 1979).

32. For more detail on qi gong and feng shui, see www.scn.org/fremont/ acu/medical_qi_gong.html and www.fengshuisociety.org.uk (both last accessed 1/30/2006).

33. Hannah is referring here to the practice of measuring women's chests before radiation and marking the radiation angles by tattooing tiny moles on women's skin.

34. Simon J. Williams and Michael Calnan, "The 'Limits' of Medicalization:

Modern Medicine and the Lay Populace in 'Late' Modernity," *Social Science and Medicine* 42 (1996): 1610.

35. Barbara E. Willard, "Feminist Interventions in Biomedical Discourse: An Analysis of the Rhetoric of Integrative Medicine," *Women's Studies in Communication* 1 (2005): 115–48.

36. For a discussion on the demographic status of women who use alternative medicine, see Lee et al., "Alternative Therapies Used by Women with Breast Cancer in Four Ethnic Populations."

37. Robert Crawford, "You Are Dangerous to Your Health: The Ideology and Politics of Victim-Blaming," *International Journal of Health Services* 4 (1977): 663–80.

38. Simpson, "Controversies in Breast Cancer Prevention."

CHAPTER 6. THE ASSAULT ON THE BREAST

1. For information on the various possible procedures that can be used in a tramflap, see Susan M. Love, *Dr. Susan Love's Breast Book* (Cambridge, MA: Perseus, 2000); Ellen Leopold, *A Darker Ribbon: Breast Cancer, Women, and Their Doctors in the Twentieth Century* (Boston: Beacon Press, 1999), 263. The procedure described here is the most common one. This is a relatively new procedure and one that doctors have perfected only fairly recently.

2. Leopold, *A Darker Ribbon.*

3. For information on average relative costs, which vary according to the exact type of procedure used, see www.smartplasticsurgery.com/reconstruction/breastreconstruction.html#CS (last accessed 5/23/06).

4. See Love, *Dr. Susan Love's Breast Book.* The two most common types of implants are silicone gel and saline. The latter are encased in silicone but do not have the same level of risk as silicone gel implants. The problem with saline implants is that they can leak and quickly go flat. In addition, they do not feel as natural and do not produce as good an appearance as silicone. The silicone gel implants were banned by the Food and Drug Administration (FDA) based on evidence of danger when they leaked. After years of controversy, the FDA has recently approved a new improved version. For a discussion of the controversy, see www.womenshealthnetwork.org (last accessed 2/15/06).

5. A keloid is a raised growth of fibrous scar tissue that forms over an area of trauma to the skin and extends beyond the area of the original injury. Keloid scars are much more noticeable than ordinary scars.

6. Amanda was one of the few women in the study who had tested positively for a breast cancer gene. This meant she was at great risk of a reoccurrence and also of ovarian cancer, a disease from which several women in her family had died. Amanda felt great pressure to develop a successful intimate relationship, to

marry, and to have children as soon as possible, because she had been advised to have her ovaries removed and to have her other breast removed prophylactically. Thus Amanda had learned to view her body as "dangerous." See Nina Hallowell, "Reconstructing the Body or Reconstructing the Woman? Problems of Prophylactic Mastectomy for Hereditary Breast Cancer Risk," in *Ideologies of Breast Cancer: Feminist Perspectives,* ed. Laura K. Potts (New York: St. Martin's Press, 2000), 153–80.

7. Carolyn Latteier, *Breasts: The Woman's Perspective on an American Obsession* (New York: Harrington Park Press, 1998); Fiona Giles, *Fresh Milk: The Secret Life of Breasts* (New York: Simon and Schuster, 2003).

8. Marilyn Yalom notes that Freud also emphasized the importance of breasts for men, describing them as "the first erotogenic zone" a child experiences. Marilyn Yalom, *A History of the Breast* (New York: Knopf, 1997).

9. Iris Marion Young, "Breasted Experience: The Look and the Feeling," in *Throwing Like a Girl and Other Essays in Feminist Philosophy and Social Theory,* ed. Iris Marion Young (Bloomington: Indiana University Press, 1990), 189–209.

10. Daphna Ayalah and Isaac J. Weinstock, *Breasts: Women Speak about Their Breasts and Their Lives* (New York: Summit Books, 1979).

11. Nora Jacobson, "The Socially Constructed Breast: Breast Implants and the Medical Construction of Need," *American Journal of Public Health* 88 (1998): 1254–61.

12. Nora Jacobson, *Cleavage: Technology, Controversy, and the Ironies of the Man-Made Breast* (New Brunswick, NJ: Rutgers University Press, 2000), 118.

13. Radiation is always recommended if a woman has a lumpectomy in order to minimize the danger of a reoccurrence of cancer in the same breast.

14. Theresa Montini and Sheryl Ruzek, "Overturning Orthodoxy: The Emergence of Breast Cancer Treatment Policy," *Research in the Sociology of Health Care* 8 (1989): 3–32.

15. Barron H. Lerner, *The Breast Cancer Wars: Hope, Fear, and the Pursuit of a Cure in Twentieth-Century America* (New York: Oxford University Press, 2001); James S. Olson, *Bathsheba's Breast: Women, Cancer and History* (Baltimore: Johns Hopkins University Press, 2002).

16. ATAC stands for Arimidex, Tamoxifen, Alone or in Combination. For a report on the 2002 Breast Cancer Symposium in San Antonio, Texas, see www.breastcancer.org/research_hormonal_120002a.html (last accessed 2/20/06).

17. See www.breastcancer.org/research_surgery_120000.html (last accessed 2/20/06).

18. Yalom, *A History of the Breast.*

19. Lisa Cartwright, "Community and the Public Body in Breast Cancer Media Activism," *Cultural Studies* 12 (1998): 117–38.

20. Raymond L. Schmitt, "Embodied Identities: Breasts as Emotional Reminders," *Studies in Symbolic Interaction* 7, part A (1986): 229–89.

21. Diana Dull and Candace West, "Accounting for Cosmetic Surgery: The Accomplishment of Gender," *Social Problems* 1 (1991): 54–70.

22. Kristin M. Langellier and Claire F. Sullivan, "Breast Talk in Breast Cancer Narratives," *Qualitative Health Research* 8 (1998): 746–94.

23. Cherise Saywell, Leslie Henderson, and Liza Beattie, "Sexualized Illness: The Newsworthy Body in Media Representations of Breast Cancer," in *Ideologies of Breast Cancer: Feminist Perspectives*, ed. Laura K. Potts (New York: St. Martin's Press, 2000), 37–62; Marcy E. Rosenbaum and Gun M. Roos, "Women's Experiences of Breast Cancer," in *Breast Cancer: Society Shapes an Epidemic*, ed. Anne S. Kasper and Susan J. Ferguson (New York: St. Martin's Press, 2000), 153–82.

24. Beth Meyerowitz, "The Impact of Mastectomy on the Lives of Women," *Professional Psychology* 12 (1981): 118–27.

25. Saywell et al., "Sexualized Illness."

26. Matushka, "Why I Did It," *Glamour*, November 1993.

27. Ayalah and Weinstock, *Breasts;* Marcy-Jane Knopf-Newman, *Beyond Slash, Burn, and Poison: Transforming Breast Cancer Stories into Action* (New Brunswick, NJ: Rutgers University Press, 2004).

28. Knopf-Newman, *Beyond Slash, Burn, and Poison.*

29. In a study of women's experiences with breast cancer, Marcy E. Rosenbaum and Gun M. Roos report that women experienced a sense of loss about losing a breast, which led to reconstruction. See Rosenbaum and Roos, "Women's Experiences of Breast Cancer."

30. Audre Lorde, *The Cancer Journals* (San Francisco: Aunt Lute Books, 1980), 58–59.

31. Jackie Stacey, *Teratologies* (New York: Routledge, 1997); Edie K. Sedgwick, *Tendencies* (Durham, NC: Duke University Press, 1993).

32. Kathy Davis, *Reshaping the Female Body: The Dilemma of Cosmetic Surgery* (New York: Routledge, 1995); Sherry Baker, "Making the Choice: What You Need to Know about Breast Reconstruction," *MAMM*, September/October 2005.

33. Dull and West, "Accounting for Cosmetic Surgery."

34. Jane Brody, "After Mastectomy, Finding the Right 'New Normal,'" *New York Times*, January 3, 2006.

35. Jacobson, *Cleavage.*

36. Jacobson, *Cleavage.*

37. Barbara Shapiro, interview by author, Philadelphia, PA, January 2000. Misshapen reconstructions are fixed with a hollow mold over the breast; for lumpectomies, a small piece can be fit inside the bra, under the bust.

38. Small breasts have been officially designated as a disease called "micromastia" by the American Society for Plastic and Reconstructive Surgeons. See

Linda Coco, "Silicone Breast Implants in America: A Choice of the Official Breast," in *Essays on Controlling Processes,* ed. Laura Nader (Berkeley: Kroeber Anthropological Society, 1994), 103−32.

39. Susan M. Zimmerman, *Silicone Survivors: Women's Experiences with Breast Implants* (Philadelphia: Temple University Press, 1998).

40. Olson, *Bathsheba's Breast.*

41. Naomi Wolf, *The Beauty Myth: How Images of Beauty Are Used against Women* (New York: William Morrow, 1991).

42. Leopold, *A Darker Ribbon.*

43. More information on Reach to Recovery can be found at www.cancer.org/docroot/ESN/content/ESN_3_1x_Reach_to_Recovery_5.asp?sitearea = SHR (last accessed 1/05/06).

44. Langellier and Sullivan, "Breast Talk in Breast Cancer Narratives."

45. Latteier, *Breasts;* Emily Martin, *The Woman in the Body: A Cultural Analysis of Reproduction* (Boston: Beacon Press, 1992).

46. Jacobson, *Cleavage.*

47. Latteier, *Breasts.*

48. Janet Lee states that breasts are rarely seen as belonging to women. Rather they are owned by men and, in this society, are commodities to be gazed at. See Janet Lee, "Never Innocent: Breasted Experiences in Women's Bodily Narratives of Puberty," *Feminism and Psychology* 7 (1997): 453−74.

49. Insurance companies rarely pay for procedures done for cosmetic reasons, and the cost of breast enhancement is in the range of five to six thousand dollars.

50. These are the mildest forms of breast cancer, which many doctors call pre-cancers rather than cancers. They are the lowest stage cancers (i.e., stage 0). DCIS is ductal carcinoma in situ and LCIS is lobular carcinoma in situ. See www .cancer.org/docroot/CRI/content/CRI_2_4_4X_Treatment_by_Stage_Breast _Cancer_5.asp?sitearea (last accessed 2/20/06).

51. There is controversy about whether these small noninvasive cancers should be removed or not. Their diagnosis is a major reason for the rise in breast cancer rates with the introduction of mammograms, since mammograms can detect small cancers that cannot be palpated manually. See Olson, *Bathsheba's Breast,* 222.

52. Of the women who had reconstruction after a mastectomy, the results were equally divided between those who were satisfied with the results and those who were unhappy about it. Two women were somewhere in the middle with a general acceptance even though they had misgivings.

53. More information about this problem can be found on the Web site of the American Cancer Society, www.cancer.org (last accessed 2/20/06).

54. A brief discussion on the topic of implants and radiation can be found at www.columbiasurgery.org/divisions/plastic/news_breast.html (last accessed 2/20/06).

55. Estimates of the rate of failures for breast implants show a range from a few months to ten or more years. See Susan G. Ferguson, "Deformities and Disease: The Medicalization of Women's Breasts," in *Breast Cancer: Society Shapes an Epidemic*, ed. Anne S. Kasper and Susan J. Ferguson (New York: St. Martin's Press, 2000), 51–88.

56. For a discussion of the controversy surrounding silicone implants, see Helen S. Edelman, "Why Is Dolly Crying? An Analysis of Silicone Breast Implants in America as an Example of Medicalization," *Journal of Popular Culture* 28 (1994): 19–32.

57. Susan Bordo, *Unbearable Weight: Feminism, Western Culture, and the Body* (Berkeley: University of California Press, 1993).

58. When a saline implant breaks, it is "harmless saline going into your body." Love, *Dr. Susan Love's Breast Book,* 449.

59. Ferguson, "Deformities and Disease."

60. Olson, *Bathsheba's Breast,* 236. Olson notes that women who sell prostheses report many women come to them asking for help after reconstruction.

61. For an account of the problems of women with silicone implants, the kind that Sheila had, see Zimmerman, *Silicone Survivors.*

62. The corset store owner I interviewed about breast prostheses told me that companies do not make very large prostheses so this could have been a problem.

63. Dorothy Smith, *Texts, Facts, and Femininity: Exploring the Relations of Ruling* (New York: Routledge, 1990).

64. Dull and West, "Accounting for Cosmetic Surgery."

CHAPTER 7. BODIES AFTER CANCER

1. Douglas Degher and Gerald Hughes, "The Adoption and Management of a 'Fat' Identity," in *Interpreting Weight: The Social Management of Fatness and Thinness,* ed. Jeffery Sobal and Donna Maurer (New York: Aldine De Gruyter, 1999), 11–28.

2. Susan Bordo, *Unbearable Weight: Feminism, Western Culture, and the Body* (Berkeley: University of California Press, 1993).

3. Naomi Wolf, *The Beauty Myth: How Images of Beauty Are Used against Women* (New York: William Morrow, 1991).

4. Judith Lorber, *Gender and the Social Construction of Illness* (Thousand Oaks, CA: Sage Publications, 1997).

5. Kandi Stinson, *Women and Dieting Culture: Inside a Commercial Weight Loss Group* (New Brunswick, NJ: Rutgers University Press, 2001).

6. Stinson, *Women and Dieting Culture.*

7. Nita Mary McKinley, "Ideal Weight/Ideal Women," in *Weighty Issues: Fat-*

ness and Thinness as Social Problems, ed. Jeffery Sobal and Donna Maurer (New York: Aldine De Gruyter, 1999), 97–115.

8. Deborah Lupton, *Medicine as Culture: Illness, Disease and the Body in Western Societies* (Thousand Oaks, CA: Sage Publications, 1994), 37.

9. Thomas F. Cash and Robin E. Roy, "Pounds of Flesh: Weight, Gender, and Body Images," in *Interpreting Weight: The Social Management of Fatness and Thinness,* ed. Jeffery Sobal and Donna Maurer (New York: Aldine De Gruyter, 1999), 209–28; Thomas F. Cash, Barbara A. Winstead, and Louis H. Janda, "The Great American Shape-up," *Psychology Today* 19 (1986): 30–37.

10. Gina Cordell and Carol Rumbo Ronai, "Identity Management among Overweight Women: Narrative Resistance to Stigma," in *Interpreting Weight: The Social Management of Fatness and Thinness,* ed. Jeffery Sobal and Donna Maurer (New York: Aldine De Gruyter, 1999), 29–48; Leanne Joanisse and Anthony Synott, "Fighting Back: Reactions and Resistance to the Stigma of Obesity," in *Interpreting Weight,* 49–72.

11. For women who have chemotherapy, tamoxifen is not commenced until this is finished.

12. This is based on my observation of them. I divided women into "slim," "medium build," and "overweight." This is personal judgment, of course, but "overweight" women were women who looked to me to be carrying at least twenty-five pounds extra weight. "Medium" was measured as between five and twenty-five pounds more than an ideal body weight and "slim" was anything less than that. Using Metropolitan Life Insurance guidelines, an ideal body weight for a woman five feet four inches in height is between 117 and 131 pounds.

13. Pierre Bourdieu, *Distinction: The Social Critique of the Judgment of Taste* (London: Routledge and Kegan Paul, 1984).

14. Erving Goffman, *The Presentation of Self in Everyday Life* (New York: Anchor Press, 1959).

15. Pamela C. Regan, "Sexual Outcasts: The Perceived Impact of Body Weight and Gender on Sexuality," *Journal of Applied Social Psychology* 26 (1996): 1803–15; S. Sitton and S. Blanchard, "Men's Preferences in Romantic Partners: Obesity versus Addiction," *Psychological Reports* 77 (1995): 1995.

16. Mary B. Harris, Laurie C. Walters, and Stefanie Waschull, "Altering Attitudes and Knowledge about Obesity," *Journal of Social Psychology* 13 (1991): 881–84; Mary B. Harris, Laurie C. Walters, and Stefanie Waschull, "Gender and Ethnic Differences in Obesity-Related Behaviors and Attitudes in a College Sample," *Journal of Social Psychology* 21 (1991): 1545–66.

17. Susan M. Love, *Dr. Susan Love's Menopause and Hormone Book* (New York: Three Rivers Press, 1998).

18. Degher and Hughes, "The Adoption and Management of a 'Fat' Identity."

19. Stinson, *Women and Dieting Culture.*

20. Lupton, *Medicine as Culture,* 38.

21. Cordell and Ronai, "Identity Management among Overweight Women."

22. Kim Chernin, *The Obsession* (New York: Harper Colophon Books, 1981).

23. Sharlene Hesse-Biber, *Am I Thin Enough Yet?* (New York: Oxford University Press, 1996); Judith Rodin, *Body Traps: Breaking the Binds That Keep You from Feeling Good about Your Body* (New York: William Morrow, 1992).

24. AC refers to Adriamycin and Cytoxan. This is currently the most common combination of drugs used in chemotherapy for breast cancer.

25. After AC treatment is complete, many oncologists move women to a second set of chemotherapy treatments using Taxotere.

26. Rose Weitz, *Rapunzel's Daughters: What Women's Hair Tells Us about Women's Lives* (New York: Farrar, Straus and Giroux, 2004).

27. Rita Freedman, *Beauty Bound* (Lexington, MA: D. C. Heath, 1986), 82.

28. Maria Scarduzio, interview by author, Drexel Hill, PA, November 1999.

29. Sandra Lee Bartky, *Femininity and Domination: Studies in the Phenomenon of Oppression* (New York: Routledge, 1990).

30. D. H. Kahane, *No Less a Woman: Femininity, Sexuality and Breast Cancer* (Alameda, CA: Hunter House, 1995); Kristin M. Langellier and Claire F. Sullivan, "Breast Talk in Breast Cancer Narratives," *Qualitative Health Research* 8 (1998): 746–94; Beth Meyerowitz, "The Impact of Mastectomy on the Lives of Women," *Professional Psychology* 12 (1981): 118–27.

31. For a discussion of the side effects of tamoxifen, Susan M. Love, *Dr. Susan Love's Breast Book* (Cambridge, MA: Perseus, 2000).

32. Carol Gilligan, *In a Different Voice: Psychological Theory and Women's Development* (Cambridge, MA: Harvard University Press, 1982); Nancy Chodorow, *The Reproduction of Mothering: Psychoanalysis and the Sociology of Gender* (Berkeley: University of California Press, 1978).

33. Francesca Cancian, *Love in America: Gender and Self-Development* (Cambridge: Cambridge University Press, 1987).

CHAPTER 8. BREAST CANCER ACTIVISM, EDUCATION, AND SUPPORT

1. Lisa Belkin, "Charity Begins at . . . the Marketing Meeting, the Gala Event, the Product Tie-in," *New York Times Sunday Magazine,* December 22, 1996.

2. For an account of some of the ways the media has presented breast cancer, see James S. Olson, *Bathsheba's Breast: Women, Cancer and History* (Baltimore: Johns Hopkins University Press, 2002).

3. Theresa Montini, "Gender and Emotion in the Advocacy for Breast Cancer

Informed Consent Legislation," *Gender and Society* 10 (1996): 9–23; Stephen Zavestoski, Sabrina McCormick, and Phil Brown, "Gender Embodiment and Disease: Environmental Breast Cancer Activists' Challenges to Science, the Biomedical Model, and Policy," *Science as Culture* 13 (2004): 563–86; Lisa Cartwright, "Community and the Public Body in Breast Cancer Media Activism," *Cultural Studies* 12 (1998): 117–38.

4. For information on National Breast Cancer Awareness Month, see www .nbcam.org (last accessed 1/09/06).

5. Quoted in Devra Lee Davis and Pamela S. Webster, "The Social Context of Science: Cancer and the Environment," *Annals of the American Academy of Political and Social Science* 1 (2002): 23.

6. Steven Epstein, *Impure Science: AIDS, Activism, and the Politics of Knowledge* (Berkeley: University of California Press, 1996).

7. Mary K. Anglin, "Working from the Inside Out: Implications of Breast Cancer Activism for Biomedical Policies and Practices," *Social Science and Medicine* 44 (1997): 1403–15; Ulrike Boehmer, *The Personal and the Political: Women's Activism in Response to the Breast Cancer and AIDS Epidemics* (Albany: State University of New York Press, 2000); Maren Klawiter, "Racing for the Cure, Walking Women and Toxic Touring: Mapping Cultures of Action within the Bay Area Terrain of Breast Cancer," *Social Problems* 29 (1999): 104–27; Sabrina McCormick, Phil Brown, and Stephen Zavestoski, "The Personal Is Scientific, the Scientific Is Political: The Public Paradigm of the Environmental Breast Cancer Movement," *Sociological Forum* 18 (2003): 545–76; Montini, "Gender and Emotion in the Advocacy for Breast Cancer Informed Consent Legislation"; Verta Taylor and Marieke Van Willigen, "Women's Self-Help and the Reconstruction of Gender: The Postpartum Support and Breast Cancer Movements," *Mobilization: An International Journal* 1 (1996): 123–42; Zavestoski, McCormick, and Brown, "Gender Embodiment and Disease."

8. Gary Alan Fine, "Public Narration and Group Culture: Discerning Discourse in Social Movements," in *Social Movements and Culture,* ed. Hank Johnston and Bert Klandermans (Minneapolis: University of Minnesota Press, 1995), 127–43.

9. Kirsten Gardner, *Early Detection: Women, Cancer, and Awareness Campaigns in the Twentieth-Century United States* (Chapel Hill: University of North Carolina Press, 2006).

10. Montini, "Gender and Emotion in the Advocacy for Breast Cancer Informed Consent Legislation"; Taylor and Van Willigen, "Women's Self-Help and the Reconstruction of Gender."

11. The term "survivor" is in itself controversial; some of the more radical organizations argue that surviving breast cancer cannot be assumed until a woman dies of a cause unrelated to her breast cancer.

12. Barron H. Lerner, *The Breast Cancer Wars: Hope, Fear, and the Pursuit of a Cure in Twentieth-Century America* (New York: Oxford University Press, 2001).

13. The American Cancer Society's Web site is www.americancancersociety .org (last accessed 1/09/06).

14. Lerner, *The Breast Cancer Wars*.

15. For the Reach to Recovery Web site, see www.cancer.org/docroot/ ESN/content/ESN_3_1x_Reach_to_Recovery_5.asp?sitearea = SHR (last accessed 1/09/06).

16. For the National Breast Cancer Coalition Web site, see www.natlbcc.org (last accessed 1/09/06).

17. The choice of stereotypically masculine symbols provides an interesting contrast to the femininity of a pink ribbon.

18. Robert N. Proctor, *Cancer Wars: How Politics Shapes What We Know and Don't Know about Cancer* (New York: Basic Books, 1995).

19. Kay Dickersin et al., "Development and Implementation of a Science Training Course for Breast Cancer Activists: Project LEAD," *Health Expectations* 4 (2001): 213–20.

20. The money went into the Department of Defense because of a restriction on other funding increases. It was introduced as a "stealth" amendment by Senator Tom Harkin. See Karen Stabiner, *To Dance with the Devil: The New War on Breast Cancer* (New York: Delta, 1997).

21. Eliot Marshall, "The Politics of Breast Cancer," *Science* 259 (1993): 616–17.

22. Zillah Eisenstein, *Manmade Breast Cancers* (Ithaca: Cornell University Press, 2001).

23. Sharon Batt, *Patient No More: The Politics of Breast Cancer* (Charlottetown, Prince Edward Island: Gynergy Books, 1994).

24. Marilyn Yalom, *A History of the Breast* (New York: Knopf, 1997).

25. Lerner, *The Breast Cancer Wars*.

26. For the Think Before You Pink campaign Web site, see www.thinkbefore youpink.org (last accessed 1/27/06).

27. Pamela L. Horn-Ross and Jennifer L. Kelsey, "Breast Cancer: Magnitude of the Problem and Descriptive Epidemiology," *Epidemiologic Reviews* 15 (1993): 7–16; Paola Pisani, "Breast Cancer: Geographic Variations and Risk Factors," *Journal of Environmental Pathology* 11 (1992): 313–16.

28. Samuel S. Epstein, "American Cancer Society: The World's Wealthiest 'Non-Profit' Institution," *International Journal of Health Services* 29 (1999): 565–78; Samuel S. Epstein, "The Stop Cancer before It Starts Campaign: How to Win the Losing War against Cancer," *International Journal of Health Services* 32 (2002): 669–707; Samuel S. Epstein, *The Politics of Cancer Revisited* (Freemont Center, NY: East Ridge Press, 1998); Samuel S. Epstein, *The Politics of Cancer* (New York: Anchor Books, 1979).

29. Roberta Altman, *Waking Up, Fighting Back: The Politics of Breast Cancer* (Boston: Little, Brown, 1996); Batt, *Patient No More;* Liane Clorfene-Casten, *Breast Cancer: Poisons, Profits and Prevention* (Monroe, ME: Common Courage Press, 1996); Ralph W. Moss, *The Cancer Industry* (New York: Equinox, 1999).

30. Barbara Ehrenreich, "Welcome to Cancerland: A Mammogram Leads to a Cult of Pink Kitsch," *Harper's Magazine,* November 2001, 43–53.

31. Theresa Montini and Sheryl Ruzek, "Overturning Orthodoxy: The Emergency of Breast Cancer Treatment Policy," *Research in the Sociology of Health Care* 8 (1989): 3–32.

32. The debate between Barbara Ehrenreich and the Komen Foundation can be found at an alternative medicine Web site: www.annieappleseedproject.org/barehar.html (last accessed 1/09/06).

33. See, for example, Barbara Brenner and Barbara Ehrenreich, "The Pink Ribbon Trap," *Los Angeles Times,* December 23, 2001. Both CNN and *USA Today* had stories on the same topic over the subsequent year.

34. www.annieappleseedproject.org/komfounresto.html (last accessed 1/09/2006).

35. Karen Springen, "Breast Cancer: A Ribbon's Far Reach," *Newsweek,* October 4, 2005; Ayelet Waldman, "Pink Is the New Black," *Salon.Com,*October 10, 2005.

36. American Cancer Society, Cancer Facts & Figures 2003–2004, at www.cancer.org/docroot/STT/content/STT_1x_Breast_Cancer_Facts__Figures_2003–2004.asp (last accessed 1/09/06). Incidence for white women is 140.8 per 100,000 versus 121.7 for black women; mortality is 35.9 for black women versus 27.2 for white women; Kaiser Commission on Medicaid and the Uninsured, *Uninsured in America: A Chart Book,* May 2000.

37. Peter C. Gotzsche and Ole Olsen, "Cochrane Review on Screening for Breast Cancer with Mammography," *Lancet* 358 (2001): 1340–42; Patricia A. Kaufert, "Women and the Debate over Mammography: An Economic, Political, and Moral History," in *Gender and Health: An International Perspective,* ed. Carolyn F. Sargent and Caroline B. Bretell (Upper Saddle River, NJ: Prentice Hall, 1996), 167–86.

38. From Maria Scarduzio, "You, Only Better," Philadelphia, PA, October 1999 (author's field notes).

39. www.annieappleseedproject.org/barehar.html (last accessed 1/09/06).

40. Anglin, "Working from the Inside Out"; Taylor and Van Willigen, "Women's Self-Help and the Reconstruction of Gender"; Patricia A. Kaufert, "Women, Resistance and the Breast Cancer Movement," in *Pragmatic Women and Body Politics,* ed. Margaret Lock and Patricia A. Kaufert (Cambridge: Cambridge University Press, 1998), 287–309.

41. Elaine Grobman, interview by author, Philadelphia, PA, November 1999.

42. Klawiter, "Racing for the Cure, Walking Women and Toxic Touring."

43. Faye D. Ginsburg, *Contested Lives: The Abortion Debate in an American Community* (Berkeley: University of California Press, 1989).

44. Taylor and Van Willigen, "Women's Self-Help and the Reconstruction of Gender," 134.

45. The National Surgical Adjuvant Breast and Bowel Project (NSABP) is a clinical trials cooperative group supported by the National Cancer Institute. Since its beginning, the NSABP has enrolled more than 100,000 women and men in clinical trials in breast and colorectal cancer. Headquartered in Pittsburgh, it has research sites at nearly a thousand major medical centers, university hospitals, large oncology practice groups, and health maintenance organizations. The NSABP was one of the first organizations to undertake large-scale studies in the prevention of breast cancer, and the Breast Cancer Prevention Trial (BCPT), which included more than 13,000 women at increased risk for breast cancer, demonstrated the value of the drug tamoxifen in reducing the incidence of the disease in this population. The second prevention trial, the Study of Tamoxifen and Raloxifene (STAR), followed more than 19,000 women to compare the effects of these two drugs in reducing the incidence of breast cancer.

46. April 2000 (author's field notes).

47. November 1999 (author's field notes).

48. Katherine S. Mangan, "Take Two Herbal Remedies and Call Me in the Morning," *Chronicle of Higher Education*, November 18, 2005.

49. From Alternative Treatments and Breast Cancer, Center for Integrative Medicine, Jefferson Hospital, Philadelphia, PA, September 1999 (author's field notes).

50. From conference on Women's Cancers at University of Pennsylvania, Philadelphia, October 1999 (author's field notes).

51. From conferences on Breast Cancer and on Breast Cancer and Diet at University of Pennsylvania, Philadelphia, January and November 1999 (author's field notes).

52. Altman, *Waking Up, Fighting Back*.

53. For an account of the NBCC story, see Maureen Hogan Casamayou, *The Politics of Breast Cancer* (Washington, DC: Georgetown University Press, 2001); Stabiner, *To Dance with the Devil*.

54. An example of this speech is one given to a training session for the Pennsylvania Breast Cancer Coalition in Valley Forge, PA, March 2000 (author's field notes).

55. Taylor and Van Willigen, "Women's Self-Help and the Reconstruction of Gender."

56. Judy Wallace, interview by author, Washington, DC, November 1999.

57. Boehmer, *The Personal and the Political*.

58. Jennifer Fishman argues that African Americans in high-risk communities

are nervous about exploitation by researchers and want to ensure that experts and others who become involved in working with the community are African American. This could explain why Shantal became such an important conduit for the community. See Jennifer Fishman, "Assessing Breast Cancer: Risk, Science, and Environmental Activism in an 'At Risk' Community," in *Ideologies of Breast Cancer: Feminist Perspectives,* ed. Laura K. Potts (New York: St. Martin's Press, 2000), 181–204.

59. From Sisters in Touch, Philadelphia, PA, November 1999 (author's field notes).

60. From a presentation on cancer and nutrition, Philadelphia, PA, September 1999 (author's field notes).

61. From board meeting of Women's Health and Environmental Network (WHEN), Philadelphia, PA, January 1999 (author's field notes).

62. Gina Kolata, "Environment and Cancer: The Links Are Elusive," *New York Times,* December 13, 2005.

63. Susan Snedeker, "Pesticides and Breast Cancer Risk: A Review of DDT, DDE, and Dieldrin," *Environmental Health Perspectives Supplements* 109, supplement 1 (2001): 35–48.

64. Kolata, "Environment and Cancer."

65. Sandra Steingraber, "The Environmental Link to Breast Cancer," in *Breast Cancer: Society Shapes an Epidemic,* ed. Anne S. Kasper and Susan J. Ferguson (New York: St. Martin's Press, 2000), 271–99.

66. Robert D. Bullard, *Dumping in Dixie: Race, Class, and Environmental Quality* (Boulder, CO: Westview Press, 2000).

67. Nurit Shein, interview by author, Philadelphia, PA, December 1999.

68. For a discussion of risk factors for breast cancer, see Olson, *Bathsheba's Breast.*

69. Boehmer, *The Personal and the Political.*

70. Susan Yadlon, "Skinny Women and Good Mothers: The Rhetoric of Risk, Control, and Culpability in the Production of Knowledge about Breast Cancer," *Feminist Studies* 23 (1997): 645–69.

71. Victoria Brownworth, *Coming Out of Cancer: Writings from the Lesbian Cancer Epidemic* (Seattle: Seal Press, 2000).

72. Montini, "Gender and Emotion in the Advocacy for Breast Cancer Informed Consent Legislation."

73. Taylor and Van Willigen, "Women's Self-Help and the Reconstruction of Gender."

74. Barron H. Lerner, "Letter to the Editor," *Harper's Magazine,* February 2002.

75. McCormick, Brown, and Zavestoski, "The Personal Is Scientific, the Scientific Is Political."

76. Klawiter, "Racing for the Cure, Walking Women, and Toxic Touring."

CONCLUSION

1. Metastatic disease is a reoccurrence of breast cancer elsewhere in the body, usually appearing in lungs, liver, or bones. For more information, see Susan M. Love, *Dr. Susan Love's Breast Book* (Cambridge, MA: Perseus, 2000).

2. Taxol (chemical name: paclitaxel) and Taxotere (chemical name: docetaxel) belong to a class of chemotherapy drugs called taxanes. See www.breastcancer .org/research_taxotere_000903a.html (last visited 1/30/06).

3. The roots of the gentian violet are sold in health food stores and recommended as an aid to digestion or to kill the mouth fungus known as thrush. It is not clear what Jo-Ellen was taking it for.

4. After the axillary (armpit) lymph nodes, bone is the most common place to which breast cancer can spread. Aredia (generic name: pamidronate disodium) is a medication used to reduce bone complications and bone pain in patients whose breast cancer has spread to the bone. See http://imaginis.com/breasthealth/bc_drugs.asp#Aredia (last accessed 1/30/06).

5. CA stands for Cytoxin and Adriamycin, two of the most common drugs used for breast cancer patients.

6. Metastasis to the bone can decrease red blood cells, white blood cells, and platelets, all of which are in the bone marrow that is harvested before this treatment. See www.cancer.gov/cancertopics/factsheet/high-dose-chemo-breast-qa (last accessed 1/30/06).

7. See http://imaginis.com/breasthealth/staging.asp#survival (last accessed 1/30/06).

8. Deborah Lupton, *Medicine as Culture: Illness, Disease and the Body in Western Societies* (Thousand Oaks, CA: Sage Publications, 1994).

9. Lupton, *Medicine as Culture;* Deborah Oates Erwin, "The Militarization of Cancer Treatment in American Society," in *Encounters with Biomedicine,* ed. Hans Baer (New York: Gordon and Breach, 1992), 201–27.

10. Susan Sontag, *Illness as Metaphor* (New York: Farrar, Straus and Giroux, 1977).

11. Erwin, "Militarization of Cancer Treatment in American Society."

12. Ibid.

13. Deborah Gordon, "Tenacious Assumptions in Western Medicine," in *Biomedicine Examined,* ed. Margaret M. Lock and Deborah Gordon (Boston: Kluwer Academic Publishers, 1988), 19–56.

14. Patrice Pinell, "How Do Cancer Patients Express Their Points of View?" *Sociology of Health and Illness* 1 (1987): 25–44.

15. Lupton, *Medicine as Culture;* Claudine Herzlich and Janine Pierret, *Illness and Self in Society,* trans. Elborg Forster (Baltimore: Johns Hopkins University

Press, 1987); Kathryn Backett, "Taboos and Excesses: Lay Health Moralities in Middle-Class Families," *Sociology of Health and Illness* 14 (1992): 225–73.

16. Lupton, *Medicine as Culture.* Michel Foucault takes the position that, in the modern world, doctors have taken on the role of surveillance over patients' bodies. Patients acquiesce in this surveillance and take pleasure in the examination of bodily faults.

17. Herzlich and Pierret, *Illness and Self in Society.*

18. Lupton, *Medicine as Culture.*

19. Gordon, "Tenacious Assumptions in Western Medicine."

20. Rosalind Coward, *The Whole Truth: The Myth of Alternative Health* (London: Faber and Faber, 1989).

21. Elliot Friedson, *Professional Dominance* (Chicago: Atherton Press, 1990).

22. Herzlich and Pierret, *Illness and Self in Society.*

23. Gordon, "Tenacious Assumptions in Western Medicine."

24. James S. Olson, *Bathsheba's Breast: Women, Cancer and History* (Baltimore: Johns Hopkins University Press, 2002), 146.

25. Barbara E. Willard, "Feminist Interventions in Biomedical Discourse: An Analysis of the Rhetoric of Integrative Medicine," *Women's Studies in Communication* 1 (2005): 115–48.

26. Herzlich and Pierret, *Illness and Self in Society.*

27. Coward, *The Whole Truth.*

28. Herzlich and Pierret, *Illness and Self in Society.*

29. Barbara Ehrenreich, "Welcome to Cancerland: A Mammogram Leads to a Cult of Pink Kitsch," *Harper's Magazine,* November 2001, 43–53.

30. Lupton, *Medicine as Culture.*

31. Barbara Ehrenreich and Deirdre English, *For Her Own Good: 150 Years of the Experts' Advice to Women* (New York: Anchor Books, 1978).

32. Peter Conrad and Joseph Schneider describe this process for a number of illnesses; Peter Conrad and Joseph W. Schneider, *Deviance and Medicalization: From Badness to Sickness* (Philadelphia: Temple University Press, 1992).

33. Elianne Riska, "Gendering the Medicalization Thesis," *Advances in Gender Research* 1 (2003): 57–87; Lupton, *Medicine as Culture.*

34. Peter Conrad, "Medicalization and Social Control," *Annual Review of Sociology* (1992): 209–32; Conrad and Schneider, *Deviance and Medicalization;* Peter Conrad and Valerie Leiter, "Medicalization, Markets and Consumers," *Journal of Health and Social Behavior* (2004, extra issue): 158–76.

35. Adele E. Clarke and Virginia Olesen, "Revising, Diffracting, Acting," in *Revisioning Women, Health, and Healing: Feminist, Cultural, and Technoscience Perspectives,* ed. Adele E. Clarke and Virginia Olesen (New York: Routledge, 1999), 3–48; Emily Martin, "The Woman in the Flexible Body," in *Revisioning Women,*

Health, and Healing: Feminist, Cultural, and Technoscience Perspectives, ed. Adele Clarke and Virginia Olesen (New York: Routledge, 1999), 97–118; Riska, "Gendering the Medicalization Thesis."

36. Eric Nagourney, "Older Women May Be Skipping Mammograms," *New York Times,* June 20, 2006.

37. Clarke and Olesen, "Revising, Diffracting, Acting."

38. Susan Love has a table showing the rates at which DCIS and LCIS become invasive breast cancer. For DCIS, the rate is 11 percent and for LCIS, 7.2 percent. Thus, most women with these precancers would never develop breast cancer if untreated over thirty years. Love calls it "a degree of risk similar to that faced by a woman whose mother and sister have breast cancer." Love, *Dr. Susan Love's Breast Book,* 264–65.

39. Gina Kolata, "Shift in Treating Breast Cancer Is under Debate," *New York Times* May 12, 2006.

40. Kolata, "Shift in Treating Breast Cancer Is under Debate"; Roni Rabin, "New Notions on Pregnant Women with Breast Cancer," *New York Times,* June 27, 2006.

41. Talcott Parsons, *The Social System* (London: Routledge and Kegan Paul, 1951).

42. Herzlich and Pierret, *Illness and Self in Society.*

Bibliography

Abrums, Mary. "'Jesus Will Fix It after Awhile': Meanings and Health." *Social Science and Medicine* 50 (2000): 89–105.

Altman, Roberta. *Waking Up, Fighting Back: The Politics of Breast Cancer.* Boston: Little, Brown, 1996.

American Medical Association. *Physician Characteristics and Distribution in the U.S.* Chicago: American Medical Association, 2003.

Angier, Natalie. *Natural Obsessions: Striving to Unlock the Secrets of the Cancer Cell.* New York: Warner, 1988.

Anglin, Mary K. "Working from the Inside Out: Implications of Breast Cancer Activism for Biomedical Policies and Practices." *Social Science and Medicine* 44 (1997): 1403–15.

Ardell, Donald B. *High Level Wellness: An Alternative to Doctors, Drugs, and Disease.* Emmaus, PA: Rodale Press, 1977.

Arnot, Bob. *The Breast Cancer Prevention Diet.* Boston: Little, Brown, 1998.

Aronowitz, Robert A. "Do Not Delay: Breast Cancer and Time, 1900–1970." *The Milbank Quarterly* 79 (2001): 335–86.

Astin, John A. "Why Patients Use Alternative Medicine." *Journal of the American Medical Association* 279 (1998): 1548–53.

Ayalah, Daphna, and Isaac J. Weinstock. *Breasts: Women Speak about Their Breasts and Their Lives*. New York: Summit Books, 1979.

Backett, Kathryn. "Taboos and Excesses: Lay Health Moralities in Middle-Class Families." *Sociology of Health and Illness* 14 (1992): 225–73.

Balshem, Martha. *Cancer in the Community: Class and Medical Authority*. Washington, DC: Smithsonian, 1993.

Bartky, Sandra Lee. *Femininity and Domination: Studies in the Phenomenon of Oppression*. New York: Routledge, 1990.

Batt, Sharon. *Patient No More: The Politics of Breast Cancer*. Charlottetown, Prince Edward Island: Gynergy Books, 1994.

Becker, Marshall H. "The Tyranny of Health Promotion." *Public Health Review* 14 (1986): 15–25.

Beisecker, Analee E., and Thomas D. Beisecker. "Using Metaphors to Character- ize Doctor-Patient Relationships: Paternalism vs. Consumerism." *Health Communication* 5 (1993): 41–58.

Blaxter, Mildred. "The Causes of Disease: Women Talking." *Social Science and Medicine* 17 (1983): 59–69.

Boehmer, Ulrike. *The Personal and the Political: Women's Activism in Response to the Breast Cancer and AIDS Epidemics*. Albany: State University of New York Press, 2000.

Bordo, Susan. *Unbearable Weight: Feminism, Western Culture, and the Body*. Berke- ley: University of California Press, 1993.

Bosk, Charles L. "Social Controls and Physicians: The Oscillation of Cynicism and Idealism in Sociological Theory." In *Social Controls and the Medical Profes- sion*, edited by J. P. Swazey and S. R. Sheer, 31–48. Boston: Oelgeschlager, Gunn, 1985.

The Boston Women's Health Collective. *Our Bodies, Ourselves: A Book by and for Women*. New York: Simon and Schuster, 1971.

Bourdieu, Pierre. *Distinction: The Social Critique of the Judgment of Taste*. London: Routledge and Kegan Paul, 1984.

Brady, Judith, ed. *One in Three: Women with Cancer Confront an Epidemic*. Pittsburgh: Cleis Press, 1991.

Brotherton, Sarah E., Frank A. Simon, and Sandra C. Tomany. "U.S. Graduate Medical Education, 1999–2000." *Journal of the American Medical Association* 284 (2000): 1121–26, 1159–61.

Brown, Phil. "Popular Epidemiology and Toxic Waste Contamination: Lay and Professional Ways of Knowing." *Journal of Health and Social Behavior* 33 (1992): 267–81.

Brown, Phil, et al. "Print Media Coverage of Environmental Causation of Breast Cancer." *Sociology of Health and Illness* 23 (2001): 747–75.

Brownworth, Victoria. *Coming Out of Cancer: Writings from the Lesbian Cancer Epidemic*. Seattle: Seal Press, 2000.

Buchanan, Sue. *I'm Alive and the Doctor's Dead: Surviving Cancer with Your Sense of Humor and Your Sexuality Intact*. Grand Rapids, MI: Zondervan Publishing House, 1994.

Bull, Malcolm. "Secularization and Medicalization." *British Journal of Sociology* 2 (1990): 245–62.

Bullard, Robert D. *Dumping in Dixie: Race, Class, and Environmental Quality*. Boulder, CO: Westview Press, 2000.

Bury, Michael. "Chronic Illness as Biographical Disruption." *Sociology of Health and Illness* 4 (1982): 168–82.

Butler, Sandra, and Barbara Rosenblum. *Cancer in Two Voices*. San Francisco: Spinster Book Co., 1991.

Cancian, Francesca. *Love in America: Gender and Self-Development*. Cambridge: Cambridge University Press, 1987.

Cartwright, Lisa. "Community and the Public Body in Breast Cancer Media Activism." *Cultural Studies* 12 (1998): 117–38.

Casamayou, Maureen Hogan. *The Politics of Breast Cancer*. Washington, DC: Georgetown University Press, 2001.

Cash, Thomas F., and Robin E. Roy. "Pounds of Flesh: Weight, Gender, and Body Images." In *Interpreting Weight: The Social Management of Fatness and Thinness*, edited by Jeffery Sobal and Donna Maurer, 209–28. New York: Aldine De Gruyter, 1999.

Cash, Thomas F., Barbara A. Winstead, and Louis H. Janda. "The Great American Shape-up." *Psychology Today* 19 (1986): 30–37.

Chernin, Kim. *The Obsession*. New York: Harper Colophon Books, 1981.

Chodorow, Nancy. *The Reproduction of Mothering: Psychoanalysis and the Sociology of Gender*. Berkeley: University of California Press, 1978.

Chopra, Deepak. *Quantum Healing: Exploring the Frontiers of Mind/Body Medicine*. New York: Bantam, 1989.

Clarke, Adele E., and Virginia Olesen. "Revising, Diffracting, Acting." In *Revisioning Women, Health, and Healing: Feminist, Cultural, and Technoscience Perspectives*, edited by Adele E. Clarke and Virginia Olesen, 3–48. New York: Routledge, 1999.

Clarke, Adele E., et al. "Biomedicalization: Technoscientific Transformations of Health, Illness, and U.S. Biomedicine." *American Sociological Review* 68 (2003): 161–94.

Clorfene-Casten, Liane. *Breast Cancer: Poisons, Profits and Prevention*. Monroe, ME: Common Courage Press, 1996.

Coco, Linda. "Silicone Breast Implants in America: A Choice of the Official

Breast." In *Essays on Controlling Processes*, edited by Laura Nader, 103–32. Berkeley: Kroeber Anthropological Society, 1994.

Cohen, Cathy J. "Contested Membership: Black Gay Identities and the Politics of AIDS." In *Queer Theory: Sociology*, edited by Steven Seidman, 362–94. Cambridge, MA: Blackwell, 1996.

Conrad, Peter. "Medicalization and Social Control." *Annual Review of Sociology* (1992): 209–32.

Conrad, Peter, and Valerie Leiter. "Medicalization, Markets and Consumers." *Journal of Health and Social Behavior* (2004, extra issue): 158–76.

Conrad, Peter, and Joseph W. Schneider. *Deviance and Medicalization: From Badness to Sickness*. Philadelphia: Temple University Press, 1992.

Cordell, Gina, and Carol Rumbo Ronai. "Identity Management among Overweight Women: Narrative Resistance to Stigma." In *Interpreting Weight: The Social Management of Fatness and Thinness*, edited by Jeffery Sobal and Donna Maurer, 29–48. New York: Aldine De Gruyter, 1999.

Coward, Rosalind. *The Whole Truth: The Myth of Alternative Health*. London: Faber and Faber, 1989.

Crawford, Robert. "A Cultural Account of 'Health': Control, Release, and the Social Body." In *Issues in the Political Economy of Health Care*, edited by John B. McKinley, 60–103. New York: Tavistock, 1984.

———."You Are Dangerous to Your Health: The Ideology and Politics of Victim-Blaming." *International Journal of Health Services* 4 (1977): 663–80.

Dally, Ann. *Women under the Knife: A History of Surgery*. New York: Routledge, 1991.

Davis, Devra Lee, and Pamela S. Webster. "The Social Context of Science: Cancer and the Environment." *Annals of the American Academy of Political and Social Science* 1 (2002): 13–34.

Davis, Kathy. *Reshaping the Female Body: The Dilemma of Cosmetic Surgery*. New York: Routledge, 1995.

Davis-Penn, Dolores. "Rural Black Women's Knowledge, Attitudes, and Practices towards Breast Cancer: A Silent Epidemic." In *African American Women's Health and Social Issues*, edited by Catherine Fisher Collins, 149–63. Westport, CT: Auburn House, 1996.

Degher, Douglas, and Gerald Hughes. "The Adoption and Management of a 'Fat' Identity." In *Interpreting Weight: The Social Management of Fatness and Thinness*, edited by Jeffery Sobal and Donna Maurer, 11–28. New York: Aldine De Gruyter, 1999.

Dickersin, Kay, et al. "Development and Implementation of a Science Training Course for Breast Cancer Activists: Project LEAD." *Health Expectations* 4 (2001): 213–20.

Diehr, P., et al. "Treatment Modality and Quality Differences for Black and

White Breast Cancer Patients Treated in Community Hospitals." *Medical Care* 27 (1989): 942–59.

Dull, Diana, and Candace West. "Accounting for Cosmetic Surgery: The Accomplishment of Gender." *Social Problems* 1 (1991): 54–70.

Edelman, Helen S. "Why Is Dolly Crying? An Analysis of Silicone Breast Implants in America as an Example of Medicalization." *Journal of Popular Culture* 28 (1994): 19–32.

Ehrenreich, Barbara. "Welcome to Cancerland: A Mammogram Leads to a Cult of Pink Kitsch." *Harper's Magazine*, November 2001, 43–53.

Ehrenreich, Barbara, and Deirdre English. *For Her Own Good: 150 Years of the Experts' Advice to Women*. New York: Anchor Books, 1978.

Eisenstein, Zillah. *Manmade Breast Cancers*. Ithaca: Cornell University Press, 2001.

Epstein, Samuel S. "American Cancer Society: The World's Wealthiest 'Non-Profit' Institution." *International Journal of Health Services* 29 (1999): 565–78.

———. *The Politics of Cancer*. New York: Anchor Books, 1979.

———. *The Politics of Cancer Revisited*. Freemont Center, NY: East Ridge Press, 1998.

———. "The Stop Cancer before It Starts Campaign: How to Win the Losing War against Cancer." *International Journal of Health Services* 32 (2002): 669–707.

Epstein, Steven. *Impure Science: AIDS, Activism, and the Politics of Knowledge*. Berkeley: University of California Press, 1996.

Erwin, Deborah Oates. "The Militarization of Cancer Treatment in American Society." In *Encounters with Biomedicine*, edited by Hans Baer, 201–27. New York: Gordon and Breach, 1992.

Ferguson, Susan G. "Deformities and Disease: The Medicalization of Women's Breasts." In *Breast Cancer: Society Shapes an Epidemic*, edited by Anne S. Kasper and Susan J. Ferguson, 51–88. New York: St. Martin's Press, 2000.

Fine, Gary Alan. "Public Narration and Group Culture: Discerning Discourse in Social Movements." In *Social Movements and Culture*, edited by Hank Johnston and Bert Klandermans, 127–43. Minneapolis: University of Minnesota Press, 1995.

Fisher, Sue. *In the Patient's Best Interest: Women and the Politics of Medical Decisions*. New Brunswick, NJ: Rutgers University Press, 1986.

Fishman, Jennifer. "Assessing Breast Cancer: Risk, Science, and Environmental Activism in an 'At Risk' Community." In *Ideologies of Breast Cancer: Feminist Perspectives*, edited by Laura K. Potts, 181–204. New York: St. Martin's Press, 2000.

Fogel, Joshua, et al. "Internet Use and Social Support in Women with Breast Cancer." *Health Psychology* 21 (2002): 398–404.

Fosket, Jennifer R. "Problematizing Biomedicine: Women's Constructions of Breast Cancer Knowledge." In *Ideologies of Breast Cancer: Feminist Perspectives,* edited by Laura K. Potts, 15–36. New York: St. Martin's Press, 2000.

Fosket, Jennifer R., Angela Karran, and Christine LaFia. "Breast Cancer in Popular Women's Magazines from 1913–1996." In *Breast Cancer: Society Shapes an Epidemic,* edited by Anne S. Kasper and Susan J. Ferguson, 303–23. New York: St. Martin's Press, 2000.

Frank, Arthur W. *The Wounded Storyteller: Body, Illness and Ethics.* Chicago: University of Chicago Press, 1995.

Freedman, Rita. *Beauty Bound.* Lexington, MA: D. C. Heath, 1986.

Freedman, Tovia G. "Prescriptions for Health Providers: From Cancer Patients." *Cancer Nursing* 26 (2003): 323–30.

Friedson, Elliot. *Professional Dominance.* Chicago: Atherton Press, 1990.

Gardner, Kirsten. *Early Detection: Women, Cancer, and Awareness Campaigns in the Twentieth-Century United States.* Chapel Hill: University of North Carolina Press, 2006.

Garro, Linda C. "Narrative Representations of Chronic Illness Experience: Cultural Models of Illness, Mind, and Body in Stories concerning the Temporomandibular Joint (TMJ)." *Social Science and Medicine* 38 (1994): 775–88.

Giddens, Anthony. *Modernity and Self-Identity.* Cambridge, UK: Polity Press, 1991.

Giles, Fiona. *Fresh Milk: The Secret Life of Breasts.* New York: Simon and Schuster, 2003.

Gilligan, Carol. *In a Different Voice: Psychological Theory and Women's Development.* Cambridge, MA: Harvard University Press, 1982.

Ginsburg, Faye D. *Contested Lives: The Abortion Debate in an American Community.* Berkeley: University of California Press, 1989.

Goffman, Erving. *The Presentation of Self in Everyday Life.* New York: Anchor Press, 1959.

———. *Stigma: Notes on the Management of a Spoiled Identity.* Englewood Cliffs, NJ: Prentice-Hall, 1963.

Goldstein, Michael S. *The Health Movement: Promoting Fitness in America.* New York: Twayne, 1992.

Gordon, Deborah. "Clinical Science and Clinical Expertise: Changing Boundaries between Art and Science in Medicine." In *Biomedicine Examined,* edited by Margaret M. Lock and Deborah Gordon, 257–95. Boston: Kluwer Academic Publishers, 1988.

———. "Tenacious Assumptions in Western Medicine." In *Biomedicine Examined,* edited by Margaret M. Lock and Deborah Gordon, 19–56. Boston: Kluwer Academic Publishers, 1988.

Gotzsche, Peter C., and Ole Olsen. "Cochrane Review on Screening for Breast Cancer with Mammography." *Lancet* 358 (2001): 1340–42.

Hallowell, Nina. "Reconstructing the Body or Reconstructing the Woman? Problems of Prophylactic Mastectomy for Hereditary Breast Cancer Risk." In *Ideologies of Breast Cancer: Feminist Perspectives,* edited by Laura K. Potts, 153–80. New York: St. Martin's Press, 2000.

Haraway, Donna. "The Virtual Speculum in the New World Order." In *Revisioning Women, Health, and Healing: Feminist, Cultural and Technoscience Perspectives,* edited by Adele Clarke and Virginia Olesen, 49–96. New York: Routledge, 1999.

Hardisty, Jean V., and Ellen Leopold. "Cancer and Poverty: Double Jeopardy for Women." In *Myths about the Powerless: Contesting Social Inequalities,* edited by M. Brinton Likes et al., 219–36. Philadelphia: Temple University Press, 1996.

Hardy, Michael. "Doctor in the House: The Internet as a Source of Lay Health Knowledge and the Challenge to Expertise." *Sociology of Health and Illness* 21 (1999): 820–36.

Harris, Mary B., Laurie C. Walters, and Stefanie Waschull. "Altering Attitudes and Knowledge about Obesity." *Journal of Social Psychology* 13 (1991): 881–84.

———. "Gender and Ethnic Differences in Obesity-Related Behaviors and Attitudes in a College Sample." *Journal of Social Psychology* 21 (1991): 1545–66.

Hartley, Heather. "'Big Pharma' in Our Bedrooms: An Analysis of the Medicalization of Women's Sexual Problems." *Gender Perspectives on Health and Medicine* 7 (2003): 89–129.

Herzlich, Claudine, and Janine Pierret. *Illness and Self in Society.* Translated by Elborg Forster. Baltimore: Johns Hopkins University Press, 1987.

Hesse-Biber, Sharlene. *Am I Thin Enough Yet?* New York: Oxford University Press, 1996.

Hobson, W. D. *Racial Discrimination in Healthcare Project—a Special Report.* Seattle: Seattle and King County Department of Public Health, 2001.

Hoover, Theresa. "Black Women and the Churches: Triple Jeopardy." In *Black Theology: A Documentary History, Volume One: 1966–1979,* edited by James H. Cone and Gayraud S. Wilmore, 293–303. New York: Orbis Books, 1993.

Horn-Ross, Pamela L., and Jennifer L. Kelsey. "Breast Cancer: Magnitude of the Problem and Descriptive Epidemiology." *Epidemiologic Reviews* 15 (1993): 7–16.

Jacobson, Nora. *Cleavage: Technology, Controversy, and the Ironies of the Man-Made Breast.* New Brunswick, NJ: Rutgers University Press, 2000.

———. "The Socially Constructed Breast: Breast Implants and the Medical Construction of Need." *American Journal of Public Health* 88 (1998): 1254–61.

Joanisse, Leanne, and Anthony Synott. "Fighting Back: Reactions and Resistance to the Stigma of Obesity." In *Interpreting Weight: The Social Management of Fatness and Thinness*, edited by Jeffery Sobal and Donna Maurer, 49–72. New York: Aldine De Gruyter, 1999.

Kahane, D. H. *No Less a Woman: Femininity, Sexuality and Breast Cancer*. Alameda, CA: Hunter House, 1995.

Henry J. Kaiser Family Foundation. *Health Insurance Coverage in America — 1999 Data Update*. Washington, DC: The Kaiser Commission on Medicaid and the Uninsured, 2000.

Karpf, Anne. *Doctoring the Media: The Reporting of Health and Medicine*. London: Routledge, 1988.

Kasper, Anne S. "Burdens and Barriers: Poor Women Face Cancer." In *Breast Cancer: Society Shapes an Epidemic*, edited by Anne S. Kasper and Susan J. Ferguson, 184–212. New York: St. Martin's Press, 2000.

Kasper, Anne S., and Susan J. Ferguson. *Breast Cancer: Society Shapes an Epidemic*. New York: St. Martin's Press, 2000.

Kaufert, Patricia A. "Women and the Debate over Mammography: An Economic, Political, and Moral History." In *Gender and Health: An International Perspective*, edited by Carolyn F. Sargent and Caroline B. Bretell, 167–86. Upper Saddle River, NJ: Prentice Hall, 1996.

———. "Women, Resistance, and the Breast Cancer Movement." In *Pragmatic Women and Body Politics*, edited by Margaret Lock and Patricia A. Kaufert, 287–309. Cambridge: Cambridge University Press, 1998.

Kavanagh, Anne M., and Dorothy H. Broom. "Embodied Risk: My Body, Myself?" *Social Science and Medicine* 46 (1998): 437–44.

King, Mary-Claire, Joan Marks, and Jessica Mandell. "Breast and Ovarian Cancer Risks Due to Inherited Mutations in *BRCA1* and *BRCA2*." *Science* 302 (2003): 643–46.

Klawiter, Maren. "Racing for the Cure, Walking Women and Toxic Touring: Mapping Cultures of Action within the Bay Area Terrain of Breast Cancer." *Social Problems* 29 (1999): 104–27.

Kleinman, Arthur. *The Illness Narratives: Suffering, Healing, and the Human Condition*. New York: Basic Books, 1988.

Knopf-Newman, Marcy-Jane. *Beyond Slash, Burn, and Poison: Transforming Breast Cancer Stories into Action*. New Brunswick, NJ: Rutgers University Press, 2004.

Knowles, John H. "The Responsibility of the Individual." In *Doing Better and Feeling Worse: Health in the United States*, edited by John H. Knowles, 57–80. New York: W. W. Norton, 1977.

Kushner, Rose. *Breast Cancer: A Personal History and Investigative Report*. New York: Harcourt Brace Jovanovich, 1975.

Lahmann, Petra H., et al. "A Prospective Study of Adiposity and the Postmenstrual Breast Cancer Risk: The Malmo Diet and Cancer Study." *International Journal of Cancer* 103 (2003): 246–52.

Lambert, Helen, and Hilary Rose. "Disembodied Knowledge? Making Sense of Medical Science." In *Misunderstanding Science: The Public Reconstruction of Science and Technology*, edited by Alan Irwin and Brian Wynne, 65–83. Cambridge: Cambridge University Press, 1996.

Langellier, Kristin M., and Claire F. Sullivan. "Breast Talk in Breast Cancer Narratives." *Qualitative Health Research* 8 (1998): 746–94.

Latour, Bruno. *Science in Action*. Cambridge, MA: Harvard University Press, 1997.

Latteier, Carolyn. *Breasts: The Woman's Perspective on an American Obsession*. New York: Harrington Park Press, 1998.

Layne, Linda L. "Unhappy Endings: A Feminist Reappraisal of the Women's Health Movement from the Vantage of Pregnancy Loss." *Social Science and Medicine* 56 (2003): 1881–91.

Lee, Janet. "Never Innocent: Breasted Experiences in Women's Bodily Narratives of Puberty." *Feminism and Psychology* 7 (1997): 453–74.

Lee, Marion M.; et al. "Alternative Therapies Used by Women with Breast Cancer in Four Ethnic Populations." *Journal of the National Cancer Institute* 92 (2000): 42–47.

Leopold, Ellen. *A Darker Ribbon: Breast Cancer, Women, and Their Doctors in the Twentieth Century*. Boston: Beacon Press, 1999.

Lerner, Barron H. *The Breast Cancer Wars: Hope, Fear, and the Pursuit of a Cure in Twentieth-Century America*. New York: Oxford University Press, 2001.

———. "Inventing a Curable Disease: Historical Perspectives on Breast Cancer." In *Breast Cancer: Society Shapes an Epidemic*, edited by Anne S. Kasper and Susan J. Ferguson, 25–49. New York: St. Martin's Press, 2000.

———. "Letter to the Editor." *Harper's Magazine*, February 2002.

Levine, Steven. *A Gradual Awakening*. New York: Anchor, 1979.

Lincoln, C. Eric, and Lawrence H. Mamiya. *The Black Church in the African-American Experience*. Durham, NC: Duke University Press, 1990.

Lorber, Judith. *Gender and the Social Construction of Illness*. Thousand Oaks, CA: Sage Publications, 1997.

Lorde, Audre. *The Cancer Journals*. San Francisco: Aunt Lute Books, 1980.

Love, Susan M. *Dr. Susan Love's Breast Book*. Cambridge, MA: Perseus, 2000.

———. *Dr. Susan Love's Menopause and Hormone Book*. New York: Three Rivers Press, 1998.

Lupton, Deborah. "Consumerism, Reflexivity, and the Medical Encounter." *Social Science and Medicine* 45 (1997): 373–81.

———. *Medicine as Culture: Illness, Disease and the Body in Western Societies*. Thousand Oaks, CA: Sage Publications, 1994.

Mangan, Katherine S. "Take Two Herbal Remedies and Call Me in the Morning." *Chronicle of Higher Education*, 18 November 2005.

Marshall, Eliot. "The Politics of Breast Cancer." *Science* 259 (1993): 616–17.

Martin, Emily. *The Woman in the Body: A Cultural Analysis of Reproduction.* Boston: Beacon Press, 1992.

———. "The Woman in the Flexible Body." In *Revisioning Women, Health, and Healing: Feminist, Cultural, and Technoscience Perspectives*, edited by Adele Clarke and Virginia Olesen, 97–118. New York: Routledge, 1999.

Martin, Paul. *The Healing Mind: The Vital Links between Brain and Behavior, Immunity and Disease.* New York: St. Martin's Press, 1997.

Matthews, Holly F., Donald R. Lannin, and James P. Mitchell. "Coming to Terms with Advanced Breast Cancer: Black Women's Narratives from Eastern North Carolina." *Social Science and Medicine* 38 (1994): 789–800.

McCormick, Sabrina, Phil Brown, and Stephen Zavestoski. "The Personal Is Scientific, the Scientific Is Political: The Public Paradigm of the Environmental Breast Cancer Movement." *Sociological Forum* 18 (2003): 545–76.

McGrath, Ellen. *When Feeling Bad Is Good.* New York: Henry Holt, 1992.

McKinlay, John B., and Lisa D. Marceau. "The End of the Golden Age of Doctoring." *International Journal of Health Services* 32 (2002): 379–416.

McKinley, Nita Mary. "Ideal Weight/Ideal Women." In *Weighty Issues: Fatness and Thinness as Social Problems*, edited by Jeffery Sobal and Donna Maurer, 97–115. New York: Aldine De Gruyter, 1999.

McMahon, Martha. *Engendering Motherhood: Identity and Self-Transformation in Women's Lives.* New York: Guilford Press, 1995.

Meyerowitz, Beth. "The Impact of Mastectomy on the Lives of Women." *Professional Psychology* 12 (1981): 118–27.

Miller, Arthur H., and Martin P. Wattenberg. "Politics from the Pulpit: Religiosity and the 1980 Elections." *Public Opinion Quarterly* 48 (1984): 301–17.

Mock, Victoria. "Body Image in Women Treated for Breast Cancer." *Nursing Research* 42 (1993): 153–57.

Montini, Theresa. "Gender and Emotion in the Advocacy for Breast Cancer Informed Consent Legislation." *Gender and Society* 10 (1996): 9–23.

Montini, Theresa, and Sheryl Ruzek. "Overturning Orthodoxy: The Emergence of Breast Cancer Treatment Policy." *Research in the Sociology of Health Care* 8 (1989): 3–32.

Moss, Ralph W. *The Cancer Industry.* New York: Equinox, 1999.

———. *Questioning Chemotherapy.* New York: Equinox, 2000.

Nahin, Richard L. "Toward Integrated Medicine." *Journal of the American Medical Women's Association* 54 (1999): 171–73.

National Cancer Institute, Breast Cancer Progress Review Group. *Charting the Course: Priorities for Breast Cancer Research.* Washington, DC, 1998.

Northrup, Christiane, M.D. *The Wisdom of Menopause*. New York: Bantam, 2001.

Olson, James S. *Bathsheba's Breast: Women, Cancer and History*. Baltimore: Johns Hopkins University Press, 2002.

Padgug, Robert A. "Gay Villain, Gay Hero: Homosexuality and the Social Construction of AIDS." In *Passion and Power: Sexuality in History*, edited by Kathy Peiss and Christina Simmons, 293–313. Philadelphia: Temple University Press, 1989.

Padubidri, Arvind N., et al. "Complications of Postmastectomy Breast Reconstruction in Smokers, Exsmokers, and Nonsmokers." *Plastic and Reconstructive Surgery* 107 (2001): 350–51.

Parsons, Talcott. *The Social System*. London: Routledge and Kegan Paul, 1951.

Patterson, James T. *The Dread Disease: Cancer and Modern American Culture*. Boston: Harvard University Press, 1987.

Pinell, Patrice. "How Do Cancer Patients Express Their Points of View?" *Sociology of Health and Illness* 1 (1987): 25–44.

Pirello, Cristina. *Cook Your Way to the Life You Want*. New York: HPBooks, 1999.

Pisani, Paola. "Breast Cancer: Geographic Variations and Risk Factors." *Journal of Environmental Pathology* 11 (1992): 313–16.

Potts, Laura K. "Publishing the Personal: Autobiographical Narratives of Breast Cancer and Self." In *Ideologies of Breast Cancer: Feminist Perspectives*, edited by Laura K. Potts, 98–127. New York: St. Martin's Press, 2000.

Proctor, Robert N. *Cancer Wars: How Politics Shapes What We Know and Don't Know about Cancer*. New York: Basic Books, 1995.

Regan, Pamela C. "Sexual Outcasts: The Perceived Impact of Body Weight and Gender on Sexuality." *Journal of Applied Social Psychology* 26 (1996): 1803–15.

Rich, Katherine Russell. *The Red Devil: To Hell with Cancer—and Back*. New York: Crown, 1999.

Richardson, Lisa C. "Treatment of Breast Cancer in Medically Underserved Women: A Review." *Breast Journal* 10 (2004): 2–5.

Richter, Donna L., et al. "Developing a Video Intervention to Model Effective Patient-Physician Communication and Health-Related Decision-Making Skills for a Multiethnic Audience." *Journal of the American Medical Women's Association* 56 (2001): 174–76.

Riessman, Catherine Kohler. "Strategic Uses of Narrative in the Presentation of Self and Illness: A Research Note." *Social Science and Medicine* 30 (1990): 1195–1200.

———. "Women and Medicalization: A New Perspective." In *Inventing Women: Science, Technology, and Medicine*, edited by Gill Kirkup and Laurie Smith Keller, 123–44. Cambridge, UK: Polity Press, 1992.

Riska, Elianne. "Gendering the Medicalization Thesis." *Advances in Gender Research* 1 (2003): 57–87.

Rodin, Judith. *Body Traps: Breaking the Binds That Keep You from Feeling Good about Your Body*. New York: William Morrow, 1992.

Rollin, Betty. *First You Cry*. New York: Harper Collins, 1976.

Rosenbaum, Marcy E., and Gun M. Roos. "Women's Experiences of Breast Cancer." In *Breast Cancer: Society Shapes an Epidemic*, edited by Anne S. Kasper and Susan J. Ferguson, 153–82. New York: St. Martin's Press, 2000.

Ruth, Sheila. "Women's Personal Lives." In *Readings for Sociology*, edited by Garth Massey, 139–49. New York: W. W. Norton, 2003.

Saltonstall, Robin. "Healthy Bodies, Social Bodies: Men's and Women's Concepts and Practices of Health in Everyday Life." *Social Science and Medicine* 36 (1993): 7–14.

Saywell, Cherise, with Leslie Henderson and Liza Beattie. "Sexualized Illness: The Newsworthy Body in Media Representations of Breast Cancer." In *Ideologies of Breast Cancer: Feminist Perspectives*, edited by Laura K. Potts, 37–62. New York: St. Martin's Press, 2000.

Schmitt, Raymond L. "Embodied Identities: Breasts as Emotional Reminders." *Studies in Symbolic Interaction* 7, part A (1986): 229–89.

Scott, Anne. "Homeopathy as a Feminist Form of Medicine." *Sociology of Health and Illness* 20 (1998): 191–214.

Sedgwick, Edie K. *Tendencies*. Durham, NC: Duke University Press, 1993.

Sherwin, Susan. "Cancer and Women: Some Feminist Ethics Concerns." In *Gender and Health: An International Perspective*, edited by Carolyn F. Sargent and Caroline B. Brettell, 167–86. Upper Saddle River, NJ: Prentice Hall, 1996.

Siegel, Bernie. *Love, Medicine, and Miracles*. New York: Harper Perennial, 1986.

Simon, Michael S., and Richard K. Severson. "Racial Differences in Survival of Female Breast Cancer in the Detroit Metropolitan Area." *Cancer* 72 (1996): 208–314.

Simpson, Christy. "Controversies in Breast Cancer Prevention: The Discourse of Risk." In *Ideologies of Breast Cancer: Feminist Perspectives*, edited by Laura K. Potts, 131–52. New York: St. Martin's Press, 2000.

Sitton, S., and S. Blanchard. "Men's Preferences in Romantic Partners: Obesity versus Addiction." *Psychological Reports* 77 (1995): 1995.

Smedley, Brian D., Adrienne Y. Smith, and Alan R. Nelson, eds. *Unequal Treatment: Confronting Racial and Ethnic Disparities in Health Care*. Washington, DC: National Academies Press, 2003.

Smith, Dorothy. *The Conceptual Practices of Power: A Feminist Sociology of Knowledge*. Boston: Northeastern University Press, 1990.

———. *Texts, Facts, and Femininity: Exploring the Relations of Ruling*. New York: Routledge, 1990.

Snedeker, Susan. "Pesticides and Breast Cancer Risk: A Review of DDT, DDE, and Dieldrin." *Environmental Health Perspectives Supplements* 109, supplement 1 (2001): 35–48.

Sontag, Susan. *Illness as Metaphor*. New York: Farrar, Straus and Giroux, 1977.

Spence, Jo. *Cultural Sniping: The Art of Transgression*. London: Routledge, 1995.

Spiegel, David, Joan R. Bloom, and Ellen Gottheil. "Effects of Psychosocial Treatment on Survival of Patients with Metastatic Breast Cancer." *Lancet* 2 (1989): 888–91.

Springen, Karen. "Breast Cancer: A Ribbon's Far Reach." *Newsweek*, 4 October 2005.

Stabiner, Karen. *To Dance with the Devil: The New War on Breast Cancer*. New York: Delta, 1997.

Stacey, Jackie. *Teratologies*. New York: Routledge, 1997.

Steingraber, Sandra. "The Environmental Link to Breast Cancer." In *Breast Cancer: Society Shapes an Epidemic*, edited by Anne S. Kasper and Susan J. Ferguson, 271–99. New York: St. Martin's Press, 2000.

Stinson, Kandi. *Women and Dieting Culture: Inside a Commercial Weight Loss Group*. New Brunswick, NJ: Rutgers University Press, 2001.

Taylor, Robert Joseph. "Structural Determinants of Religious Participation among Black Americans." *Review of Religious Research* 30 (1988): 114–25.

Taylor, Verta, and Marieke Van Willigen. "Women's Self-Help and the Reconstruction of Gender: The Postpartum Support and Breast Cancer Movements." *Mobilization: An International Journal* 1 (1996): 123–42.

Thomas, Stephen B., et al. "The Characteristics of Northern Black Churches with Community Health Outreach Programs." *American Journal of Public Health* 84 (1994): 575–79.

Thurer, Shari L. *The Myths of Motherhood: How Culture Reinvents the Good Mother*. New York: Penguin, 1994.

Turner, Bryan S. *The Body and Society*. Oxford: Basil Blackwell, 1984.

———. *Medical Power and Social Knowledge*. London: Sage, 1987.

Walters, Richard. *Options: The Alternative Cancer Therapy Book*. New York: Avery, 1993.

Wanebo, H. J., et al. "Bilateral Breast Cancer: Risk Reduction by Contralateral Biopsy." *Annals of Surgery* 201 (1985): 667–77.

Weis, Joachim. "Support Groups for Cancer Patients." *Support Cancer Care* 11 (2003): 763–68.

Weiss, Marisa, M.D., and Ellen Weiss. *Living beyond Breast Cancer: A Survivor's Guide for When Treatment Ends and the Rest of Your Life Begins*. New York: Random House, 1997.

Weitz, Rose. *Rapunzel's Daughters: What Women's Hair Tells Us about Women's Lives*. New York: Farrar, Straus and Giroux, 2004.

West, Cornel. *Race Matters*. Boston: Beacon Press, 1993.

West, Hollie I. "Down from the Clouds: Black Churches Battle Earthly Problems." *Emerge* 1 (1990): 48–56.
Willard, Barbara E. "Feminist Interventions in Biomedical Discourse: An Analy-
  sis of the Rhetoric of Integrative Medicine." *Women's Studies in Communica-
  tion* 1 (2005): 115–48.
Williams, Gareth. "The Genesis of Chronic Illness: Narrative Re-Construction."
  Sociology of Health and Illness 6 (1984): 175–200.
Williams, Simon J., and Michael Calnan. "The 'Limits' of Medicalization: Mod-
  ern Medicine and the Lay Populace in 'Late' Modernity." *Social Science and
  Medicine* 42 (1996): 1609–20.
Wolf, Naomi. *The Beauty Myth: How Images of Beauty Are Used against Women.*
  New York: William Morrow, 1991.
Yadlon, Susan. "Skinny Women and Good Mothers: The Rhetoric of Risk, Con-
  trol, and Culpability in the Production of Knowledge about Breast Cancer."
  Feminist Studies 23 (1997): 645–69.
Yalom, Marilyn. *A History of the Breast.* New York: Knopf, 1997.
Yardley, Lucy. "Introducing Material-Discursive Approaches to Health and
  Illness." In *Material Discourses of Health and Illness*, edited by Lucy Yardley,
  1–24. New York: Routledge, 1997.
Young, Iris Marion. "Breasted Experience: The Look and the Feeling." In *Throw-
  ing Like a Girl and Other Essays in Feminist Philosophy and Social Theory*, edited
  by Iris Marion Young, 189–209. Bloomington: Indiana University Press, 1990.
Zavestoski, Stephen, Sabrina McCormick, and Phil Brown. "Gender
  Embodiment and Disease: Environmental Breast Cancer Activists'
  Challenges to Science, the Biomedical Model, and Policy." *Science as Culture*
  13 (2004): 563–86.
Zimmerman, Susan M. *Silicone Survivors: Women's Experiences with Breast
  Implants.* Philadelphia: Temple University Press, 1998.
Zola, Irving Kenneth. "Medicine as an Institution of Social Control." *Sociological
  Review* 20 (1972): 487–504.

Index

1 in 9 (organization), 211

Abrums, Mary, 102–3, 108
Abzug, Bella, 228
AC. *See* Adriamycin (drug), with Cytoxin
Activism: abortion, 217; AIDS, 17, 73, 139, 252. *See also* Women's health movement
Activism, breast cancer, 11, 230; fund-raising in, 206, 208–9, 210, 230; individual responsibility in, 208, 210; Kushner's, 16, 47, 207n8; mainstream, 213; militant, 28, 210–11, 215; radical, 227; survivors', 7l, 28, 205–6; types of, 207, 212, 217. *See also* Breast cancer movement
Activists, breast cancer, 6, 19; African American, 224–26, 231, 250; alternative experts, 214, 227–28, 231, 252; biomedical experts, 214, 218–24, 230–31, 248; feminist, 16–17; interviews with, 8; Jewish, 8; on one-step procedure, 47; religious responders, 110, 120, 224–26, 231, 250; white, 224

Acupuncture, 144, 238
Adriamycin (drug): with Cytoxin, 190, 218, 236, 272n31, 284nn24–25, 290n5; hair loss with, 191
African American community: access to health care, 103–4; breast cancer activism in, 224–26; breast cancer organizations in, 289n58; religious faith in, 101–3; risk factors in, 229, 288n58
African American women: breast cancer education for, 110–11, 217, 226; risk factors for, 229. *See also* Breast cancer patients, African American
AIDS: activism, 17, 73, 139; drug trials for, 28; public visibility of, 14
Alternative experts (responders): acceptance by, 147; activists, 214, 227–28, 231, 252; agency of, 251; alienation from society, 142; anger of, 125, 231, 232; anxieties of, 150–51; and biomedicine, 125, 127, 129–30, 135–39, 142, 146, 151–52, 250–51; and

307

Text	10/14 Palatino
Display	Palatino
Compositor	BookMatters, Berkeley
Indexer	Roberta Engleman
Printer and binder	Sheridan Books, Inc.